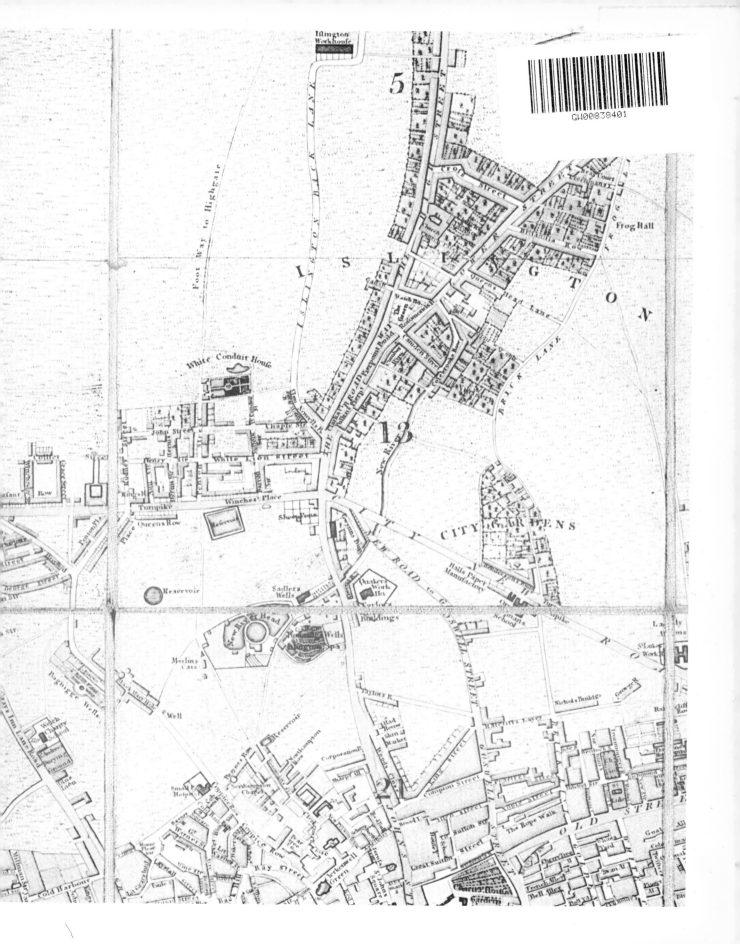

THE
ROYAL VETERINARY COLLEGE
LONDON
A Bicentenary History

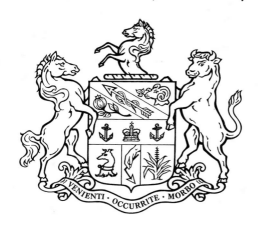

VENIENTI · OCCURRITE · MORBO

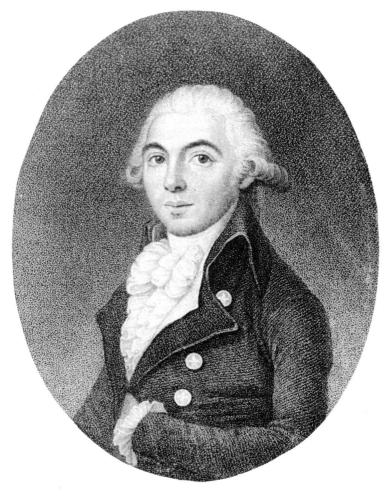

Charles Vial, first Professor of the Veterinary College, engraved from a
portrait owned by his widow. Note the signature: Vial De Saint Bel.

THE
ROYAL
VETERINARY
COLLEGE
LONDON

A Bicentenary History

BY

Emeritus Professor
ERNEST COTCHIN DSc FRCPath FRCVS

EDITED BY
VALERIE CARTER

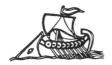

BARRACUDA BOOKS LIMITED
BUCKINGHAM, ENGLAND
MCMXC

PUBLISHED BY BARRACUDA BOOKS LIMITED
BUCKINGHAM, ENGLAND
AND PRINTED BY
THE DEVONSHIRE PRESS LTD
TORQUAY, ENGLAND

COLOUR PLATES PRINTED BY
RAVEN PRINT LTD
BRACKLEY, ENGLAND

JACKET PRINTED BY
CHENEY & SONS LTD
BANBURY, OXON

BOUND BY
CHARLES LETTS LTD
DALKEITH, SCOTLAND

LITHOGRAPHY BY
CAMERA GRAPHIC LTD
AMERSHAM, ENGLAND

COLOUR LITHOGRAPHY BY
SOUTH MIDLANDS LITHOPLATES LTD
LUTON, ENGLAND

DISPLAY SET IN BASKERVILLE
AND TEXT SET IN 10½/12pt BASKERVILLE BY
KEY COMPOSITION
NORTHAMPTON, ENGLAND

ISBN 0 86023 476 2

CONTENTS

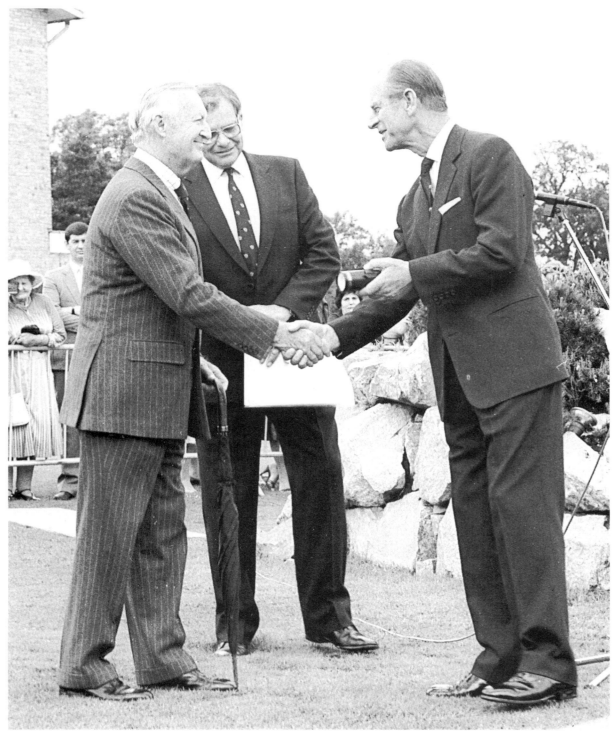

The Duke of Edinburgh with Paul Mellon (left) and Dr Alan Betts at the
unveiling of the bronze cast of Duncan's Horses, 1985.

8

For a people who pride themselves on their love of animals, and considering the age-old human dependence on animals for food and work and as pets, it seems strange that a college to train veterinary surgeons in this country was only established two hundred years ago in response to a plan proposed by a Frenchman. The credit for founding the College goes to the Odiham Agricultural Society, but, as so often happens, it was the demands of war that gave the College the initial impetus. In the following hundred years, between Waterloo and Sarajevo, the health of animals in agriculture and transport became the chief concern of the College.

The industrial revolution changed the scene dramatically and animals for transport gave way to horses kept for sport and pleasure while the success of veterinary surgeons in raising the health standards of agricultural animals ensured that their services would remain in demand. It is an irony that in this mechanical age the Royal Veterinary College is probably as secure as it ever has been, while the scientific and professional challenges become ever more complex.

The College and its staff and graduates have made many significant contributions to the science and practice of veterinary medicine and I am delighted that this history has been written to coincide with its bi-centenary. The story has its ups and downs. Great practical achievements jostle with the expected financial and administrative problems but throughout it is a story of people doing their very best to improve the health and welfare of animals of all shapes and sizes and in all circumstances. I hope that all who read this book will join me in wishing the Royal Veterinary College a successful and rewarding third century.

1990

INTRODUCTION

I have prepared this history of the Royal Veterinary College, the oldest veterinary school in the English-speaking world, as a contribution to the celebration of the College's bicentenary in 1991. In reading it, it may be helpful to bear in mind the generalization that the life of the College falls broadly into two epochs each lasting almost exactly one century. In the first century of its existence the Royal Veterinary College was inadequately provided with staff and with funds, and was mostly concerned with diseases of the horse. Forward-looking College principals in the third and fourth quarters of the 19th century — Simonds, Robertson, Brown — tried with some success to widen the curriculum to include domesticated animals other than the horse. In 1892, with the appointment of McFadyean as dean (he became Principal in 1894) there began, on the foundations laid by his predecessors, a second century showing a remarkable transformation which led to a marked expansion of the numbers of teaching staff, to a greater development of the staff's research activities, and to the full incorporation of the College into the country's university system.

In 1906 the College became a school of the University of London, with recognised teachers, and could prepare candidates for the university's BSc (Veterinary Science) degree as well as carrying out its basic function of training candidates for the diploma of membership of the Royal College of Veterinary Surgeons. In 1949 the College achieved full status as an integral school of the university. Training is now provided for the BVetMed degree, entitling graduates to be registered as members of the Royal College of Veterinary Surgeons, which confers on them the title of veterinary surgeon and the sole right to practise as such.

The major line of development of the College has thus been its transformation from a teaching school attached to an equine infirmary, to a fully fledged university school in which teaching at undergraduate level and research of high standing encompass the whole range of domesticated animals, and where postgraduate courses meet the increasing demands of specialisation in such subjects as animal health, pathology and laboratory animal science.

This history is not intended as an exhaustive one. Unfortunately a great deal of early archival material has been lost, particularly in the upheaval caused by the wartime evacuation of the College from Camden Town to Berkshire in 1940, but especially during the complete rebuilding of the College in Camden Town in the 1930s. I would also stress that I do not claim any special archival expertise. This history should be looked on as my attempt to explore the history of the College so as best to understand why it has become what it is today.

I have divided the chapters in a way reminiscent of the old histories of the Kings of England, and I often refer to the 'reign' of a particular Principal. This biographical approach has its weaknesses, but it is one that an amateur often finds easy to handle.

The establishment of the College, and the early days of its life, were described by an anonymous writer in 1793 in *An Account of the Veterinary College from its Institution in 1791;* this is largely a transcript of early College minutes. (The secretary, Mounsher, lost the original minute books on 10 May 1794. He thought he had them with him in the coach when going to the College, but did not see them again. He said the fair copies were *bona fide* and accurate.)

Towards the end of the 19th century, in 1894, former College Principal James Beart Simonds published in his old age a series of biographical sketches of some College teachers he had known. A brief, and perhaps unduly euphoric historical note, probably written by J.G. Wright (then professor designate of surgery) was included in the brochure prepared for the opening of the present buildings in Camden Town by King George VI and Queen Elizabeth in 1937.

A detailed account of the first half-century of the history of the College, up to the foundation of the Royal College of Veterinary Surgeons, which took over the College's examining functions in 1844, was given by Leslie Pugh (1895-1983) in his book *From Farriery to Veterinary Medicine,* published by Heffer of Cambridge in 1962. The books by Iain Pattison on the development of the veterinary profession, and on Principal McFadyean, are invaluable sources of information. There is also much useful information about members of the College staff in the 19th century in Sir Frederick Smith's *Early History of Veterinary Literature.* From these various works, from the College's minute books, and from veterinary periodicals, I have constructed what I hope is a reasonably coherent narrative of the College's life. I have arbitrarily chosen to finish my biographical accounts in 1988, when the Principal, Dr Alan Betts, retired.

Throughout the book I have referred to the Royal Veterinary College simply as 'the College', when no possibility of ambiguity is involved. Similarly, I have referred to the Royal College of Veterinary Surgeons as 'the Royal College' where again the context makes the matter clear.

Ernest Cotchin.

ACKNOWLEDGEMENTS

The manuscript on which Ernest Cotchin had been working for so many years was unfinished and unrevised when he died in September 1988. A few months after his death, I was asked to act as editor of this bicentenary history of the Royal Veterinary College, and I am proud to have been one of the team that has produced a book which I hope does justice to the author and to the College.

The story has been brought up to date with a challenging final chapter by Professor Lance Lanyon, Principal of the College. Sherwin Hall has contributed introductions that add a historical perspective to parts II and III. Professor Clifford Formston has vividly described the Hobday debacle, and the period when the College was based at Streatley on Thames. I am particularly grateful for his generous help with photographs, historical records and advice.

I am indebted to the College librarian, Linda Warden (who compiled the index) and to the library staff for their unfailing help with records and pictures, to Anna John who typed the manuscript, to David Gunn for photography and to Benita Horder, librarian of the Royal College of Veterinary Surgeons' Wellcome Library for historical material and illustrations.

Many members of the veterinary profession sent the author information and photographs for inclusion in this history. Their names were unfortunately not recorded, but their assistance has been greatly appreciated.

Valerie Carter

The Rev.ᵈ Thomas Burgess delivered a Memoir on several topics (which was ordered to be entered in the correspondence book) and made the following motions.

That Farriery is a most useful science and is so intimately connected with the Interests of Agriculture; that it is in a very imperfect neglected state and highly deserving the attention of all friends of Agricultural economy.

That Farriery as it is commonly practised is conducted without principle or science and greatly to the injury to the noblest and most useful of our animals.

That the improvement of Farriery established on a study of the Anatomy diseases and cures of cattle, particularly Horses, Cows, and Sheep, will be an essential benefit to Agriculture and will greatly improve some of the most important branches of national commerce such as Wool and Leather ——

Whereupon it was Resolved,

That the Society will consult the good of the community in general and of the limits of the Society in particular, by encouraging such means as are likely to promote the study of Farriery upon rational scientific principles.

Extract from minutes of the Odiham Agricultural Society, 19 August 1785. (RCVS)

PART I

The First Veterinary Surgeons

THE FOUNDING OF THE COLLEGE

The establishment of the College in 1791 marked a crucial stage in the separation of the functions of farrier and veterinaran. Farriers were basically shoeing-smiths who had acquired a rudimentary knowledge of equine diseases, which led them to become 'horse-doctors'. Most of them, according to contemporary accounts, were still using the same crude methods and homely remedies that were popular 100 years before.

With the advent of the College, veterinarians increasingly took over the treatment of horses and cattle. Students of the College called themselves veterinary surgeons, and in time this became an accepted designation. Good evidence of the use and meaning of the term is contained in a report, in the second issue of *The Veterinarian*, of a meeting held on 22 July 1829 to consider the method of examination adopted at the College. One of the speakers, a Mr Sibbald, who had studied at the College and obtained his certificate, said 'My father was a farrier. He was intimate with the greatest practitioner of his day, Layton, who was not a veterinary surgeon, but was farrier to the King. The term "veterinary surgeon" arose with the College. There is honour attached to it. I have obtained it, and I prize it.'

The process of separation and demarcation was not a rapid one, and considerable ambiguity in the use of the term 'farrier' and 'farriery' persisted for many years after the establishment of the College, reflecting the degree to which the occupation of farrier and veterinarian overlapped. As late as 1815, in his *Treatise* on the management of draught horses, especially those in the coal trade in London, Higgs was pleading for a clear detachment of the veterinary surgeon and the farrier from each other. This was also eloquently urged by Taplin in 1803. On the other hand, in 1806 no less a person than James Clark, farrier to the King in Scotland, in his *First Lines of Veterinary Physiology and Pathology* wrote that the healing art, and the art of shoeing, would and should necessarily continue as two linked aspects of a country veterinary practitioner's work.

Why the foundation of the London Veterinary College so notoriously lagged behind the foundation of the French, and then of other continental veterinary schools, remains unexplained. There had for a long time been publicly expressed unease in the United Kingdom about the unsatisfactory training of people treating the diseases of animals, whether they were farriers in the sense of being shoeing-smiths acting as horse-doctors, or were medical practitioners — physicians, or more especially surgeons — who had, partly or completely, left human medicine for the less crowded and potentially more lucrative (if less socially acceptable) field of animal medicine. In view of the number of working and pleasure horses in the kingdom, when the phrase 'horsepower' meant literally just that, and the concentration of dairy cows around and even within the metropolis, and also the growing number of pets in middle-class households, it is strange that the demands of so many animal owners, some wealthy or even extremely rich, had not led to the development of a proper profession competent to deal with animal diseases, just as the professions of physician, surgeon and apothecary had burgeoned to meet public demand at the end of the 17th and the beginning of the 18th centuries.

Formal veterinary instruction began in France in 1762, when the world's first veterinary school opened in Lyons, where a 24-year-old named Laurent Gaillard became the first pupil on 16 February. It was established by Claude Bourgelat (1712-1779) with a grant of 50,000 livres from Louis XV. This was soon followed by the establishment of the larger veterinary school at Alfort near Paris, thanks to the interest of Bourgelat's friend Henri-Leonard Jean-Baptiste Bertin (1719-1792) who was Louis's comptroller general of finance, and later a minister of state whose portfolio covered agriculture. Bourgelat was clearly an intelligent man. He was a friend of d'Alembert, and contributed to Diderot's seminal *Encyclopedia* (published in 35 volumes in 1750-1780) an article (1764) on equine maladies. The year 1762 is one for all veterinarians to remember. In that same year, the celebrated naturalist Buffon, echoing Burdon, felt advantages would accrue if some physicians should turn from human medicine to study veterinary medicine.

In a letter in the *Gentleman's Magazine* of 1790, 'Philippos', identified by Pugh as Granville Penn, who was to play a central role in the foundation of the London Veterinary College, wrote that he 'had often lamented the failure of the plan which the late ingenious M Bourgelat had formed for establishing a veterinary school in England'. It has been speculated by Smith that this idea might have been suggested to Bourgelat by the Earl of Pembroke (1734-1794), a cavalry officer in the Seven Years' War. Had it succeeded, we would have been enriched by those labours which he afterwards devoted to his native country and which laid the first regular foundation for the science of veterinary medicine in Europe. The deduction seems warranted that, prior to the establishment of the Lyons and Alfort schools, Bourgelat had a plan to establish one in England. It is interesting, in view of later criticism of Edward Coleman's reported preference for the sons of farriers and grooms as students, that Bourgelat preferred his veterinary students to be young men of good morals and behaviour, vigorous and robust, and of *souche terriere;* he only occasionally sought out men of more 'exalted' origin.

After the establishment of the French veterinary schools, other continental schools followed in quick succession. Those founded before 1791 included Turin, Padua and Parma in Italy; Dresden, Hanover, Freiburg-im-Breisgau, Karlsruhe, Berlin and Munich in Germany, and schools in Vienna, Budapest, Copenhagen and Sweden. The Berlin school deserves special mention. In 1787 Frederick William II commissioned Count von Lindenau to establish a veterinary college in Berlin. A physician, Naumann, was sent along with a farrier to see what went on at Alfort; Sick, a surgeon, again with a farrier, was sent to Vienna, and an apothecary, Ratzburg, was sent to Leipzig to fit himself for teaching botany and chemistry. Had such an enlightened scheme been followed in London, it might have been more immediately successful than the one adopted. The high promise of the Berlin school, officially opened on 1 June 1790, was unfortunately not immediately fulfilled, the teachers appearing somewhat lax in the discharge of their duties.

Meanwhile in 1766, Edward Snape, farrier to George III and to the second troop of Life Guards, published a proposal to establish in London what might be called a 'teaching hospital' for instruction on the diseases of horses. This hospital was apparently established in Knightsbridge in 1778, but it survived only a short while, Snape having been left in the lurch by noblemen who promised financial support. According to Smith, Snape must nevertheless be given credit for being the first to project, and actually found, a veterinary school in this country.

The same year saw the foundation of the veterinary school in Hanover. This was done with government support, and our own King George III's name appears on the decree establishing the school, in his capacity as King of Hanover. As Principal Buxton, Ernest Gray and others have noted, no account seems to have been taken in government circles in London of the plan for the Hanover school, although Vial, the College's first professor, does mention it in his

Preliminary Discourse. The possibility of establishing a veterinary college in London with government money was one way its promoters considered financing it, but this was unfortunately dismissed in favour of raising funds from students' fees and subscribers' contributions. This was to the fundamental and long-term detriment of the financial base of the College.

In 1776, John Mills FRS had joined those who deplored the absence of a veterinary school in this country. He referred to the school at Lyons, and indeed knew Bourgelat personally.

It is thus amply clear that, while surgeons like Taplin and physicians like Prosser turned to the financially rewarding field of veterinary medicine, there was widespread dissatisfaction with the state of veterinary science in the United Kingdom. Yet nothing was done until decades after the need was recognised. Pugh suggests: 'The explanation probably lies in the customary contrast between the benevolent despotism of the Continent and the *laissez-faire* regime of eighteenth century England'. More prosaically, the army farrier was less in demand in England than on the oft-warring Continent, and our island country was only sporadically, even if at times seriously, exposed to the ravages of epidemic disease in its animal stocks.

David Everett, in *Lines Written For a School Declamation,* memorably observed that 'tall oaks from little acorns grow'. The acorn which resulted in the foundation of the College was obscurely and unwittingly planted when, in 1783, at a meeting on 16 May at the George Inn in the small market town of Odiham in Hampshire, there was established, on the proposition of William Terry of Yately, a 'society for encouraging Agriculture and Industry in the said Town and its Neighbourhood'. It is now generally accepted that this meeting was the first step on the unpremeditated road which led to the establishment of the London Veterinary College. The chair was taken by Sir Henry Pawlett St John Bt of Dogmersfield and, in addition to Mr Terry, the others present were Thomas Hall of Preston Candover, Rev William St John of Dogmersfield, George Green of Weston, and George Small, also of Weston. James Huntingford, an attorney of Odiham, was appointed secretary; he was later to become secretary of the London committee, an executive offshoot of the Odiham Agricultural Society which was eventually to undertake the actual institution of the London Veterinary College, of which he was the first secretary.

The list of 47 subscribers to the Odiham Society includes the name of Rev Thomas Burgess of Oxford, later to play a key role in the London committee of the society. It was said of him that 'the untiring perseverance with which he prosecuted his researches for evidence in any particular subject was inconceivable'. Burgess (1756-1837) became Bishop of Salisbury in 1825. He attended meetings of the London committee on 3 November 1790 and in 1791.

The Odiham Society continued to grow, having 100 members in 1784, owing to the devoted exertions of Huntingford. On 7 January 1785 the society set out its principal objectives: to promote the good of the community by encouragement of industry and ingenuity; to excite a spirit of enquiry which may lead to improvements not yet known; and to fix knowledge and art upon the certain test of accurate experiment.

Three weeks later, Lord Rivers (later to be a vice-president of the College) was elected the Odiham Society's president. From the minutes of the meeting of 15 January, it seems that the society was already in touch with correspondents all over the United Kingdom.

Matters developed slowly in the Odiham Agricultural Society. On 19 August 1785 the following motion was proposed by Rev Thomas Burgess: 'That Farriery is a most useful science and intimately connected with the interest of Agriculture; that it is in a very imperfect and neglected state, and highly deserving of the attention of all friends of Agricultural economy. That Farriery as it is commonly practised is conducted without principle or science, and greatly to the injury of the noblest and most useful of our animals. That the improvement of Farriery established as a study of the Anatomy, diseases and cure of cattle, particularly

Horses, Cows and Sheep, will be an essential benefit to Agriculture and will greatly improve some of the most important branches of national commerce such as Wool and Leather'. (It is clear that Burgess in the term 'farriery' meant to include the treatment of the diseases of farm animals as well as of the horse). Whereupon it was resolved: 'That the Society will consult the good of the Community in general and of the limits of the Society in particular, by encouraging such means as are likely to promote the study of farriery on rational scientific principles. That it be referred to the meeting in October to consider what means may be most likely to encourage the study of scientific farriery. That it be referred to the same Meeting to open a voluntary subscription to forward such means as may be thought most likely to promote the study of scientific Farriery. . .'.

On 7 June 1786 the society noted that it still lacked information on which to base any specific resolution for the encouragement of scientific farriery and the matter was put aside. Huntingford confirmed on 14 March 1788 that (for reasons not given) he had resigned the post of secretary, being succeeded on 14 April by Mr Raggett, another attorney of Odiham. The society obviously accepted that the resigning secretary acted in good faith, for a month later it passed a vote of thanks to Huntingford for 'his unremitting zeal in extending the extra connection of the Society, and in soliciting the correspondence of other Agriculture Societies and Individuals, and his Diligence in forwarding the attendance of Committees, in preparing the business of all meetings and in arranging the correspondence and other Communications to the Society'.

At that time, powerful support for the establishment of a veterinary college came from Arthur Young, FRS (1741-1820), the younger son of the rector of Bradfield, Suffolk (Speaker Onslow's chaplain). He took a farm of 100 acres at North Mimms in 1766 — 'a hungry, vitriolic gravel' — leaving there in 1777. Young contributed largely to *Annals of Agriculture*. He travelled in France in 1788, 1789 and 1790 and founded the Farmers' Club in 1794. Breakfasting at Bradfield Hall on one occasion, the agriculturalist Duke of Bedford found him surrounded by pupils from Russia, France, America, Naples, Sicily and Portugal.

In October 1787, Young (who was once bluntly described as the best writer on agriculture and the worst farmer) was shown round the Alfort veterinary school by the director, Chabert. Young was impressed by the fact that the school had a farm, a facility lacking at the London College for over 150 years (it would be interesting to know if the College later unwittingly purchased his North Mimms farm). He was also impressed by the school's four professors (in contrast, the London College was to start with only one professor). Young wrote of the Alfort school that 'the establishment does honour to the Government of France. There are at present over 100 pupils from every country in Europe except England, a strange exception considering how grossly ignorant our farriers are'.

Again in 1788, James Clark of Edinburgh, in the preface to his *Treatise on the Prevention of Diseases Incidental to Horses* wrote: 'In France, a regular academy for the Instruction of young Farriers has been instituted. The attempt is laudable and worthy of imitation. The Physician and Surgeon enjoy the greatest opportunities for receiving instruction in their professions, by a regular education. The analogy between the diseases of the human body and those to which the horse is liable is very great. Hence it must be obvious that the cure of those diseases must depend on the same principles as the former: from which it is likewise evident that a regular education is necessary to the Farrier'.

In June 1788 Charles Vial, the Frenchman who was to become the first Professor of the London Veterinary College in 1791, arrived in England with letters of introduction from Pierre-Marie Auguste Broussonet (1761-1807) to Sir Joseph Banks PRS (1743-1820), Samuel Foart Simmons MD, FRS (1750-1813) and Dr P.D. Layard MD, FRS (1721-1802). Sir Joseph, botanist and explorer, with an interest in plants of agricultural importance, was president of the Royal Society for 42 years. Dr Simmons was physician-extraordinary to George III, and was called to treat the King in his 'mad' periods. Dr Layard, physician to the Princess Dowager of Wales, was the author of a book on *Contagious distemper among horned cattle*.

In September, Vial published proposals for the creation of an English veterinary school. It is assumed that, having married an Englishwoman, he returned to France in December 1788 at the end of his six months' leave. He was back in England by February 1789, when he directed and possibly assisted Edmund Bond in his dissection of the magnificent racehorse Eclipse which, like his grandsire Regulus, was never beaten.

At meetings in May 1788, March and June 1789, the Odiham Society, in its leisurely way, resolved to advertise its intention to educate two or more boys 'at the great School of Farriery in the neighbourhood of Paris, where children from every part of Europe are taught the business of Farriery scientifically and practically, and solicit the contributions of the Public at large'. The matter was to be brought more closely to the notice of 'noblemen, gentlemen and farmers' by a circular letter signed by the society's treasurer, Rev William St John, calling for subscriptions. The name of Granville Penn first appears in the Odiham Society minutes of 5 August 1789, as a subscriber to this farriery fund.

While the Odiham Society has earned and received its fair share of credit, it must be concluded that this modest proposal, so long in incubation, was likely even if put into effect, to have had only a marginal impact on the situation it was meant to remedy — as the society soon realised.

In October 1789 Charles Vial announced proposals to deliver lectures in England on the veterinary art. On the 9th of that month, James Clark of Edinburgh was elected an honorary and subscribing member of the Odiham Society. This was the same Clark who had stressed that a regular education was necessary for a farrier. Whether the preface to his treatise in which this comment was made was ever actually read by the society's members is not known, although they did order two copies of his 'two publications on Farriery'. The Odiham Society knew of Clark, and could have known of his views on the education of farriers, before it received copies of Vial's plan on 5 August 1790.

The 25 May 1790 Odiham minutes refer to a London committee, of which Huntingford was secretary, and which met at 10 Welbeck Street. The meeting of the Odiham Society on 5 August 1790 was of crucial significance. Among the seven people present (including the secretary, Mr Raggett) was Rev Thomas Burgess. The society now moved from the rather passive position of regretting (as it did on 5 August 1789) that 'there was no appropriate educational establishment in England for the desired improvement of farriery (in this context comprehending the medical treatment of horses, cattle and sheep) by a regular education in that science on medical and anatomical principles', to a positive position of recommending such an institution as had been established in France, Germany and elsewhere on the Continent, as being necessary in this country. They now recognised that their plan to send some intelligent lads for education in farriery to such continental schools would be at best a rather feeble stopgap measure, while in any case the revolutionary situation in France was not favourable to the original Odiham plan. All the same, the plan to send two or more lads to Alfort was not yet finally abandoned, and subscriptions were still called for, to be sent to Odiham or to the London committee. To that committee were nominated Lord Rivers (still president of the Odiham Agricultural Society), Granville Penn, the Earl of Dartmouth, Sir James Tilney Long, Sir Thomas Miller, Henry Maxwell, George Ross and Henry Peters, with Huntingford as secretary.

A further significant motion at the meeting on 5 August 1790 called for provision to be made under Parliamentary authority for placing the profession of farriery (as practised by shoeing-smiths) on a more respectable footing, by forbidding farriers from practising unless licensed, by preventing, after a limited time, any person from practising farriery who had not served seven years' apprenticeship under a licensed farrier, and so on.

At this same meeting it was reported that Charles Vial had presented 10 copies of his plan of 19 March 1790, for establishing an institution to cultivate and teach veterinary medicine, for which thanks were to be transmitted by the secretary. This plan is given in full in Appendix 3 of Pugh's book. The salient features were:

'An institution for the purpose of cultivating this art (of veterinary medicine) similar to those which have been established some years in France, Germany, Piedmont, Sweden, Denmark, etc. would afford an exhaustless fund of amusement to independent persons, as well as of precious instruction to all. The means by which establishments have been effected in this country are: by Royal or Parliamentary institution . . . or by a general subscription . . . or by subscriptions of substantial sums . . . subscribers become governors or directors of their own establishment . . . this latter seems to be the proper method to be adopted in the present case . . . A college . . . should provide a school . . . and the subscribers, becoming Governors of the new institution, should proceed to choose a President, Vice-Presidents, Treasurer, Secretary, and such other officers as should appear convenient . . . to institute their Veterinary Professor . . . that His Majesty, and His Royal Highness the Prince of Wales, be humbly prayed to take it under their joint patronage: and, the Master of the Horse, the President of the Royal Society, the President of the Royal College of Physicians, and the President of the Society for the Encouragement of Arts, Manufacturers and Commerce, should be each invited to a government of the college . . . Our College would serve: to collect and deposit the variety of sound veterinary knowledge which floats dispersedly in the kingdom . . . to collect and arrange whatever the labours and experience of other nations have furnished on this subject; to improve on this extensive stock . . . correspondencies and communications should be encouraged . . . Evening meetings, weekly, or more frequently . . . should be held; and, every year, the transactions of the college, including those of the school, should be published . . . The members of the college should . . . be increased by ballot . . . and it may perhaps be advisable, to divide the members into three different classes, perpetual governors . . . annual governors . . . members . . . The lectures should treat fully and amply of anatomy and physiology; of the veterinary pharmacopoeia; of chirurgical operations; and of the structure, geometrical proportions, mechanic powers, beauty, defects and age of the horse . . . Lectures should also be read to students on botany and pharmacy, and on natural philosophy and chemistry . . . Whenever a student should have regularly attended an entire course of study, and should have passed an examination before the college and its Professors, he should obtain a certificate . . . an infirmary, in which diseased horses and other cattle might be received . . . a forge for farriery would be equally necessary . . . Finally, when the college has obtained its full consistency, it be incorporated by Charter . . . by the name of, The Royal Veterinary College'.

On reading this plan, one is left with a feeling of sadness. The concept clearly was meant to establish a College in the broad sense of a learned foundation, whereas what emerged almost inevitably, from the actual circumstances of its establishment and funding, degenerated into what was to remain for a century basically and predominantly a horse infirmary.

On 5 October 1790 a letter from Clark of Edinburgh to the Odiham Society was read, in which he proposed the establishment of a veterinary school in that city, under his direction. This school was to have been patronised by some of the first noblemen and gentlemen of the country, and Clark had the fullest assurance that the government would aid and support his venture. (If government would support a veterinary school in Edinburgh, why did it not do so in London, or was it simply not asked?). However, the proposed Edinburgh school was not established at that time, a fact which Clark attributed, somewhat obscurely, to 'the political situation'. At the same meeting Vial was elected an honorary and subscribing member. On 26 October Josiah Brookes, surgeon, FRS, was elected an honorary member of the society and a member of the London committee (his museum rivalled Hunter's). On this committee, any three members of the Odiham Society were to form a quorum.

The fulcrum of action now shifted from the society to the committee in London. The first minuted meeting of that committee was held in the Prince of Wales coffee house, Conduit Street, Hanover Square, on 3 November 1790. Those present were Josiah Brookes and Rev T. Burgess, along with secretary Huntingford. The minutes and resolutions of the Odiham Society respecting farriery, from meetings between 19 August 1785 and 26 October 1790, were read and ordered to be entered into the minutes of the London committee. Then followed a list of members of the Odiham Society resident in London, including Granville Penn. The list of honorary and corresponding members included gentlemen living in 30 English counties, and at a few places in Scotland and Wales. These members included Robert Bakewell of Leicestershire, Rev Dr Priestley of Birmingham, Mr Raikes of Gloucester, and Arthur Young of Bradfield Hall, Suffolk. There is also a list of 19 subscribers to the fund for the improvement of farriery which includes four members of the London committee (Rivers, Long, Penn and Maxwell).

One of the committee members active in founding the College was Granville Penn (1761-1844). He was the grandson of William Penn, the founder of Pennsylvania, who purchased an estate in Stoke Poges Park in 1760. Granville eventually inherited the estate and his connection with Stoke Poges may be of more than usual significance. In Joan Wake's book *The Brudenells of Deene* one reads that 'not the least of John, Duke of Montagu's many attractive qualities was a love for animals, which led him to maintain a hospital for sick dogs at his house in Ditton Park in Buckinghamshire'. This was the second Duke, 1690-1745. Ditton is a hamlet of Stoke Poges, and the park was owned by the Montagus from the end of the 17th century. Perhaps Granville Penn knew of this hospital by tradition.

Having placed these matters on record in its minutes, the London committee proceeded to its own business: (i) a prize of 10 guineas was offered for the best description of not more than 20 cases of glanders; (ii) the circularisation of honorary and subscribing members, asking for their 'communications on the veterinary art'. The committee then adjourned to meet at the Blenheim coffee house, New Bond Street, on 12 January 1791.

During 1790, while these meetings were taking place, an important series of letters appeared in *The Gentleman's Magazine*. Three letters were written over the pseudonym of 'Philippos of London', two were signed by 'Zoophilus of Birmingham', one by John Elderton of Bath, one by 'S' of London, and one by J.H. (undoubtedly Huntingford). Pugh attributed the Philippos letters to Granville Penn, and he considered him also to be the likely author of the Zoophilus letters (a possible alternative author might be Dr Priestley of Birmingham). The object of these letters was to bring Vial's plan of 18 March 1790 to the notice of the influential readers of *The Gentleman's Magazine*. It is not at all clear why the author(s) of the Philippos and Zoophilus letters chose to write under pseudonyms. Nor is it clear in what way Penn (if he was indeed Philippos and/or Zoophilus) became interested in Vial's plan. According to Pugh, Penn had seen and admired the veterinary schools in France, and had read Clark's treatise with approval. Pugh suggested three ways in which Penn may have become aware of the Odiham Society's initiative before he became a member of the society. He may have met Burgess at Oxford; Lord Rivers, who was also a graduate of Magdalen College, and was president of the Odiham Society, may have discussed the society with him; or Penn may simply have read the society's advertisement of its intention to send two lads to Alfort for training.

The letters are set out in Appendix 4 of Pugh's book and some are summarised here:
1. Philippos, 5 March 1790. The art of veterinary medicine had been, surprisingly, neglected

in this country, and consigned to the hands of incapacity and ignorance. The art was a practical application of sure and scientific principles to the preservation of health in domestic animals, and to the cure of their diseases. The science on which the art was grounded comprised the natural history, anatomy, physiology and pathology of those animals, together with those portions of the vegetable and mineral kingdoms providing either aliment or remedy. Farriery was wanting in that fundamental science. Veterinary schools had been established in France, Germany, Denmark and Sweden.

2. Zoophilus, 7 September 1790. Zoophilus had not been able to acquire a copy of Vial's plan, but he put forward a plan of his own for an animal hospital, for a regular set of teachers forming a school, and provision for receiving living subjects in various states of disease. The hospital, for instruction and for receiving cases, would be a large and handsome structure, erected by subscription at a little distance out of town. It should have wards or stalls for larger animals, and pens for small animals such as sheep or dogs. There should be a house or hall, containing, besides dwelling-apartments for the servants and assistants, a common lecture room, an anatomical theatre and a museum, a laboratory, and a medicine-shop. Lectures would be regularly delivered, and dissections made, twice a year. Each course would last at least three months, and would cover one of five subjects — anatomy, physiology, pathology, *materia medica* and therapeutics. The professors would have fixed salaries, the pupils' fees being added to the funds of the establishment. Pupils would receive a certificate on completion of the course, and gentlemen in general should only call in certified practitioners. Farriery, in the strict sense of the term, would be left to shoeing-smiths. It was envisaged that such animal hospitals would be opened in all the principal towns of the kingdom. The patronage and support of the medical profession, and of the great and rich, and protection from the Heir Apparent, would help meet the great expense of such an institution. Subscribers would have the usual privilege of sending in one or more subjects for treatment, proportional to their subscriptions.

3. Philippos, 21 October 1790. The groundwork of the veterinary art was medical science; farriery was no art, but a mere practice, habit or routine. The arguments in favour of the cultivation of veterinary medicine were principally two — the excellence of the art, and the importance of the subjects of its operation. Farring, farriery or farrier were words of origin from the Latin, signifying the shoe and shoer of a horse. Great Britain was almost the only remaining State which had not extended its protection to this important art. The genius of the nation, remarkable for its activity and its jealousy; the general excellence of our education; the universal influence of science; our experience in agriculture; and the number of horses and cattle, all these were earnests that would abundantly secure the success of the measure, if we should ever decide to adopt it. It was announced that the un-named author [Vial] of the plan intended to deliver a course of public lectures in veterinary medicine that winter.

4. Philippos, 11 November 1790. The writer knew the author (still not named) of the plan (which was publicly available) and had occasionally acted as his interpreter. The plan had been more laboriously considered than that of Zoophilus, and the school was to be formed under the protection of enlightened citizens. The author describes himself as 'a man of no profession, and following this and every other pursuit through a general and independent love of science, and a desire of substituting its just authority in every part of science to the offensive usurpation of ignorance and imposture'.

Why Philippos and Zoophilus failed to name Vial as the author of a plan to form a veterinary school is unknown. Vial is said to have published his proposals for a veterinary school in September 1788, and also in October 1789, and he had issued his plan (perhaps as revised by Granville Penn) in March 1790. He had sent 10 copies to the Odiham Society in August 1790, so his name was already widely known.

From the beginning of 1791 the London committee held a series of meetings at the Blenheim coffee house which led to the foundation of the Veterinary College on 8 April.

At the meeting of 12 January 1791 there were present Granville Penn (chairman), Sir William Fordyce, Rev T. Burgess, Vial and Huntingford. It was resolved that 'the immediate objects of the Society are to establish a Fund by subscription, for collecting by premiums [prizes] well-authenticated facts relating to the diseases in horses, cows and sheep, their treatment and cure: — for establishing an extensive communication with foreign veterinary societies: — for the speedy and general circulation of such memoirs on the diseases of horses, cows and sheep as may be communicated to the Society; — for providing an hospital for diseases in horses, cows and sheep: — and for promoting the science of Farriery by the regular education in it, on medical and anatomical principles'.

It was resolved to publish an advertisement in the *Morning Post* and *English Chronicle* soliciting subscriptions, and to circulate a letter, also soliciting subscriptions, addressed to noblemen, gentlemen and others likely to be interested in the improvement of farriery in its several branches. Copies of the resolutions were to be sent to the society in Odiham, to subscribers to that society's farriery fund, and to members of the society resident in London. It is clear at that stage the London committee envisaged funding its proposed activities by subscriptions, and that it intended to concern itself with the diseases of cows and sheep as well as horses.

At the next meeting of the London committee, on 28 January, Sir William Fordyce (chairman), supported by John Burgess, Mr Benezek, Vial and Huntingford, agreed on the terms of the proposed public advertisement. Members of the Odiham Society resident in London 'and all friends of the Institution' were requested to attend the next meeting. The minute book contains a list of subscribers (presumably to the London committee's funds) including Lord Rivers and Granville Penn, and three gentlemen were nominated as members — Edward Topham (1751-1820) proprietor of *The World,* Peter Benezek and Reuben Smith. The committee already had prematurely exalted views of its importance, for it deferred to the next meeting the question of how to apply to the King for royal patronage — patronage of an institution which had no actual existence. Penn, Topham, Burgess and Benezek were asked to deal with any proposals that might be made to the committee regarding a building that would be suitable as a hospital, and Messrs Shepperson and Reynolds of Oxford Street were appointed (for what immediate purpose is not clear) booksellers and stationers to the institution. Consideration of rules and regulations was deferred to the next meeting.

At a meeting on 11 February, Granville Penn (chairman) supported by William Fordyce, Dr A. Crawford, John Gretton, William Stone and James Huntingdon, again deferred consideration of the rules and regulations, and of the patronage, to the next meeting. It was reported that an offer had been made of leasehold premises in Oxford Street, between Rathbone Place and Newman Street, lately occupied by Mr Burr, stable-keeper, consisting of a dwelling house, yard, nine coach houses, 14 stables containing 51 stalls, and a covered ride. This was held for an unexpired term of six years 'from Christmas last' at £140 per annum; it was offered (fortunately unsuccessfully) by the new proprietor, Mr Collier, for £600. Certain noblemen and gentlemen from the topmost ranks of society were named as subscribers, including the Marquess of Titchfield and Sir T.C. Bunbury, steward of the Jockey Club.

The committee was seriously convinced of the benefits that must result from an institution to cultivate and teach veterinary medicine; the object of this committee's concern, and that of Vial, were one and the same; and it was greatly to be desired that the two plans — that of the Odiham Agricultural Society and that of Vial — (which may be termed the Alfort plan) should be consolidated into one. Since several gentlemen had already subscribed towards furthering Vial's proposals, Penn, Stone and Gretton were asked to discuss with Vial the best way of amalgamating the two plans.

On 18 February 1791 Granville Penn (chairman) supported by Rev Mr Cook, John Gretton, William Stone, Edward Topham and Huntingford, received information from Vial (who had been confined to bed with a cold and fever, and had been unable to meet the committee's delegation) that he supported the amalgamation of the two plans, and that he would consult his patrons and subscribers accordingly. Then followed a resolution naming the London committee 'The Veterinary College, London', and separating it from its parent, the Odiham Agricultural Society. 'This meeting, having taken into consideration the proceedings of former meetings, and being informed that many respectable persons delay giving their names as subscribers while the proceedings of the committee are subject to be reported to the Odiham Society, and are under the controul [sic] thereof, find it expedient to detach themselves from that Society, the work on which they are engaged being of so considerable importance, the reformation and improvement of Farriery, requiring that it should be confined to that purpose and use alone, and be under the sole management and control of its own members. It was resolved that from this day forward they shall be called by the name of the Veterinary College, London. That Vial be appointed Professor of the College. That the Transactions of the College be published annually, and a copy thereof delivered, gratis, to each subscriber'. A general meeting would be held at the Blenheim coffee house on 8 April to appoint a president, vice-presidents, directors, and other officers. Annual members would subscribe two guineas per annum, and life members 20 guineas. Advertisements of the above resolutions were to be published in the press, including *The Times* and Topham's *World,* and copies were to be sent to members of both Houses of Parliament, to other noblemen and gentlemen, and also to high sheriffs, to be laid before grand juries (composed of men of substance) at the ensuing assizes. The secretary was ordered to write to the Odiham Society, recording these changes.

At a meeting on 25 February (Stone, chairman, with Crawford, Vial, Huntingford), the following advertisement was reported published in the *World:* 'Veterinary College, London. For the Reformation and improvement of Farriery. The public are respectfully informed, that the Committee appointed by the Odiham Agriculture Society to consider the best method of improving the Art commonly called Farriery, have, in pursuance of that design, and feeling themselves unable to act with due energy and effect in the capacity of a Committee, found it expedient to detach themselves from that respectable Society, and to erect themselves into the present form. The object of the Institution is, to reform, and bring into a regular system, that important branch of medicine which regards the treatment of diseases incidental to horses and other cattle, and which has hitherto been neglected and much abused in this country . . . M. Vial, for some years Professor of Veterinary Medicine in the Royal School of Lyons, and of Comparative Anatomy at Montpellier, a gentleman well-known for his anatomical skill and knowledge in every part of this Art, is appointed Professor to the College'. Vial accepted the office of Professor, and reported that his 'friends and subscribers', the Earl of Morton, Earl of Grosvenor and Lord Belgrave, approved of the union of the two plans, Odiham's and Vial's.

The College having been named, the secretary was directed (it might be thought, somewhat late in the day) to draw up statutes for its constitution and organisation.

Meetings were now held every week. On 4 March (Topham, Crawford, Stone, Huntingford, Vial) further noblemen and gentlemen became subscribing members. On 11 March (Penn, Vial, Huntingford) the Duke of Northumberland was nominated for membership, and thanked for his 'bounty' of 50 guineas. Vial was asked to draw up regulations for the school and infirmary, keeping in mind the example of the foreign veterinary schools. These College regulations, based closely on those in the French veterinary schools, although reduced in number and somewhat ameliorated, set out for resident pupils a pretty strictly regimented way of life, against which they occasionally rebelled.

A week later, on 18 March (Topham, Penn, Vial, Huntingford) Dr Daniel Peter Layard became a honorary member. The Earl of Pembroke had intimated to Vial his intention to become a member of the College. Other members nominated included the Duke of Montrose (Master of the Horse). Sir George Baker, Sir Joseph Banks and John Hunter were elected honorary and subscribing members. At a meeting on 25 March (Penn, Crawford, Stone, Topham, Vial, Huntingford) further members were nominated, including James Burton, later architect to the College. The secretary was directed to write to the Master of the Horse, asking leave to nominate him as president of the College at the forthcoming general meeting. At a meeting on 1 April (Stone, Gretton, Penn, Topham, Vial, Huntingford) it was reported that the Master of the Horse had declined 'as such' being president. The secretary was therefore directed to write to the Duke of Northumberland, asking permission to nominate him as president. The Prince of Wales and the Duke of York gave in their names (but not their money) as 'Subscribers and Promoters'. The statutes, and Vial's scheme for the internal order and regulation of the College, were read, and sent forward to the general meeting.

Finally, the great day dawned. The first general meeting of the College was held at the Blenheim coffee house on 8 April 1791, under the chairmanship of Granville Penn, supported by Sir William Fordyce, Wm Stone, E. Topham, G.M. Ascough, J. Gretton, G.F. Steward, W.G. Brown, Dr A. Crawford, Dr Wm Drew, Richard Burton, James Burton, Francis Steward, John Baynes, Mr Grosvenor, Mr Peake, Mr Rivers, Mr Reuben Smith.

The Duke of Northumberland was unanimously chosen to be president. Eight vice-presidents were appointed: Earl Grosvenor, Earl Morton, Earl Orford, Lord Rivers, Sir George Baker, Sir T.C. Bunbury, Sir Wm Fordyce, and John Hunter. Twenty directors were appointed for the current year, including Granville Penn and Rev T. Burgess. A permanent committee for the current year comprised Dr Crawford, Dr Drew, Penn, Stone, Topham, Gretton and Baynes. Messrs Ransom, Morland and Hammersley acted as treasurer. A small audit committee was elected and the appointments of Vial as Professor and Huntingford as secretary were formally confirmed.

A number of overseas honorary and corresponding members were appointed, most from France. Granville Penn presented to the College 44 publications on the veterinary art and science. The statutes for the constitution and organisation of the College, and Vial's plan for its internal order and regulation, were unanimously approved.

A choice of dates is available from which to reckon the life of the College: 18 February 1791, when the London committee decided to call itself The Veterinary College, London, and 8 April 1791, when the president, vice-presidents and directors were elected and the statutes and regulations were approved. The date generally chosen is 8 April 1791. On the coat of arms over the main entrance of the College in Camden Town the dates shown are 1785-1937: the latter refers to the year in which the new Camden Town buildings were royally opened. Why the date 1785 was used is uncertain; it was said by Professor J.G. Wright to commemorate the meeting of the Odiham Agricultural Society when the first mention of the idea of improving farriery was made, but the strong possibility remains that it was originally meant to be 1875, the year the College received its Charter of Incorporation and adopted its coat of arms, and that someone corrected what was wrongly assumed to be an error.

On 8 April 1791 the College had no pupils and no land or buildings. It had only one professor. Its origin, and its method of financing, almost inevitably led to it becoming effectively a horse infirmary.

The received opinion among veterinary surgeons who have given any thought to the role of John Hunter in the early life of the Veterinary College agrees with the statement expressed in 1831 by Youatt, that Hunter was the 'life and soul' of the founding and development of the London Veterinary College. Edward Coleman, second Professor (Principal) of the College, said Hunter was one of the best friends the College ever had. Pugh may be nearer the truth. He points out there is no evidence that Hunter was connected with the College before he was nominated an honorary member in March 1791, and that he did not attend any meetings of the College before December 1791. Pugh feels that Hunter's responsibility for the early affairs of the College has been overrated. He had given up lecturing in 1790, apparently due to the angina which troubled and eventually killed him. His contributions were nevertheless important. He lent prestige to the young veterinary profession by telling Moorcroft that he would, if he were a young man, follow a veterinary career himself. He served as a vice-president of the College. He treated Vial leniently in his committee's report, but failed to press for the early appointment of the necessary second professor. By getting his colleagues to admit pupils to their lectures after Vial's death, apparently waiving the customary fee of 10 guineas, he helped the College over a difficult patch, but may unwittingly have set an unfortunate precedent which suggested that preclinical veterinary teaching could be done as well in a medical as in a veterinary context.

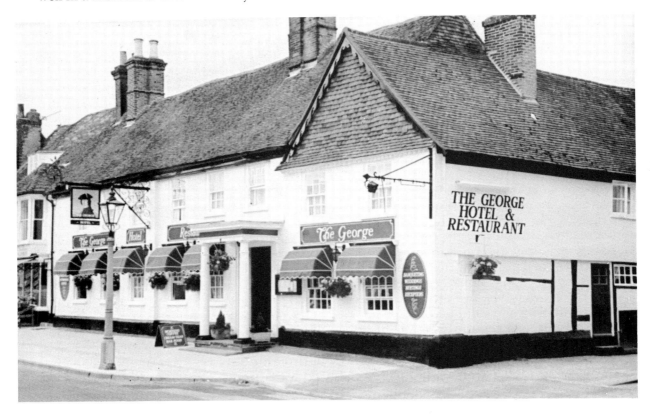

The George Hotel, Odiham, meeting place of the Odiham Agricultural
Society from 1783-1791.

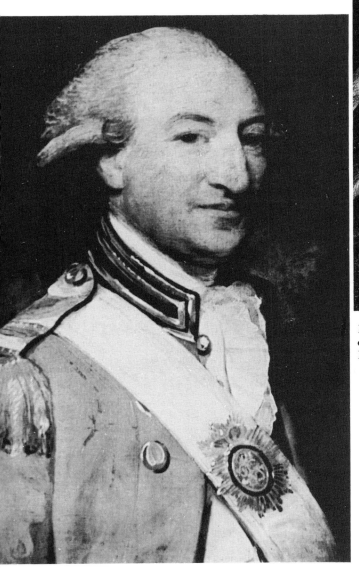

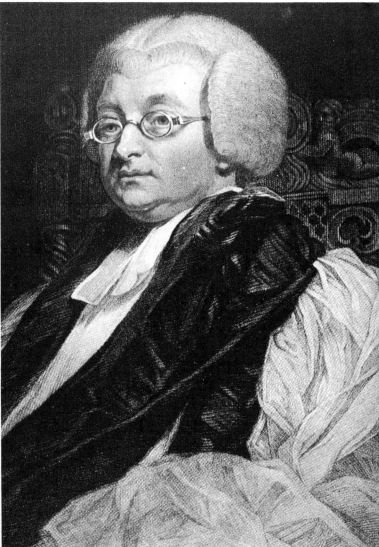

LEFT: Hugh, 2nd Duke of Northumberland, first president of the Veterinary College. RIGHT: Thomas Burgess DD FRS, initiator of the move within the Odiham Society which led to the foundation of the Veterinary College.

Wednesday. Jan.ʳʸ 12. 1791.

Sir

I beg the favour of you to inform the gentlemen of the Odiham Society, that I have but just been informed of the notice they were pleased to take of the letter, & plan, which I had the honour of conveying to them in the Summer; & that the letter they addressed to me in Leicester Square, never reached me, on account of my having left that place, & being in the Country. They will be so candid as to ascribe to this, & to no other cause, my not acknowledging the honour they were pleased to confer upon me; & to believe, that I shall be at all times happy to unite my labours to their exertions, in favour of Veterinary Medicine.

I have the Honor to remain, Sir;
Your Obed.ᵗ & Humble Ser.ᵗ
Vial DeSainbel

Mr Huntingford
Secret.ʸ of the Odiham Society.

Letter from Vial to the Odiham Society, to whom he had sent 10 copies
of his plan for forming a veterinary college. (RCVS)

BENOIT CHARLES MARIE VIAL

Professor 1791-1793

The College's first Principal (or Professor, as he and his more immediate successors were called) published his first proposals for a veterinary school in England in 1788, but it was not until two years later that he made contact with the Odiham Agricultural Society. In April 1791 he was appointed Professor of the London Veterinary College — a college in name only. From the start, the College was hampered by shortage of funds, an inappropriate site, and a lack of suitable staff. A lucrative system of 'subscribers' was introduced; shortly before Vial died there were 900, but only 14 students were enrolled. His early and unexpected death was a cruel setback which left the College floundering in indecision over the choice of a suitable successor.

Vial (1750-1793) was sometimes known as Vial de Saint Bel. In August 1769, eight years after it was opened, he enrolled as a student at the veterinary school in Lyons. About 1773 he became junior professorial assistant to the professor of anatomy at Alfort veterinary school. He left this position in circumstances which are unclear, having incurred the strong displeasure of M Bourgelat, the inspector-general of veterinary schools. After a spell in private practice, Vial was made equerry to Louis XVI and *chef de manège* of the Lyons riding academy, a post he apparently held for some years, but could not retain.

Vial made many attempts to be reappointed at Alfort after Bourgelat died in 1779, but was unsuccessful. On the advice of M Broussonet MD FRS, perpetual secretary of the Royal Society of Agriculture in Paris, he took the momentous step of obtaining six months' leave of absence to visit England. He had, he claimed, been superseded in a promotion which he thought he had a right to expect from the Master of the Horse. Vial arrived here in June 1788, armed with letters of introduction (without which no serious traveller went abroad) to Sir Joseph Banks, Dr Simmons, Dr Layard and others. His stated object was to examine the different breeds of horses and cattle, and to observe the condition of rural economy in this country. Broussonet had also suggested he should put forward proposals for the creation of a veterinary school in England, an idea possibly prompted by the visit to the Alfort school of Arthur Young a few days earlier.

In 1788, his published proposals for forming a veterinary school here having met with no success, Vial married an English lady 'of great accomplishments', and returned to Paris with her, his knowledge of the English language no doubt showing some improvement as time passed. In due course, finding that national discontents and factious habits of thinking were spreading rapidly in that city and throughout France, he obtained leave to visit England again, under the pretext of buying horses for his sovereign's stud. Fortunately for him, but more so for this kingdom, he was in this country at the onset of the Revolution and the destruction of the Bastille. In this first commotion he lost his guardian and friend, M de Flesseille, 'who fell the second victim to that unjust, indiscriminate vengeance, of the enraged people'. Vial thus lost his annuity from Flesseille, and he was deprived of his other appointments. His patrimonial estate (if it ever existed) was confiscated because, as he claimed, he was now an *emigré*, having failed to return to France in the prescribed period.

On his return to England, Vial was available to guide the dissection of the racehorse Eclipse, obtaining (in true Vial fashion) many noble and zealous patrons in the process, including Lords Grosvenor, Morton and Belgrave. This was probably the most famous and least useful dissection of a horse ever undertaken.

The following account is largely drawn from Sherwin Hall's article in *Veterinary History* (Summer 1984). Bred by the Duke of Cumberland (1721-1765) at Windsor, by Marske (a third generation descendant of the Darley Arabian) out of Spilette (a granddaughter of the Godolphin Barb on the sire's side) Eclipse was born on the day of a solar eclipse, 1 April 1764. After the death of the 'Butcher' Duke on 31 October 1765, the stud was sold and the yearling Eclipse was bought by a Leadenhall merchant and grazier, one Wildman, for 75 guineas. Eclipse's first race was a Fifty Guinea Plate at Epsom in May 1769. In 18 races, Eclipse was 'first, the rest nowhere', being either unbeaten, or walking over.

Eclipse, put to stud in 1770, was now owned by Denis O'Kelly of Canons, Edgware, who had bought a half-share for 650 guineas after Eclipse's second race at Ascot in 1769, buying the other half for 1100 guineas. O'Kelly died in 1787, and Eclipse died of a 'violent colic' 14 months later, at 7 pm on 27 February 1789. Vial was invited to supervise the autopsy, which was performed (whether in part or as a whole is not clear) by Edmund Bond (later to be the first pupil to obtain a certificate from the medical examining committee of the London Veterinary College in 1794). Also present were Bracy Clark and his elder brother, Henry.

Bracy Clark (1771-1862) was the brilliant son of a Quaker living in Chipping Norton. Leaving school at the age of 14 to study medicine, he was apprenticed to a surgeon in Worcester. His elder brother, Henry, urged Bracy to go to the London College, which Bracy entered in 1792, gaining his certificate in 1794. He had been elected a fellow of the Linnean Society in 1793. After a two-year tour of the Continent, he returned to England in 1799 and started a veterinary practice at 17 Giltspur Street, mainly among brewery horses and those of a similar type. He devised a set of heavy draft horse casting hobbles which are now outmoded but still bear his name.

Bracy Clark was a prolific writer. One critic said that no man, perhaps, ever wrote so learnedly or so much, to so little purpose. His hobbies were horse-shoeing and cricket — he established the first cricket club in Worcester. When he retired from practice, probably in 1828, he and others produced a veterinary periodical called the *Farrier and Naturalist,* which was devoted to attacks on Professor Coleman, and ran for three years. He was elected vice-president of the Royal College in 1857.

Clark's paternal grandmother, Margaret Bracy, was the last representative of a family long settled in Long Compton in Warwickshire. A family of cow doctors worked in this region for over three centuries; this family is now represented by Dr John Walker, who has a veterinary practice in Hook Norton, near Long Compton.

The dissection of Eclipse was continued until only the skeleton, still with its ligaments, was left. Vial pronounced the cause of death to be (unspecified) disease of the kidneys, with violent inflammation of the bowels. He claimed he had taken the measurements of Eclipse during life, and wished to satisfy his curiosity by trying them on the dead subject. His objectives were to give a guide to the better choice of an animal; to establish the true conformation of the racehorse, setting a standard for an ideal animal to achieve maximum speed, and at any given time to discover whether the breeds had improved or degenerated.

The peculiarity of the proportions (published in French and English in 1791 in an essay dedicated to the Prince of Wales) is that the measurements are not given direct but are based on the head, divided into 22 equal parts (according to Percivall, Eclipse stood 16½ hands high and the head measured 22 inches). Joseph Gamgee says that Vial's measurements were thoroughly at variance with the skeleton as he knew it.

A few years after the dissection, it is believed that Philip O'Kelly, brother of the deceased Denis, gave the skeleton to Bond, who kept it in his premises in Upper Brook Street until his death. At some time Bracy Clark had lent £500 to Bond, and his widow, unable to discharge the debt, gave the skeleton to Clark and it remained in his study until shortly before his death. The Royal College of Surgeons offered him 60 guineas for it, but he sold it to John Gamgee in November 1860 for 100 guineas. It was taken to the New Veterinary College in Edinburgh by John's father, Joseph, and there it was first mounted as a complete skeleton. Presumably it was brought to London when John Gamgee moved his college there as the short-lived Albert Veterinary College. In 1871 the Gamgees gave the skeleton to the Royal College in Red Lion Square. The request by the National History Museum for the loan of the skeleton in 1902 was turned down, but it was eventually presented to that museum when the heavily criticised RCVS museum was closed in 1921. In 1983 the skeleton was transferred to the National Horseracing Museum at Newmarket.

In 1790 Vial made contact with the Odiham Agricultural Society and he was appointed Professor at the London Veterinary College on 8 April 1791. It has been said that Vial was quite unsuited for the post of founding Professor. Delabere Pritchett Blaine (1770-1845), a medical man, had been recommended to assist Vial by demonstrating anatomy and helping with the translation of Vial's lectures. The recommendation came from Dr Heighton, whom Blaine had assisted in making dissections and physiological experiments to illustrate the union of divided nerves and the nature of the interposed substance. In 1802, a few years after his short service with Vial, Blaine said the latter was an ingenious man, who probably understood the *manège,* and who was indefatigable in promoting the interests of the College. It was a matter of surprise to Blaine that the College was ever established at all, with Vial as its head. Youatt, in 1839, wrote that the appointment of Vial as Professor was a flagrant and irreparable error, for he knew nothing of the diseases of cattle and their treatment. More recently, the appointment of Vial has been attributed to the influence of Granville Penn, who seems to have taken the Frenchman uncritically at his own valuation.

Vial did not apparently introduce for some time any regular system of instruction which would have concentrated the labours of the students. Soon after it was founded, the College ran into financial difficulties because of an improper management of funds. The death of some, and the secession of others of the College's founders and original supporters was bound, Blaine felt, to trouble Vial's mind, which was not well equipped to struggle with disappointments. However he considered that Vial 'was a man of such good natural abilities that when his mind was at ease, he had so much application that his deficiencies, had he lived, might have been in a great measure made up'.

As regards Vial's personality, Bracy Clark noted that he was polite and easy in his manners, and often a stickler for etiquette and punctilio, believing, reasonably enough, that his office as Professor of the College required it. He was recognised to be highly jealous and irascible. He was always on the watch for an affront, which he would often imagine even when it had not been intended, an easy thing for a Frenchman at a politically sensitive time. This irascible trait naturally served to increase his enemies. Even suspecting the pupils of plotting against him, Vial, according to Bracy Clark, would spy on them and eavesdrop, yet he was apparently much beloved by some. His vanity was exemplified by his taking a house at 36 Little St Martin's Street (once Sir Isaac Newton's, and later rented by the celebrated Dr Burney and his daughter Frances, Madame D'Arblay, author of the once popular novel *Evalina*) which was far beyond his means.

Vial's scanty publications have been analysed at length by Smith, who pronounced: 'In summing up Vial's practical knowledge one is compelled to estimate it as not very wide. He seems to have had a good acquaintance with the theory and practice of shoeing, though we cannot admit his claim to originality. He is, excepting in one respect, admirable on glanders.

His knowledge of sprains is not good . . . He understood the various causes of colic, but his practice was dilatory and generally out of date'.

An anonymous writer (possibly Simonds or Hunting) in the *Veterinary Record* of 1891 said that Vial was undoubtedly a man of intelligence and force of character. He had immense difficulties to overcome, partly because of the average Englishman's prejudice against foreigners (especially perhaps the French) and partly because of the then prejudice of society against a science — veterinary medicine — which was not yet established as respectable. The anonymous author goes on to say that while Vial was not a highly educated veterinarian, even for those times, he was far in advance of the general practitioner in this country, who had usually no training whatever in anatomy or medicine. Had his life been prolonged, the writer thought it probable that he would have left a deeper mark on the science of the profession.

What did Vial look like? The familiar doll-like figure in the engraving (said to have been taken from a portrait in the possession of Mrs Vial) is stated by Bracy Clark to bear little resemblance to Vial. He was described as a tall, bony man with much black hair, a dark complexion, a deep jaw, prominent cheekbones, dilated nostrils, and altogether an open and manly countenance.

The College having been founded, it was necessary to give it premises and students. It was also necessary formally to sever its links with the Odiham Agricultural Society so, on 19 April 1791, a letter was sent to the Society, saying that the College would not now persist in the Odiham plan of sending youths to France to be trained. The Society responded gracefully on 3 May, transferring its farriery fund and relevant papers to the College. The Professor's salary, and that of secretary Huntingford, were fixed at £100 per annum. A month later, it was resolved that a proper place should be provided for the Professor's dissections and lectures, and advertisements were placed accordingly in publications including the *Morning Post* and the *Daily Advertiser*. Several premises were then brought to the notice of the College. Mr Carr's at Brompton; Mr Saunder's of East Smithfield; premises in Tottenham Court Road; Mr Haygarth's ground near the end of Gray's Inn Lane; Mr Jacob Leroux's of Somers Town; Mr Cook's near Draper's Gardens. None was thought suitable.

A significant step was taken on 6 September 1791 at a meeting at the Crown and Anchor tavern in the Strand. The following memorandum was presented by Vial, and read by the secretary: 'When the Members of the Veterinary College were occupied by objects to which I was in no wise competent I was absolutely silent — but now that it is a question to chuse [sic] a convenient situation for the establishment of the College, I think it a duty incumbent on me to give my advice on this important point.

'A healthy situation should be the first object that ought to fix the attention of the Society — because there is no person but is very well convinced that a marshy and low Ground exhales very unwholesome and putrid vapours which affect the bodies of individuals that may be exposed to their action either through the pores or attracted by the breath, or otherways by the Food and Drink — if these particles will affect healthy bodies, their effect must be much more pernicious on diseased animals, therefore the Veterinary Infirmary should not be established in an atmosphere continually charged with particles destructive to health. Independent of this physical cause there exists always one more or less contrary evil to the cure of maladies in any Hospital whatever which results from the great number of sick assembled in one place, the bodies of which occasion emanations which alters more or less the wholesomeness of the air, but this cause may in some manner be done away with by the great cleanliness of the Stables and fumigations that might be performed from time to time. . . .

'It will now be necessary to observe that animals are more frequently attacked by epizootic, endemic and contagious diseases than the human species because we are protected from these casualties by our Houses, Clothing and manner of Living, in short by all the precautions that reason dictates, whilst animals are deprived of all these recourses and are constantly exposed to dangers which we avoid by the above-mentioned precautions, besides their food and drink is constantly the same, which often is the cause of a fermentation in their blood which generally terminates in stubborn and fatal diseases.

'It would be useless to enter more largely on this subject to demonstrate the absolute necessity of chusing the most healthy situation for the establishment of the Veterinary College. We must not add to the execution of this plan — physical obstacles to moral difficulties, for it will be enough to fight through prejudice and ignorance.

'I will now beg leave to make some observations on the distance of the Veterinary College from the Town — first — because the Society has no rival to dread in an establishment of this nature — secondly — whether the Infirmary is situated a Mile further or nearer it will not prevent people of sense from sending their Horses there — thirdly — the resident pupils being distant from places of dissipation, it will protect their morals and they will employ their time in study. It may perhaps be objected that the distance may prevent the pupils of the Hospitals from attending the Lectures of the Veterinary Professor — I will first answer to that — that it would be dangerous for the progress of the Veterinary science to give them too free admission into the College — because it might give a disgust to the residing pupils from their application to the Veterinary Medicine and many of them would change their mind and apply themselves to the anatomy of the human body, thinking that it would be more honorable for them to cure the human species than Animals, this happened in France and the best Veterinary pupils are now Physicians and Surgeons to the human species — this prejudiced ideal would inculcate itself into the minds of young men, the more so as the Veterinary Science is still in its Infancy in this Country, and in an abject state, for this reason it would be equally dangerous to permit residing pupils to attend medical or anatomical lectures, of the human body, or to frequent Hospitals: Therefore a certain distance from the Town would be more useful than otherwise for the progress of the Veterinary Science.

'For to obviate the inconveniencies that might result from the too frequent communication with the out pupils the Professor will demonstrate to the latter only what might be useful to them as Surgeons and Physicians to the human body, such as the most important demonstrations of comparative anatomy as likewise experiences [experiments] on several animals, which could not be attempted on Man without imminent danger, and lastly, a comparison between epidemical and epizootic diseases — therefore the out pupils ought to be considered by the Society [College] as a separate Class: the consideration of which ought not to have any influence as to the situation of the establishments.

'As the intention of the Society is to form Veterinary Physicians and Surgeons intended to be dispersed throughout the Kingdom to exercise usefully their art, the Professor will teach the residing pupils only the most important difference between the two medicines — that of the human body, and that of Cattle — he will confine himself strictly to the teaching of the Veterinary Science.' (Note the phrase 'Veterinary Physicians and Surgeons'. This is an early use of the implied term 'Veterinary Surgeon', which was not established as a title until about 1796 when it was introduced as an army designation).

'It will be useless to observe to the Society that it is of the greatest importance to procure a place as soon as possible, if the Professor is not enabled to begin his Lectures by Christmas (1791) the establishment will be put off for one year — the Zootomy being strictly the first part he is to begin to teach to the pupils, which everyone knows could not be attempted in the Summer — and it would be feared too long a delay might hurt the success of the establishment.'

It was ordered that this memorandum should be entered in the minutes, but there is no indication that it was considered or discussed.

31

Vial urged that the College could be located, with benefit and without detriment, some way (say two miles) out of London. Yet the first indications that London was soon to show explosive growth were already present, and it did not need much foresight to see that it would not be long before any green-field site chosen near London for the location of the College would soon be engulfed in bricks and mortar, which would sweep away hay- and grazing-fields, market gardens and brickfields alike.

There is no surviving record that Vial, or indeed anyone concerned, had made a detailed study of what would be needed to establish a College with adequate ensured finance, premises and staff, nor is there any indication that his interest extended beyond the horse, to include other domesticated animals.

At the same meeting at which the Vial memorandum was read, on 6 September 1791, a letter to the secretary from Messrs Kirkman and Hendy (who were present) was produced: 'Sir, In consequence of your Advertisement we beg leave to inform you, that we have contracted with Lord Camden for about 100 acres of building land, near [Old] St Pancras Church, abutting on the Turnpike Road leading to Kentish Town, which is intended to be called Camden Town conceiving the situation eligible for your truly valuable Institution we request you will lay this our proposal before the Society — We hold this Land under his Lordship for 99 years from Michaelmas last, the three first subject to no Ground Rent, our proposal is, that Lord Camden does and he will under our direction grant the Society a lease for 99 years from that time, the three first subject to no rent but for the remainder of the term an Annual Rent of thirty pounds per acre, should this proposal meet with approbation, the Society have only to direct their Surveyor to make out any quantity of land and in what position they conceive will best answer their purpose'.

(Charles Pratt, 1714-1794, Attorney General and Lord Chancellor in the reign of George III, was in 1765 created Baron Camden of Camden Place in Kent. He derived his title from his seat at Chislehurst, formerly the residence of the historian William Camden, author of *Britannia*.)

The letter concluded: 'We will only add this land is on an eminence with plenty of fall for water with a small Rivulet running through the same, is not subject to any Tax for paving, cleansing and lighting but is lighted and watched at the expense of the Turnpike Trust and the Kings Tax in the parish of Saint Pancras is only two pence in the pound — these circumstances so favourable to building need no comment. We are Sir Your obedient Serv Kirkman & Hendy, Upper Gower Street, Bedford Square, September 6th 1791.'

This is a somewhat disingenuous letter. The eminence referred to is not a striking local geographical feature, and the 'small Rivulet' is presumably the Fleet River, which was so often flash-flooded as to give the area towards Battle Bridge (Kings Cross) the name of 'Pancras Wash'. The line of Pancras Way (once known as Longwich Lane, then as King's Road) follows the pack-horse track on the banks of the river Fleet.

It has always seemed a bit of a mystery that the College chose its present Camden Town site. Kirkman and Hendy, the Earl of Camden's agents, may merely have responded to the College's advertisement, but another explanation for their involvement seems possible. Pugh lists Horatio, Earl of Orford, as a foundation member of the Society for the Encouragement of Arts, Manufactures and Commerce (called later the Royal Society of Arts) along with others who were members of that society and also foundation members of the College in 1791. At the same time, the College minutes (said to be a *bona fide* copy of the lost original) show that the Earl of Orford was elected a vice-president of the College on 8 April 1791. The difficulty is that the Earl of Orford, who did not die until 5 December 1791, was named George, while his uncle who succeeded him as fourth Earl was named Horatio, although he disliked this name, and called himself Horace Walpole instead. This famous author of 3,000

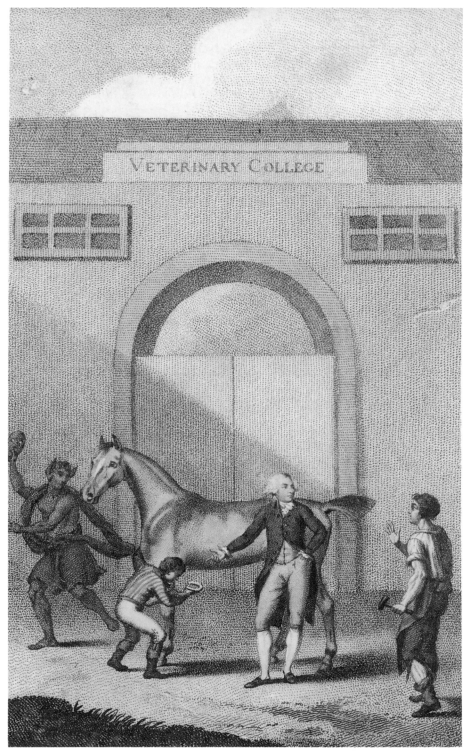

Engraving published in 1795, showing Vial demonstrating to a shoeing-smith in front of the Veterinary College, with 'Ignorance' in flight on the left.

'incomparable' (Byron) letters, among other largely dilettante activities, showed by a letter written to Sir Horace Mann on 8 June 1791 that he knew of the 1788 Kentish Town Act, which freed the Earl of Camden to build 1,400 houses in Kentish Town. Although there is no evidence that Horace Walpole (who died on 2 March 1797) ever attended College meetings, it is pleasant to think that he may have formed the undiscovered link between Lord Camden and the as yet unlocated Veterinary College.

On 13 September, at a house taken for the College near the Elephant & Castle tavern, close to St Pancras Church (which became Old St Pancras Church when St Pancras New Church was built by the Inwood brothers in 1819-1822) the proposal from Messrs Kirkman and Hendy was approved. The area of ground selected was described somewhat imprecisely as: 'All that piece of ground situate north of Fig Lane [now Crowndale Road] St Pancras extending northwards from thence 650 feet on average abutting Eastwards on the Church path leading to Kentish Town and is in a parallel breadth 270 feet abutting Westward on other Ground intended and agreed to be used as Garden Ground by the said Messrs. Kirkman and Hendy or the Undertenants and no buildings to be erected thereon which shall raise more than 12 feet above the present surface and nearer than 80 feet to the ground hereby lett and that they will reserve a Street or way 60 feet wide at the least at the northern extremity of the said ground and that the said Messrs. Kirkman and Hendy do engage to lett to the Veterinary College a piece or any part of their ground at any time within twelve months which they the College shall determine upon a ranging line with the north extremity of the piece already described at and after the rate of £30 per acre nett which are the same terms as the ground described and mentioned are lett at and also at and upon the same reservation of the pepper corn Rent.' Present at this meeting was James Burton, the Scottish developer, who was to be concerned with erecting the early College buildings. At the same meeting Vial was asked to move into the house, and to procure such temporary assistance as necessary to prepare for reading lectures in October.

On 20 September 1791, trustees for taking up the Camden lease were appointed. Taplin offered (unsuccessfully) to become superintendent general of the College, combining the offices of clerk and steward. An offer of the skeleton of a horse, by a Mr Longbottom, was declined. Students were to be taken in as boarders, having been recommended by a respectable person who knew them or their families. The admission fee was 20 guineas, and board and lodging were 30 guineas per annum, for a course planned (on paper at least) to last three years. Age limits of 15 and 22 years on entry were fixed.

On 27 September Mr Burton was asked to prepare, in conjunction with Vial, a plan for a building for the College, and to superintend any temporary erection or alteration in the premises engaged for the College. James Burton has been acclaimed as 'the most important London builder to appear since Nicolas Barbon'. By 1800 he was involved in the development of the Bedford estates and the Regent's Park terraces.

Soon, a watchman was provided for Vial's house and the College land, at nine shillings a week, and labourers were paid £5 8s 6d for clearing the bed of the Fleet. A Mr Portier was offered five guineas to translate the first part of the Professor's lectures on 'The Bones'. On 1 November it was decided to hand copies of the proposed College regulations to stagecoach proprietors for distribution. Notice boards were set up on the College house, and at the corner of the road.

On 8 November Mr Jones of Stamford offered himself as a pupil, as did Mr Bloxam of Alcester. On 22 November Mr Nash of Pampisford (near Cambridge) asked for information on pupillage. Mr Burton produced his plans on 6 December. Vial had by now postponed his lectures to Wednesday, 4 January 1792; they were given in the College house to four pupils. The course, intended to occupy three years, was manifestly beyond the power of one single professor, no matter how well qualified. The subjects of the first year of this proposed course would be anatomy, physiology, conformation and external diseases; in the second year, surgery, *materia medica,* pharmacy and botany as relating to veterinary medicine; in the third year, pathology, epizootic diseases, treatment and prevention of disease, hospital practice and shoeing.

There was growing pressure on the College to receive the diseased horses of subscribers, but as yet no stables were ready. A resolution of 22 March 1792 provided for the erection of temporary stabling for 50 horses, to which were to be added later a lecture theatre and a dissecting room. An additional piece of land was taken from Messrs Kirkman and Hendy, making a total of six acres, lying between the new College Place on the west, the Fleet on the east, Crowndale Road on the south and College Grove to the north. To raise funds for the buildings, it was resolved that 'friends of the Institution should be requested to lend money on interest at three per cent per annum — the principal to be repaid as soon as funds of the College were found sufficient for that purpose'.

On 26 April 1792 it was agreed that Messrs Howell and Russell should build the stables for £2,850. The Professor was told he was allowed to see diseased horses of subscribers only between one and three o'clock, and he was also told to avoid giving an opinion on any proposed purchaser of horses. To this meeting the Professor presented a surprising memorandum in which he stated that he had been calumniated both with respect to his private character and his professional abilities, and requesting that committees should be appointed immediately to enquire into the matter and report. A committee, comprising John Hunter and 15 (eventually 17) professional gentlemen was appointed to examine Vial (one year after his appointment) as to his abilities in the office of veterinary Professor. The Earl of Morton (one of Vial's earliest patrons in this country) and 12 other gentlemen were appointed to deal with the calumny aspect.

The reports from these committees were presented at a special general meeting on 17 May, as follows:

1. 'Veterinary College May 9th 1792 — At a meeting (held at the Crown & Anchor Tavern in the Strand) of a committee of Physicians and Surgeons appointed at the request of the Veterinary College, for the purpose of investigating the medical and chirurgical abilities of Mr C.B. Vial the professor of the above Institution, Present: John Hunter, Esq., Sir George Baker, Bart., Doctor Crawford, Doctor Packwood, Everard Home, Esq., Mr Cline, Mr Vaux, Mr Peake and Mr Thos. Sheldon, The following Resolutions wre unanimously agreed to:- The treatment of Horses and other Animals (serviceable to mankind) divides itself, in the Opinion of the Committee into three Branches — similar to the treatment of Man — that is to say — internal and external diseases — We know that, in the practice of Medicine, where we have our Intelligence from patients; both Professions are too much for one Man to undertake and much less to practice and teach. We think, therefore, that it is absolutely necessary in order to carry on the Business of this Establishment, as perfectly as possible, that two such Characters should be appointed — and we, in consequence suggest, that altho' each be as much as possible qualified in both Departments, yet if one were to devote himself to one Branch and the other to the other branch — the College would be much more usefully directed — for, if one Professor were fully qualified for both — yet so arduous a task could not possibly be executed by one Man only. The Committee after minute Examination, do recommend Mr Vial as properly qualified for one of the professors — and they do further observe that if the Members of the College coincide in this Opinion, they are ready to investigate the merits of any other Candidate. John Hunter, Chairman.'

2. 'Veterinary College, London. Crown & Anchor Tavern, Strand 17th May 1792. At a meeting of the Committee appointed to enquire into the Complaints made by the Officers of

this Institution. Earl of Morton in the Chair. That it appears to this Committee that the Secretary (Mr Huntingford) has propagated reports injurious to the character of the Professor and that his conduct appears highly culpable in having spread such reports after he had reason to be satisfied that they were groundless.

'That it appears to this Committee that the conduct of the Secretary has been highly culpable in inspecting and exposing the contents of papers of a private nature belonging to the professor which had by accident fallen into his (the Secretary's) hands.

'That it appears to this Committee that the conduct of the Secretary has been highly improper, in suppressing a Letter addressed to the general Committee.

'That this Committee having inspected various Documents produced by the Professor Mr Vial, are satisfied of their Authenticity and of the fairness of his Character — and that he did actually hold in France the situations of professor of the Veterinary School and of Ecuyer du Roi at Lyons and of professor of comparative anatomy at Montpellier. Morton, Chairman, Heathfield, James Murray, John Julius Angerstein [1735-1823, whose collection of pictures formed the basis of the National Gallery], Alexr. Hendy, John Baynes, John Ingilby, J. Butt, Wm. Baker, W. Walcot.'

The special general meeting then resolved 'that from the report of the medical Committee consisting of John Hunter Esq. Chairman &c. this meeting is perfectly satisfied that Mr Vial is properly qualified for the Office of Veterinary Professor in this College. Resolved that this meeting concurs in Apinion [sic] with the said Committee — that it will be necessary to carry on the Business of this Institution as perfectly as possible, that there should be two Professors appointed & that as soon as the proposed plan for the College is executed, which, from the Encouragement already given, 'tis hoped will be speedily accomplished — The members will avail themselves of the Offer made by the Committee and refer the Merits of Candidates for the second professorship to their investigation. Resolved that, from the report of the Committee consisting of the Earl of Morton, Chairman, &c this meeting is perfectly satisfied with the Character & Conduct of the Professor Mr Vial and is of opinion that the conduct of the Secretary Mr Huntingford is highly culpable in having propagated reports injurious to the Professor Mr Vial after he had reason to be satisfied the [sic] were groundless.'

Mr Stone then left the chair, and was succeeded by Mr Walcot. 'Resolved that in consequence of the report of the Committee last mentioned and the charges now exhibited against the said Secretary — this meeting is of the opinion that his conduct has been highly injurious to the Interests of the College and that he be immediately dismissed.' The secretary was then called in, and after a serious address from the chairman, he was informed of the resolution of the general meeting, and that he was dismissed from the service of the College. This was not welcomed by all the students, some of whom left the College after the secretary's dismissal, causing it to issue an advertisement calling on clients not to employ them as farriers.

From these reports, it seems that Huntingford at least was not satisfied that Vial was all he claimed to be. Hunter's committee clearly thought that Vial on his own could not conduct the course, while Morton's committee appear to have accepted Vial's claims regarding appointments which apparently he had never held. There is a curious statement in the minutes of the general meeting, that William Stone left the chair before sentence of dismissal was pronounced on Huntingford. Stone was arrested on a charge of high treason on 3 May 1794 and was taken to the Tower of London. He remained imprisoned and untried for nearly two years, eventually being found not guilty after a trial on 28 January 1795. On 10 May 1794, Huntingford wrote to the Speaker of the House of Commons (who had himself been elected a vice-president of the College) as follows: 'Honble Sir, I should not have taken the liberty of troubling you on the subject of the Veterinary College did not the recent business of Wm Stone who stands charged with High Treason prove the cause of his exerting himself to my prejudice in favor of M Vial the late Professor, to be that he might establish a French Connection in that Institution in order that he might through the channel carry on his correspondence with the enemy. I am much induced to believe that from an examination of the foreign correspondence of that Society (of which W. Watson of Bartlett's Buildings is sollicitor) [sic] some traces might be found which might lead to discover some of Mr. Stone's accomplices. I have the honor to be with great respect and esteem Honble Sir Your most Obedient humble Servant, J. Huntingford'.

Thus Vial got the support he asked for, and Huntingford, to whose untiring efforts the establishment and early functioning of the College was in very great measure due, was ignominiously dismissed.

At the end of May 1792 the College decided it had no further occasion for the service of Blaine, who had been assisting Vial as demonstrator in anatomy. Blaine says he was let go because he had found Vial in error on anatomical matters. William Mounsher was appointed College secretary in succession to Huntingford on 1 July, when a smith was also appointed. At the end of July, the College decided to build lecture and dissecting rooms and enclosing walls. In August, the forge was open for the reception of subscribers' horses, at one shilling per shoe. Among the 913 subscribers in 1793 were Members of Parliament, lords, knights, doctors, clergymen, dukes, earls, viscounts, marquesses, one margrave (of Anspach), barons, military men, and a number of fellows of the Royal Society. The names of women subscribers appeared in 1793 and later years. In 1793 there were Mrs Wood of Lime Grove, Putney; Mrs Codrington of Davies Street, Berkeley Square; Lady Elcho of Queen Anne Street, Westminster; in 1822, Mrs Boucherett at J. Angerstein's House, Pall Mall; Miss E. Corbett of Wimpole Street; Lady C. Denys at the Pavilion, Hans Square; Lady Mary Eyre of Mortlake; Mrs J. Franks of Charles Street, Berkeley Square; Countess Glengall, Lower Grosvenor Street, Mrs Arabella Rainley, Chesterfield Street; Mrs Rougement of Clapham; Mrs Shepherd of Wimpole Street. It is clear that these women subscribers lived in the best parts of London.

An important move in September 1792 was the appointment of a medical experimental committee, consisting of Sir George Baker, Sir William Fordyce, Dr Crawford, Dr Scott, John Hunter, Mr Cline and Mr Houlston. Their task was to suggest experiments that might be carried out in the College, and to act as an examination committee for awarding certificates after pupils had completed the course.

Edmund Bond (the dissector of Eclipse) became a resident pupil. A young entrant was Mr Eldred, aged 15, of King's Lynn. Another resident pupil admitted was Bracy Clark of Worcester. A residence was acquired for the secretary, and a water supply was sought from the Hampstead and New River Companies. There was extensive building work — the excise duty on 441,515 bricks is recorded as £23 18s 4½d.

The infirmary for the reception of diseased horses was opened on 1 January 1793, the first horse being led in by Bracy Clark. Percivall, in his 1834 introductory lecture, says one of the first operations performed by Vial at the College was the excision of two redundant or accessory feet which grew from the fetlocks of the forelegs of a foal. Vial operated on one leg at a time. In the first operation, which he performed 'with considerable anxiety', fearing that the superfluous digit communicated with the fetlock joint, he was assisted by John Hunter. Hunter, seeing Vial remove the part without preserving a flap of skin to cover the wound, advised Vial, the next time he operated, to provide for this. The consequence of this 'friendly and useful' advice was that the parts healed in half the time after the second operation as they did after the first. It seems that Hunter's observations on thrombosis in veins were supplemented by noting the local effect of phlebotomy in the horse.

At the time there were some 900 subscribers to the College (a number seldom subsequently exceeded) and 14 pupils. The staff consisted of the Professor (Vial) secretary (Mounsher) collector (Reuben Smith) an assistant to the Professor (Prosser, engaged in November 1792) a porter, three smiths and five grooms. There were about 50 diseased horses in the infirmary. There was an interval at the beginning of 1793 when lectures had to be suspended — owing to the 'very disagreeable and offensive state of the dissecting room' — until the new theatre was ready in June. In March, George Dance Junior (1741-1825) was asked to examine the College's buildings regarding their solidity and the quality of the materials used. A week later, Dance reported satisfactorily, and he subsequently received five guineas for his trouble. In May, Burton was asked to make a path in lieu of the church path to Kentish Town which crossed the College grounds. At that time, too, the Professor complained (not for the first time) about the students' conduct.

In July 1793 — over a year after the Hunter committee had made its recommendations — Mr Butt gave notice that he would be asking the next general meeting to consider the propriety of appointing another professor to help Vial, whose duties were beyond the competence of any one individual. However, the death of Vial shortly afterwards threw everything into confusion. To quote the memoirs: '. . . on Sunday the 4th August 1793, after having finished the morning duty he always performed in person, of visiting, prescribing for, and superintending the dressing of the wounds of the horses in the infirmary, he sat down to continue his treatise on the outward conformation of the horse, a work he intended for publication: in a short time he informed Mrs. Vial that he felt himself extremely ill, complaining of cold to a degree of shivering, attended with a violent headach [sic], and great thirst. She administered to him some wine diluted in water. By this finding himself relieved, he again resumed his studies until the hour of dinner, when the disorder again attacked him so violently that it produced a fainting fit, which held him till the evening; he went soon after to bed, and passed a very uneasy, restless night. The next day Dr Crawford was called to him. Under the care of this gentleman he remained near a week; when, not finding that relief he hoped for, Dr Scott was requested to assist Dr Crawford, but with no better success, for, notwithstanding the united efforts of these eminent physicians, the fevers and faintings encreased [sic] till they ended in delirium and death on the 21st, being seventeen days after the first attack'.

According to Smith, the illness was described in the language of the day as a putrid fever with buboes on the face and body, which caused Dr Crawford to compare it to the plague. (Subsequent opinion — Hunting, Smith — is that the disease was glanders). No one was to be allowed to approach the body, although Bracy Clark, with the assistance of a London artist (though to be Flaxman, 1755-1826) took a plaster of Paris death cast of his face. Many years later, in 1861, at a meeting in the Freemasons' tavern on 23 February, the proposal was made that a marble bust of Vial should be made for the Royal College. The whereabouts of Flaxman's death mask was not known, and nothing came of the suggestion. Vial was buried (at the expense of the College, as a mark of respect) in the chapel in the Savoy — Vial's wife was of the Lutheran faith. The service, which cost £49 7s, was conducted in German and attended by staff, governors and pupils. Smith could not trace Vial's tomb; the chapel was later pulled down, and the bodies buried there were transferred to the Great Northern Cemetery in New Southgate where, on the western side, shaded by yew trees, huge vault slabs cover the remains of the dead removed from the Savoy chapel in the Strand.

The death of Vial left his widow in parlous straits. For many years the College did not provide pensions for members of staff, let alone dependents. Mrs Vial was given a grant of ten guineas to purchase mourning dress, and was made, for a very short time only, a grant of 60 guineas per annum. In July 1794, the students presented a petition to the College for some assistance for the distressed widow.

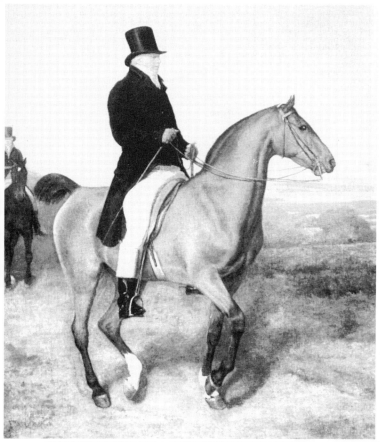

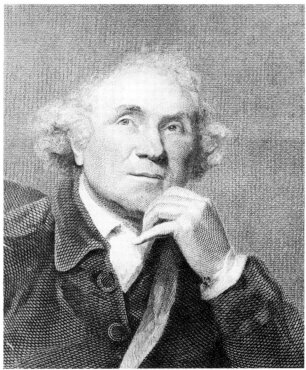

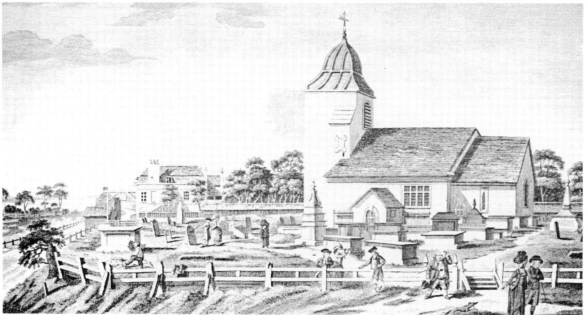

Lord Heathfield (1750-1813) was actively involved in founding the Veterinary College and (later) what was to become the Royal Army Veterinary Corps. From a painting by Jacques-Laurent Agasse (1767-1849) whose works include several made at the College. RIGHT: John Hunter FRS (1728-1793), elected vice-president of the Veterinary College in April 1791. BELOW: Old St Pancras Church, with the Adam and Eve Inn on left.

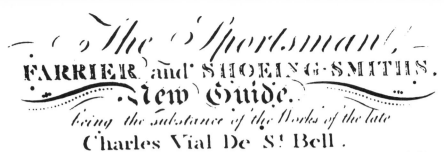

The Sportsman,
FARRIER and SHOEING-SMITHS.
New Guide.

being the substance of the Works of the late

Charles Vial De St Bell.

Professor of Medicine at the Veterinary College or Hospital for the Diseases of Horses,

St Pancras, London.

With Plates.

to which is prefixed a short Account of his Life & the Origin of the College
Also, an Appendix, containing valuable Extracts from the most
Approved Veterinary Writers.)

——— By John Lawrence. ———

Late of Lambeth Marsh, Surrey.

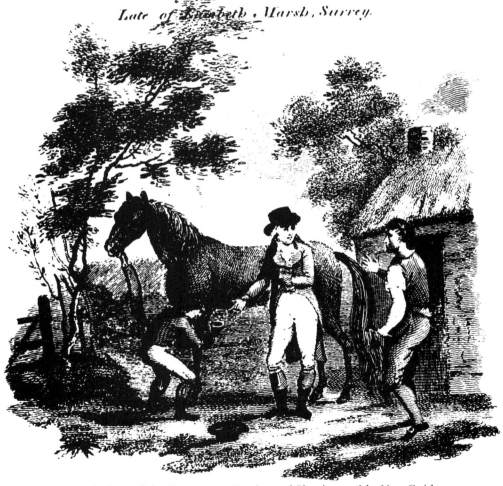

Frontispiece of 'the Sportsman, Farrier and Shoeing-smiths New Guide,
being the substance of the Works of the late Charles Vial De St Bell,
Professor of Medicine at the Veterinary College or Hospital for the
Diseases of Horses'.

INTERREGNUM

August 1793-February 1794

Following the death of Vial it was decided, on 24 August 1793, to leave the infirmary in charge of the pupils. They were placed under the supervision of a senior student, Richard Lawrence of Birmingham, who was to have one guinea a week and board and accommodation at the expense of the College. On 3 September a letter was received from William Moorcroft offering his temporary services, it was not followed up, on the ostensible grounds that it was a private letter addressed to Sheldon and not to the College committee in general. It was now once again resolved that two professors should be appointed, and the medical committee was asked to arrange a plan for their appointment and to define their duties. On the Sunday following, John Hunter chaired a meeting at the Crown & Anchor tavern, those present being Houlston, Crawford, Cline and Scott. Accepting that eventually two professors would be necessary, the meeting felt that in its then poor financial state the College might have to make do with one professor plus one subordinate teacher. In the event, two professors — Moorcroft and Coleman — were appointed, but only for a brief period.

Nine days later, on 17 September 1793, Hunter said that Fordyce, Baillie and Home would receive pupils recommended by the medical committee at their lectures. Later, students could attend lectures at the Royal Institution by Michael Faraday (1791-1867) who was himself the son of a blacksmith farrier. A letter had been received from E. Coleman, surgeon, of Palsgrave Place, Temple, but this was held in abeyance until 7 January 1794, A week later, Clark of Edinburgh, who had been offered the post of professor, was asked to make his mind up, whereupon he declined the appointment.

Having looked again at Coleman's letter of the previous September, the committee had some discussion with him, and eventually proposals prepared jointly by Coleman and Moorcroft were referred to a meeting, which they both attended, on 10 February 1794. On the 17th the medical committee (Cline, Crawford, Sandeman and Houlston) interviewed the two candidates separately. Coleman apparently refused the offer of the professorship unless Moorcroft became his colleague, and the two were appointed joint professors of the College on 18 February (proposed by Stone, seconded by Perkyns).

As we learn from Alder's book, *Beyond Bokhara*, William Moorcroft (1767-1825) was born in Ormskirk, Lancashire, the illegitimate son of Anne, daughter of Richard and Dorothy Moorcroft. Mother and son lived with her father. In the early 1780s William became a pupil of Dr John Lyon, one of the surgeons at Liverpool infirmary. While still a pupil there he was selected, along with Mr Wilson, reputedly the ablest farmer of the day, to investigate an epidemic disease in horned cattle; this is a curious echo of the student days of Vial. Moorcroft was subsequently encouraged by John Hunter to acquire a training at the veterinary school in Lyons. Lyons was chosen because it was believed to offer a more practical training than Alfort (especially in the control of cattle plagues) and was presumably a safe distance from revolutionary Paris. He was enrolled on 8 March 1790, paying six months' fees in advance, and completed his training on 7 March 1791. The Lyons course was scheduled to last four years, but few pupils stayed much more than a year. His Lyons school record says of him: 'A model of work and application, sharp and intelligent; he possesses remarkable knowledge for his years, has rapidly acquired our language and technical information'.

Moorcroft returned to England in 1791, and in the spring of 1792 he began to conduct a veterinary practice. As Smith commented, it is incomprehensible that Moorcroft does not appear to have been considered for appointment as the first Professor of the London College. In 1789 Moorcroft, of Russell Court, Half Moon Street, surgeon, had become a member of the future Royal Society of Arts. He was sponsored by William Houlson, surgeon, of Chancery Lane. He was presumably known to at least some of his fellow members — who themselves became foundation members of the Veterinary College — in particular the Duke of Northumberland, first president of the College; Granville Penn, active in the establishment of the College, who became a member of the Society of Arts in 1788 and was in 1791 a steward; the Earl of Morton (one of Vial's patrons); Thomas Pitt FSA, subsequently to be one of the most assiduous attenders of meetings of the College governors, and last, but not least, Arthur Young, a member of the Society of Arts since 1769.

In this context, Thomas Eccleston of Scarisbrick Hall is important; he is described as active in scientific farming and agricultural improvement, and seems to have treated Moorcroft as a son. On 20 January 1789, Eccleston concluded a letter to the editor of the *Transactions of the Society of Arts* with a postscript: 'Mr Moorcroft is a young man of the greatest abilities, and has agreed to turn his thoughts from the practice of physic and surgery, entirely to that of farriery in every branch, provided he can meet with sufficient and certain encouragement in the establishment of a Veterinarian School. If you can point out any method likely to raise a subscription for such a purpose, you will confer a singular favour on all in the farming line'.

Moorcroft and Coleman were appointed joint professors after an interregnum of seven months, but only a few weeks later, on 4 April, Moorcroft resigned. His reasons have been variously stated to include a wish to avoid undue interference by his College work with his private practice, and temperamental incompatibility with Coleman, who was only two years his senior. It is also said that Moorcroft was shocked to find that his co-professor was wholly ignorant of all veterinary matters; yet Moorcroft and Coleman had negotiated the terms of their joint appointment, and it is inconceivable that Moorcroft could have remained unaware of his future colleague's lack of veterinary knowledge. Moorcroft's letter of resignation refers to his ill health, but speaking 40 years later, Coleman said: 'I could see no ill health [in Moorcroft] at all. He also pleaded interference with his duty to those by whom he was employed in a private practice of considerable extent, but his time at the College had been clearly specified — two hours for consultation by subscribers with sick horses on three days a week, with little or no call upon him for attendance at uncertain hours.' (Moorcroft would also have had to prepare public and student lectures.) 'I confess I felt myself rather ill-used. I felt it would be presumptuous, perhaps dishonourable, for me, so little versed in veterinary matters, to superintend the interests and growth of the infant school'.

Ill-health does not appear to have been a long-lasting problem, for, with John Field, Moorcroft soon established a flourishing practice, eventually with stabling for 63 sick horses, in Oxford Street, and a further 20 stalls at a branch in Hammersmith. It has been estimated that in 16 years he acquired a fortune of £40,000, despite apparently losing a lot of money in a project for the commercial manufacture of seated cast-iron horseshoes.

Moorcroft was employed to manage the East India Company's stud in Essex, and to select breeding stock for their stud in Bengal. In 1808, at a salary of £3,000 a year, he became superintendent of the stud in India, where he was successful in controlling diseases and improving management (he is said to have introduced the cultivation of oats into India). He considered that the breeding of the company's horses could be improved by, for example, crossing Turkestan sires with Hindustan mares. He also became interested in the breeding of goats to provide wool for shawls. This led him to numerous adventures in penetrating to Kabul and beyond, which have been described by Smith, Barber-Lomax, and especially Alder, who studied much of the terrain, in enthusiastic detail.

Moorcroft, the first Englishman to cross the Himalayas, is something of a hero for veterinary historians, and the Veterinary History Society has marked the site of his practice in Oxford Street (now Littlewoods store) with a commemorative plaque. He was an outstanding veterinary surgeon, and obviously a man of enormous enterprise, daring courage and strong will.

According to one account, Moorcroft caught a fever and died near Ladakh (now in north-western Afghanistan) in 1825, while Smith says he was murdered on 27 August 1825, 'doubtless by the "cup of medicated tea" that he had so frequently described as being his destined end'.

Of Moorcroft's veterinary knowledge and skills, Smith has written at length. Of his short time as joint professor at the Veterinary College, no certain information has survived.

A contemporary magazine report of a horse infirmary near Coventry reflects some light on the College in Moorcroft's time. In the *Sporting Magazine* for March 1794, there appears a 'picturesque view of Palfrey's Infirmary' said to be about a quarter of a mile west of Coventry. The account describes the 'hospitals and open stables for the reception of diseased and sick horses in the first stage of their complaints' . . . 'more pure stables, which are taken up by horses in physic, or patients whose complaints are not contagious' . . . stocks where 'all operations are performed without the trouble or hazard of casting . . . a perfect skeleton of a horse, to refer to in cases of lameness, fractures, etc . . . various paddocks, some with and some without water for the better accommodation of horses of different descriptions, whose complaints require open air, or grass, for their perfect recovery'. The report concludes: 'In short, we believe it to be the most complete undertaking, (the Veterinary College excepted) of the kind in the kingdom'.

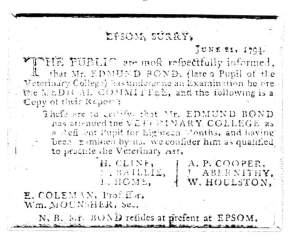

Newspaper announcement, June 1794: 'The public are most respectfully informed that Mr Edmund Bond (late a Pupil of the Veterinary College) has undergone an Examination before the Medical Committee, and the following is a Copy of their Report: These are to certify that Mr Edmund Bond has attended the Veterinary College as a Resident Pupil for Eighteen Months, and having been examined by us, we consider him as qualified to practise the Veterinary Art. H.Cline, M. Baillie, E. Home, A.P. Cooper, H. Abernithy, W. Houlston, E. Coleman, Professor Wm Mounsher, Sec. N. B. Mr Bond resides at present in Epsom.

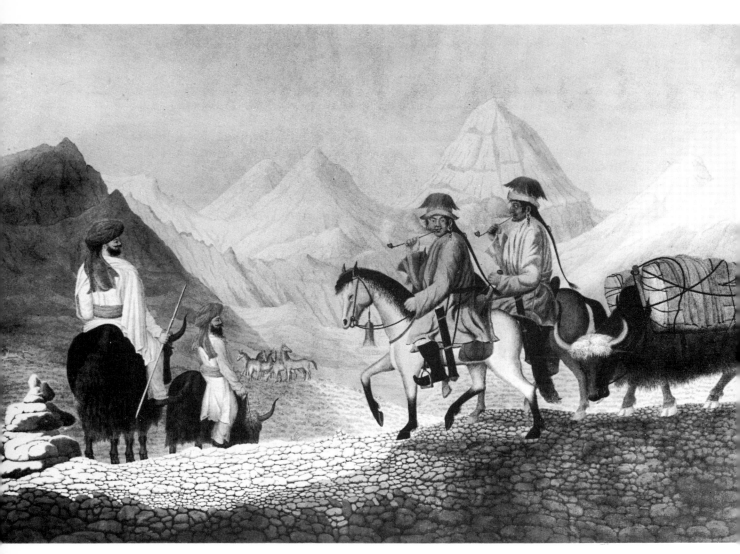

Hyder Hearsey's painting of Moorcroft (extreme left) and himself in Tibet, 1812. William Moorcroft, the first Englishman to cross the Himalayas, was professor at the College in 1794.

EDWARD COLEMAN

Professor 1794-1839

When Moorcroft resigned in April 1794, Coleman also proffered his resignation but was persuaded to continue in office. The recommendation by Hunter's committee that two professors were desirable was forgotten. Restricted finances allowed only one appointment, that of Coleman, who became sole Professor at the age of 28. The College was hampered by shortage of funds throughout Coleman's 45 years as Professor. Veterinary historians still differ sharply about the effect his long spell in charge of the College had on the emerging profession. Coleman, a surgeon with no veterinary training or experience, drastically reduced the length of the course of instruction. The buildings remained inadequate and the establishment was under-staffed. To augment the tuition at the College, students had to traipse all over London to attend lectures at medical schools, and to hear additional veterinary lectures on private premises in the evening. To gain experience in practical work, they went on their own initiative to slaughterhouses or the knacker's yard; horses were still almost the only animals seen at the College. Yet by the 1830s, some 50 students a year were gaining their qualifying diploma (after an oral examination, conducted exclusively by medical men) and the profession was steadily gaining recognition and status.

Soon after Coleman was appointed Professor, he was given two assistants: Sewell, who was later to succeed him as Principal, and Stockley.

William Stockley (1776-1860) was one of the six foundation students of the College, becoming a resident pupil in January 1792 on the recommendation of Lord Rivers. His certificate was dated 5 July 1794. He was assistant to Coleman until September 1795, and in that year, with the support of Lord Heathfield, he was sent to a regiment of cavalry to test the utility of introducing veterinary surgeons into the army and to justify the granting of public funds to the College.

Two conflicting assessments of Edward Coleman have been made — a favourable one by Principal James Beart Simonds, his one-time pupil at the College, in a biographical sketch published in his own old age, and an unfavourable one by Sir Frederick Smith in his *History of the Royal Army Veterinary Corps*. Smith said bluntly that Coleman's long life was an unmitigated evil (has anyone ever lived such a life?). This extreme view was not even sustained by Smith himself, although it has been repeated at intervals by people who should have known better. Coleman, of course, is 'indifferent to blame or praise, bribe or threat'. But, since he was Professor (or, as we would now call him, Principal) at the Veterinary College for over 45 years, and Principal Army Veterinary Surgeon for nearly 43 years, and since in these positions he inevitably greatly influenced the development of our College and profession, an attempt at a balanced re-appraisal seems worthwhile.

Smith expressed his typically extreme view that the appointment of Coleman was the greatest calamity the veterinary profession ever experienced. Coleman, he wrote, a struggling surgeon 'condescended' (why condescended?) 'to come to our only veterinary college and to teach that of which he had absolutely no knowledge or experience'. However, Coleman's reported disclaimer at that time should be remembered: 'I am come to learn and not to teach'.

Youatt said the bust of Coleman by Sievier (among whose other works is the bust of Edward Jenner in Gloucester cathedral) was a lifelike portrayal. The presentation to Coleman of the bust took place on 10 March 1835, and was suggested by two Lancashire practitioners, Byron and Hollingworth. Coleman, whose three surviving daughters sat opposite him, was noticed to be in some pain (he suffered from gout in his later years). A number of copies of the bust was made. One is in the College, one was presented to Astley Cooper and one, with the toga'd bust in reverse, is in the Royal College historical library. At the College there is an engraving of Coleman as a younger man, probably under 40, which is reproduced on the magnificent certificates of the London Veterinary Medical Society.

Thomas Mayer, with fellow students Youatt and Turner, founded the London Veterinary Medical Society at the College in 1813. It met every week from 7-9pm at a tavern in Marchmont Street, and was said to have 'risen like a phoenix' from the ashes of an earlier society. In 1814 Sewell became its president, and a little later Coleman, who had earlier declined an invitation to be president, became its patron.

The history of the society up to 1828 appears to have been almost entirely lost. In that year, a separate society of practitioners was formed, which did not become amalgamated with the College's society. This practitioners' society functioned until 1835, when it was dissolved because of poor attendance by its members, while the College's society continued to exist. Richard Vines was its librarian, but he was removed from office after six years and, after he had openly burned his certificate of membership of the society, he was voted to be a non-member. In March 1836 a group of student members demanded that Vines be restored to the society, and formed themselves into a committee of management, upon which all the officers resigned. The society apparently ceased to exist in 1837. However, on 12 September 1836 a number of practitioners met at the Freemansons' tavern, and decided to unite practitioners and students in a new association. The Veterinary Medical Association so formed, familiarly known since then as the VMA, received permission to hold a meeting in the College theatre on 22 November 1836. Coleman was elected patron, Sewell chairman, Morton secretary and Youatt treasurer.

The disruptive activities of Richard Vines (1794-1865) were in accord with his reputation as a trouble-maker. He qualified at the College in 1824, being rather older than most of the students, and was appointed demonstrator in anatomy by Coleman. He was something of an experimentalist, being particularly interested in glanders (he claimed success in some cases from treatment with cantharides) and in the circulatory system. Rush's paper in March 1836 to the Veterinary Medical Society on *The Blood Circulation in the Foetus and Adult, and the changes it undergoes during Respiration* was challenged by Vines as an unacknowledged copy of his own work. Vines, as a non-member, was directed to retire from the meeting, but he was apparently responsible for some insurrection among the student members. Vines resigned from the College in 1838, setting up private practice at 13 Great College Street, the third house up from the College. He died there in April 1865, aged 71.

Over the years, the VMA gradually became a students' association and at the first general meeting of its 45th session, on 19 October 1880, John H. Steel, the secretary and librarian, announced 'the Veterinary Medical Association, while having wide sympathies with its members who have become qualified practitioners, is now the Students' Society of the largest British Veterinary School'. Less than two years later the students asked the new Principal,

Professor Robertson, for help in forming a medical society — 'one in the government of which students, being constituent parts of the Society, should have a voice and vote'. Thus was founded the Royal Veterinary College Medical Society, later known as the RVCVMA, and now the RVCMA.

In 1936, despite considerable controversy among veterinary historians about when the association was founded, the RCVMA decided to celebrate its centenary. The association was resuscitated in 1976, after a lapse of 10 years, by Professor Richard Penny, Ruth Layton being elected the first 'new' president. Ten years later, in May 1986, the RVC Medical Association celebrated its sesquicentenary. The occasion was marked by the unveiling of a commemorative plaque in the hall of the College in Camden Town by Professor Clifford Formston.

In 1834, the pseudonymous Paul Pry observed of Coleman, now 'stricken with years', that

'Time has laid his temples bare
And turned to white his once dark hair.'

According to the same writer, Coleman was a little below middle height. His features were irregular, but gave a strong impression of intellectual energy. Unfortunately most of what we know about Coleman is related to the last decade or so of his life. He had then become an object of often severely critical interest to the *Veterinarian*, the journal founded in 1828 by William Percivall to reform, it said, certain alleged abuse in the College.

Coleman had a powerful personality, and Smith admitted that he was also a man of great charm, adding (on unstated evidence) that 'he had all the cleverness of a woman at turning that advantage to account'. In old age, he quietened somewhat — 'I want only social comfort and good feeling' — but he was not afraid to meet his critics on occasion. In the face of many attacks, he continued imperturbably on his way — the dogs barked, but the caravan moved on — and this steadfastness seems to have aroused his critics to further ineffectual fury.

In temperament, Coleman appears to have been somewhat mercurial, and he could be despondent, as he was understandably at the time of his wife's illness. Bransby Cooper (Sir Astley's nephew) who knew Coleman personally for many years, said it seemed impossible not to love one so agreeable, kind-hearted, and blessed with all those qualities which endear man to man. Coleman lived on cordial terms with his assistant, William Sewell, for over 40 years. He charged Sewell with the maintenance of discipline in the College (which led to Sewell recommending the expulsion of only one pupil, although some students paid too much attention to tavern and skittle-ground). Smith, true to form, condemned this entirely usual and reasonable delegation of disciplinary authority to the second-in-command as being Coleman's method of avoiding any loss of popularity with his students. This popularity was undoubtedly great, and their affection was fully reciprocated by Coleman. He frequently referred to the students when they were at College, and for long after, as his 'children'.

Sir Benjamin Brodie, in an obituary address to the Royal Medicochirurgical Society (of which Coleman had been a member) said he though Coleman's intellect was of a high order, and even gave indications of genius. 'He had obtained little knowledge from books, but he had been an original observer, and had reflected much on all he had observed, and drew his own conclusions. Hence it was that in many subjects he was behind the knowledge of the day. However, he had a peculiar knowledge of his own, and could give information such as no one else could impart.'

Coleman's superior natural talents were admitted by his bitterest critics, and there are many tributes on record to his powers as a teacher. He delivered up to 90 lectures in a session in the College theatre. If this resembled (as seems likely) in the closing years of Coleman's life what it had become in 1846, when an anonymous member of the Royal College visited it, the word theatre was a grandiloquent description of an ignoble room. At the time, we are told by

'MRCVS' that the College buildings were low and plain, and bleak even to bareness, suggesting a warehouse, barracks or mews rather than a seat of learning (the brick front facing College Street was not stuccoed until much later). The main entrance was through an archway, the folding gates of which were kept closed, necessitating entry even for horses through an inconvenient wicket gate. Under the archway one of a pair of glass doors led to a room, estimated (wrongly?) by MRCVS as being about 10 feet long and six feet wide; this was the combined consulting room for the Professor and the College library. The un-named visitor thought the whole scene, complete with students buying oranges and nuts from an old man under the archway, was one of 'painful vapidity'. (Incidentally, oranges and nuts seem to have occupied in the social life of those days the place soft drinks and ice cream occupy today, being consumed in great quantities even in the most dignified circles.)

The students had no room in which to wait between lectures, but it was suggested to MRCVS that students who lodged near enough might go home if they wanted to, or more usefully spend their non-lecture time in the dissecting room or in the stables, although the Bell & Crown inn, with a good fire, was close at hand.

Along a short passage, the visitor came to the locked theatre door (the same door whose creaking had sometimes disturbed Coleman in his introductory lectures, when old students who had come to pay their respects, arrived after he had begun). The theatre was estimated to measure about 10 feet in height, 15 in breadth, and 20 in length (can these measurements be correct — classes sometimes numbered 70 or more students?). The theatre had two windows, between which was a table. In front of this table were four rows of benches, slightly raised one above the other. The lecturer stood between the table and the wall — the worst possible position. The room was badly ventilated, and the floor was strewn with nut shells and orange peel. It is reported that the window blinds had been indecently defaced wih coloured chalk. It sounds most depressing.

Supplementing this account of the College shortly after the Coleman regime comes one written late in life by Principal Simonds, describing the College and its environs in 1828-1829, when he was a student there. He notes that: 'the Institution was built in a Quadrangle Form, having now in the centre a large lawn or grass plot surrounded by posts and chains, and that between the Buildings and these a broad Pathway had been left, partly paved with stones . . . used chiefly for testing the freedom from lameness of Horses sent for examination prior to purchase; as well as for ascertaining the progress of those under treatment in the Infirmary for lameness arising from various causes.

'In the central part of the Lawn, a Mound, planted with trees and shrubs, concealed from view a large Water-tank, protected by a strong iron grating. From this source the water — needed by the whole Institution — is drawn, the supply to the tank being furnished by the New River Company.' (This tank, filled with concrete, still exists beneath the main hall of the College in Camden Town). Simonds goes on to describe the general layout in some detail, including 'a long stable, well lighted (by windows and oil lamps) and ventilated. It is filled with horses mostly affected with lameness. At the furthermost end of it, a door opens into the Upper Paddock. We . . . turn to the right and find a long line of Loose Boxes extending to the Forge . . . Passing out of the entrance to these boxes into the Quadrangle, we observe a residence on the opposite side corresponding in elevation to that of the Forge. It is the one in which Assistant Professor Sewell resides. We now walk along a covered way called the Ride, designed for exercising Infirmary Patients, and also for testing for freedom from disease or otherwise of the Respiratory Organs of horses prior to purchase. Reaching the end we observe that, adjacent to the Assistant Professor's house, another series of Loose Boxes . . . are erected. These with some stalls intervening, we saw reached to the furthermost end of the main building, a wall separating them from the Museum and also from College Street.

'Returning now to the Long Stable, we enter the Upper Paddock, and first observe a hot-water apparatus, so arranged as to supply practically a constant supply. Here a wide entrance, guarded by boarded doors from the street provides for the bringing in of Corn, Hay, Straw, &c . . . receptacles for soiled litter and stable sweepings are provided. On the north side of this Paddock a low wall separates it from some buildings occasionally used for canine patients, but chiefly as a Storage . . . Erected on its south, east, and west sides we also observe several lean-to Infirmary Sheds . . . From the Upper we enter (eastwards) the Middle Paddock, which is also surrounded by similar Sheds; at the north-west corner . . . a brick-built Loose Box, for the reception of Equine patients suffering from glanders and other special diseases. From Middle Paddock we pass (still eastwards) into the Lower one . . . Here the Dissecting-room . . . also a similar detached Loose Box . . . The Fleet Ditch here forms the boundary of the College ground . . . we, Students, in my days, now drawing near to seventy years since, too often left the study of Anatomy, during the absence of Mr Vines, to try our powers as Athletes by jumping over, not, however, infrequently into, the Ditch — unto a narrow road on the other side — the frontage to some half-dozen cottages. This road we also notice leads from King's Road [Pancras Way] as a back entrance to Professor Coleman's residence and garden, and to his stable, coach-house and kennel for his dogs — which, however, we understood he rarely used except in the shooting season.

'His [Coleman's] House, doubtless was the one originally occupied by Vial, there being no other in the immediate neighbourhood of sufficient size for his family and resident Students. Being situated on the opposite side of the Fleet, it was approached from the College buildings by a strongly-built Rustic-bridge which spanned the river just in front of the Forge at the north end of the Ride . . . It may here also be explained that after the main source of the Fleet was diverted, the portion of it which originally formed the boundary of the site granted for the building of the College, became a stagnant Ditch, which in process of time dried up, and that, with the addition of gravel and earth, a dry path from the College to the Professor's house was thus constructed. There being now no necessity for the bridge, it was removed . . . about the year 1834. A Gate was now fixed at the entrance to the garden, which as a rule was kept locked — a necessary precaution . . . when so many young men were located near thereto.

'The Professor's garden, however, was not only protected originally on the College side by the Fleet Ditch, but by a Thorn-planted Hedge, which extended onwards to the Bridge in Fig Lane [Crowndale Road] thus also enclosing the 'Green' at the back of the Elephant & Castle Inn. About the same date [1834] a range of Loose Boxes and Stalls were erected in the Lower Paddock near to the Ditch. The reserved ground around them, together with some addition subsequently gained by filling up of the Ditch, thus provided for a back entrance to the College from King's Road. This entrance was protected by a boarded fence and gate sufficiently wide to admit carriages. Professor Sewell had a square building erected, open on each side, so that operations, requiring the casting of the patient, could be performed under shelter in any state of the weather'. (Morton occupied Coleman's house after the latter's death, until he retired in 1860. The house then reverted to its owners, who erected a wall separating their premises from those of the College).

The environs of the College in 1828-1829 are described by Simonds in *A ramble from the Royal Veterinary College to Battle Bridge and back*. He starts by entering College Grove. 'First on our way (east) we crossed the old Fleet Ditch by a wooden bridge, rather rudely constructed. Looking to our right we recognised the Cottages with the road in front of them close to the ditch; also our Professor's stable, coach-house and dog kennels, with the back entrance from the road to his garden . . . we were soon in King's Road [Pancras Way] which we found to be well studded with trees on each side . . . to our left the Country residence of Counsellor Agar [builder of Agar's Town] . . . we turned to the right and first took notice of the front of our Professor's house with its large garden protected from the pathway and road by a brick wall.

49

A little further on we passed the Elephant & Castle Inn [in Pancras Way, near to the workhouse of 1809] kept by Mr Wrench, who is reported to be very strict in his management of the Inn. Many of the students go here to dine, and are also accustomed to assemble together in the evening. Father Wrench, however, as he is sometimes called — will never allow more than a proper quantity of either ale, wine or spirits . . . We here crossed to the other side of the road, near to the Workhouse, and soon passed (on the left) a row of small houses called Cook's Row, and a little further on another row — Church Row — at the nothern end of which stood the Adam & Eve Inn with its attached Tea gardens. The place looked inviting, nevertheless we do not enter'.

The site of these gardens is now St Giles-in-the-Fields burial ground, north of Old St Pancras Church, which is built on a natural or embanked hillock. The tavern, we learn from Walford, originally had attached to it some extensive pleasure grounds.

Simonds notes that 'Nearly opposite to St Pancras Church stood a Toll-Bar, and to prevent horsemen avoiding payment, some posts were erected on the footpath, between which we had to pass. No demand, however, was made on us by the gate-keeper, the authorities being so liberal as not to charge persons for walking either on the roads or footpaths.

'Being quit of this obstruction, we were soon on the Bridge . . . We learned, however, that highway robberies in past days were very common in the district of both Camden and Kentish Town; and on more than one occasion we had heard Professor Sewell state that a Hampstead stage coach . . . was stopped and the passengers robbed near to St Pancras Church . . . With further reference to the Toll-gate, it may be stated that the general traffic on the road, even in 1828-9, was but little, and that scarcely on any occasion was the Keeper required to sit up late. An exception to this has to be mentioned, viz., that Professor Coleman was accustomed, unless prevented by some special cause — to visit Sir Astley Cooper in the evening of one day in the week during the winter half of the year, to indulge in a game of whist. Thus, his return was often late, much to the annoyance of the Gatekeeper. To soften his feelings, however, we learned that the Professor from time to time gave him a fee which far exceeded the amount of the toll . . . just by the Bridge, turnstiles admitted foot-passengers to pass by different paths, intersecting the large extent of open ground, some of this led to Somers Town, Red Lion Street, etc . . . here and there, especially at the lower portion of the [College] ground, walls were standing, some of them being eight or ten feet high.' (Part of the wall facing College Street, at the lower limit of the pathology building, has unaccountably survived.)

'. . . for many years after the time named in this Ramble, Great College Street — beyond the terrace of houses extending to the entrance of Messrs. Goodall's existing premises — was totally impassable even as a footpath in the winter. At length, however, the Parish authorities saw fit to properly put this also into repair, and extend the Street to Camden Road.'

Paul Pry described an introductory lecture given to nearly 80 students (20 per bench) in the closing years of Coleman's life. The Professor, he tells us, was some time in making his appearance, but suddenly the noise and bustle of conversation were stopped by his entrance. His walk, attitude and gestures were those of a self-confident man, a little addicted to be indifferent to others, and far more disposed to lead than to follow. He lectured on the anatomy, physiology and pathology of the horse, and clearly took enormous pleasure in communicating knowledge. Those who heard him lecture remarked on the way he seized on and illustrated the most interesting parts of his subject, so that he was intelligible to the novice and listened to with pleasure by even the best informed, generally leading his class unresistingly to the desired conclusion. His lectures on the eye, the foetal circulation, and especially on the foot, would never, it was claimed, be forgotten by those who had the good fortune to hear him.

In the elucidation of disease and its treatment, while the patient was standing by, Coleman was said to be even more successful. The two, sometimes three, hours spent in the College quadrangle when, we are told, the Professor would courteously listen and give an intelligible answer to every question, and when the instruction he communicated was stamped on the memory by the good temper and joke and repartee with which it was accompanied, these were periods which an old student liked to call to memory, for they were hours pleasantly and usefully passed.

The rest of the College, like the theatre, seems in Paul Pry's day to have run to seed. The museum, said to be about 30 feet long, was the largest room. A few years after Coleman's death it contained dried specimens under an accumulation of discoloured varnish, plus an incomplete horse skeleton, but there was no catalogue. The pupils were said to have no right of entry into the museum (nor, it was said, did they have access to a certain 'necessary article'). The stables were well built but badly ventilated (surely not be expected in Coleman's time, for he was the arch-exponent of adequate ventilation) a duct-blocking luxuriant vine having been trained against the outside wall of some loose boxes.

There were three dissecting rooms, containing carcasses of donkeys purchased wholesale. On an open piece of ground with no privacy, the donkeys were destroyed, horses slaughtered, and operations performed. It is alleged that, through the hedge, the local boys and girls could see 'the most disgusting sights'. Even so, the College buildings, although in a damp locality and a badly chosen situation, were thought to have 'capabilities' if the spirit and inclination for improvement existed.

The animals coming into the infirmary were almost entirely horses. In 1828, for example, there were admitted 869 horses, one ass and 16 dogs. Many of the horses were lame. The College pharmacopoeia consisted largely of aloes, calomel, copper sulphate and croton oil. No regular warning was given to students of the time of operations. There appears to have been some slackness in staff discipline in that teachers were often late for, or even absent from, lectures.

What on Hunter's initiative had been a saving grace for the College on Vial's death — the admission of veterinary students to lectures by surgeons and physicians — later became a source of complaint. Students spent a lot of time travelling (walking and even running) from one lecture to another in various parts of London, and it was increasingly demanded that they should find within the walls of the College all that they required, or that they should at least pay a fee that would entitle them as of right, rather than for charity's sake, to enter medical lectures. For some time, however, teaching was supplemented, with the College's approbation, in three main fields. Charles Spooner, from 1834, gave anatomy lectures at his house in College Street. Morton gave lectures on chemistry and *materia medica* in the evenings; Youatt lectured in Nassau Street on animals other than the horse, with the blessing of London University.

One of the major preoccupations of the young veterinary profession was a search for public recognition of its respectability, the gaining of which has now been crowned by the secular apotheosis of James Herriot. Right from the start, the College included men of the highest aristocratic or professional standing among its governors and subscribers. The Prince Regent is reported as a subscriber on 2 May 1811, having expressed the view that the College 'held forth the expectation of much public benefit'. In 1818, on the death of the Duke of Northumberland, the Duke of York became president. Since then, the College has enjoyed continuous royal patronage, the title of the office having been changed from 'president' to 'patron' in 1956, following the different system of government resulting from the College's new Charter. The Duke of Gloucester, appointed in 1932, became the last president and first official patron of the College, and the Duke of Edinburgh agreed to become patron in 1975 following the Duke of Gloucester's death.

51

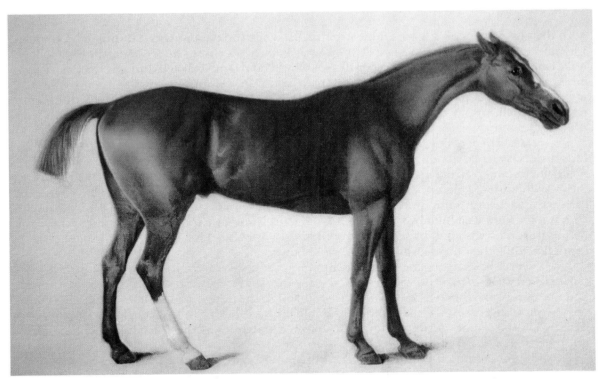

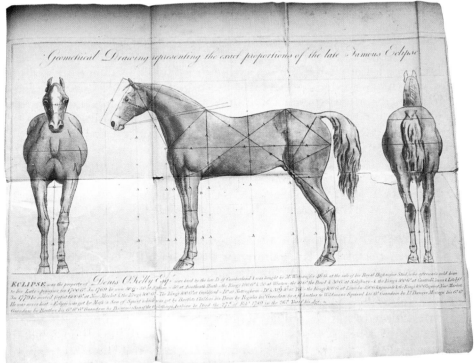

ABOVE: Eclipse, by George Stubbs, reputedly the only painting of this famous horse to have been made from life. BELOW: 'Geometrical Drawing representing the exact proportions of the late Famous Eclipse' from the Essay published by Vial, 1791.

The casual unauthorised assumption of the word Royal into the College's title is generally thought to have occurred in about 1828. George IV became patron on 27 May 1827 and the College minutes, which referred to the Veterinary College on 25 May 1828, used the title Royal in June. However, *The Lancet* referred to 'the Royal Veterinary College' as early as 22 December 1827. The *Farrier and Naturalist* for 1828 has a frontispiece showing the Royal Veterinary College. In the early part of the April issue, it refers to the Veterinary College, but in the later part to the Royal Veterinary College. Curiously enough, an unidentified author (William Nesbit?) in the second (1818) edition of *Authentic Memoirs, biographical, critical and literary, of the most eminent physicians and surgeons in Great Britain,* included Coleman as 'Royal Veterinary Professor' and refers to the College as 'the Royal Veterinary College, Pancras' (for many years of its life, the College was known as the St Pancras School, the term 'Camden Town' coming into use much later).

Coleman claimed that his greatest contribution to the young veterinary profession was that he played a major role in securing that from 1796 appointments as veterinary surgeons (a term used by the Standing Board of General Officers) in the cavalry, and eventually (1805) in the artillery, were by commission rather than by warrant. Even so, Coleman did not attempt the then unachievable, and claim equality with the medical profession. He said bluntly that he was a great advocate of a proper observance of status and rank. The veterinary surgeon should not claim a higher place for his profession than the public thought it had earned, and was willing to give it. Human surgery and medicine would always be superior to a profession where the education was less expensive, the difficulties of the courses of instruction were fewer, emoluments were smaller, and the sanctity of life was not a determinant of treatment.

Smith, who has set out Coleman's army career in detail, concurred with the opinion of F.C. Cherry (who succeeded Coleman as Principal Army Veterinary Surgeon on Coleman's death, thus blighting the hope of assistant professor Sewell that he might follow Coleman in that post) that Coleman was 'the greatest enemy that the profession has ever had in its highest ranks'. This is frankly unbelievable. Coleman would have had to be a man of superhuman cunning and stupidity to have served for over 40 years fighting the very thing he was engaged in creating. It is obvious that Smith's assessment is coloured by his self-revealing remark that 'Coleman had never done a day's soldiering in his life, and for that reason alone was incapable of leading and directing'.

In *A History of the Royal Army Veterinary Corps*, Smith has described Coleman's relationship with the establishment and development of the army veterinary service. It appears that on 19 February 1796 the Deputy Adjutant-General of Artillery reported to the Board of Ordnance on a disease affecting artillery horses in Kent. The board directed Coleman to investigate the disease, and he diagnosed the condition as glanders. In his report, Coleman suggested that the 'prodigious loss of horses was due to expert advice not having been sought when the outbreak started'. Representation was made to the board that an appointment securing Coleman's attendance would quickly pay for itself.

Coleman, in a letter of 17 February, proposed that an infirmary should be prepared in part of the Woolwich stables, where he could attend once or twice a week. He also suggested that a College pupil should be in residence at Woolwich, to remain there until the farriers were 'sufficiently instructed in the treatment of disease'. The assistant was John Percivall, who qualified in 1795.

On 3 March the Adjutant-General of the army directed a standing committee of general officers to report *inter alia* whether the instruction at the College was such as to furnish the means of improving the present practice of farriery. The committee reported, and it was agreed on 24 May that a veterinary surgeon should be attached to each regiment of cavalry. It was hoped that medical men would be attracted to take the College course, and then be commissioned as veterinary surgeons in the cavalry. The first and only veterinary surgeon appointed to the army in 1796 joined the 11th Light Dragoons on 25 June that year as a warrant officer, but was commissioned the following year. He was John Shipp, the elusive subject of devoted study by Dr Ernest Gray.

In the artillery, veterinary surgeons served on warrants issued by the Master General of the Ordnance, receiving the right to commissions in 1805 when Thomas Peall (who qualified in London in 1796) and others addressed the Commander-in-Chief about this anomaly. (It was this Thomas Peall who, while still at College in 1795, produced glanders in an ass by placing the discharge from a farcy ulcer inside the nostrils).

By commission dated 21 September 1796 Coleman became Principal Veterinary Surgeon to the cavalry, and was also appointed veterinary surgeon to the artillery in a civil capacity, holding these posts until his death. His duties included the preparation of a handbook of *Instructions for the use of farriers attached to the British Cavalry and to the Honourable Board of Ordnance*. There was a second edition in 1803, bearing Coleman's name. The first edition, dated 1796, apparently contained the notorious instruction, in the treatment of 'staggers', of having the 'hair clipped off the pasterns as high as the fetlock, and boiling water poured on the part twice a day'.

Coleman had been lecturing to officers of the army medical staff at Woolwich, and Dr Rollo and the officers of the medical staff signed a memorial, suggesting Coleman's appointment as veterinary surgeon to the Ordnance. 'Coleman's duties with the Ordnance were to examine for soundness all "recruit" horses, advise on the treatment of disease, inspect at outstations, bringing in such cases as he thought necessary for treatment at Woolwich, to lecture occasionally to the officers, artillery cadets and farriers, and to direct the shoeing.' Smith wrote that Coleman 'improved the health of army horses beyond recognition . . . what we have to thank him for more particularly is the lessons he taught on the prevention of disease'. In five years, Coleman had provided 44 veterinary surgeons (how many were medical men is apparently not known). Coleman received the right to supply the cavalry with drugs and surgical appliances, but he lost this contract later.

Smith said that Coleman was a dictator and monopolist, ruling with an iron hand in military and civil life. Certainly, Coleman and no other was the route of entry into the College and into the army veterinary service. His only potential rival — William Dick of Edinburgh — was too far away to be effective. In the autumn of 1817 Dick (son of a smith and farrier in Edinburgh) came to the Veterinary College, rooming in Somers Town. He attended Coleman's lectures, and obtained his diploma on 21 January 1818 after three months' study. He set up his school in Edinburgh and in 1838 graduates of that school were made eligible to serve as army veterinary surgeons. None was admitted so long as Coleman was alive. Smith, well in character, says 'It is difficult to find sufficiently restrained language to express the wickedness of this attitude'. A report on the unsatisfactory nature of the examinations at the Edinburgh School a little later suggests that Coleman may have had much right on his side.

John Gamgee gave a considered opinion of Coleman in 1855: 'Coleman was by education, character and deportment, a fair example of an English gentleman . . . By the urbanity of his almost patrician deportment, Coleman tended greatly to raise the standard of the profession in public esteem, and he powerfully contributed to obtain for veterinarians the grade of commissioned officers in the army. By his intimate connection with the greatest men of the day in the medical profession, he obtained for his pupils the privilege of their teaching free of expense, and thus it is that a considerable number in the ranks of our profession are pupils of Abernethy, Astley Cooper, Charles Bell, Brodie, Faraday and Brand. By imparting his enthusiasm to his pupils, impressing them most earnestly with the importance of their calling, he sent them out into the world with a store of self-respect which greatly contributed to uphold their position, and gave them an impetus to endeavour to raise its standard, which was often crowned with the most happy success'. However, Gamgee was not all praise. He stated that 'experimental committees, public reports on the workings of the institution, legal injunctions of the council, were soon assigned to the ominous alphabet of dead letters . . . he enjoyed the privileges of undivided authority, nay, of despotism and great wealth'.

According to Smith, Coleman had an inordinate love of money. He quotes Gamgee: 'He toiled for lucre and not for the advancement of veterinary science'. It is worth noting that some men in veterinary practice at that time became far richer than Coleman (who was worth £47,000 at his death). Coleman got his fees and salary from the College, a daily retainer from the army, and for a time money from the sale of drugs provided for the College and the army. He said he got no money from private practice.

Coleman would probably have claimed that one of his greatest contributions to veterinary practice was the ventilation of stables. The initial defects of his system, depending on the introduction of fresh air at a high level and its extraction at a low level, were corrected by Karkeek of Truro. Karkeek, who died aged 55 in 1858 following an accident to his gig, qualified on 1 December 1834. He was a prolific writer of learned articles in the *Veterinarian* of which he was for a time co-editor, and his classical education is reflected in his thoughtful commentaries. As Percivall noted in 1843 'One of the Professor's projects was crowned with signal success; and for this his name must be handed to posterity with no ordinary éclat — I mean his introduction of Ventilation into stables and other places used as the habitations of horses and cattle. Before his time, it was the practise of grooms . . . with a view of keeping their horses as warm as possible by the exclusion of air, to close up every chink and cranny through the wall or boarding of the stable, not omitting even the keyhole . . . The first to assent to the Professor's new doctrine were the Cavalry . . .'

Coleman's passion for fresh air never left him. He noted that two shirts were warmer than one overcoat, and he obviously enjoyed his open air sessions on the clinic rounds in the College yard. Bransby Cooper says that 'I have sometimes suffered from the Professor's love of cold air; for if ever he could manage at his parties to have a window left open unperceived, he was delighted; and many a time when I have dined with him I have said "Pray, Mr Coleman, have your ventilators shut or I shall be blown out of the room", at which he laughed and had the direction of the current changed by stealth so as to apply the breeze upon some other visitor less sensitive than myself'.

Bransby Cooper continues: 'I was with my dear old friend twenty-four hours before his death; I call him my friend, for such he always was. He was pallid, and with every mark of approaching dissolution, excepting loss of spirits. He was lying on a bed, placed between two open windows, his head being without any cap or covering of any sort, while his grey locks were literally floating in the wind, for, although in July, it was cold and blowing weather. Acquainted as I was with his peculiar notions on the subject, I could not help saying, "My dear sir, you must be cold, thus exposed", and he said "No, I have plenty of clothes on my bed, a large fire in my room, and with this pure air passing freely to my lungs, I shall live a few hours longer: but to-day, I think, is my last. The scene of life, Bransby", continued he, "is drawing to a close: although my career has been a most happy one, I feel much less regret than I expected in leaving it, for I have full confidence in the mercy of God." ' (The last phrase is omitted in Smith's quotation of this passage, which omission somewhat alters its significance.) 'His enunciation proved prophetic, for in less than twenty-four hours he was no more.' Coleman was buried at St James Church, Hampstead Road, where was laid also the animal and genre painter, George Morland (1763-1804).

Coleman's will, dated 1 July 1839, provided for the founding of a Coleman prize: 'Also, I give to the Royal Veterinary College, at the expiration of three years from my decease, the sum of one hundred and sixty-six pounds thirteen shillings and fourpence, 3 per Cent. consolidated Bank Annuities, with the dividends thereon accruing and to accrue, due at and from that time only, at and after my decease, for the purposes hereafter declared concerning the same'. He directed that the governors of the College should 'apply the interest and proceeds thereof annually for ever in the purchase of a Medal to be given Annually to the author of the best dissertation on the Anatomy, Physiology, or Pathology of the foot of the horse, or the principles and practice of shoeing horses (to be decided by Examiners, viz. either Veterinary examiners or Veterinary surgeons, to be appointed by the Governors at their annual meeting)'. He gave detailed instructions for the procedure to be followed if no suitable dissertations were submitted, concluding: 'But if no such dissertations, worthy, in the opinion of the said Examiners, of any such reward as aforesaid should be offered for seven years, then a Medal, to be purchased with the said accumulations, shall be offered for the best dissertation on any Veterinary subject thought worthy by the said Examiners of such reward, but at all times the Foot of the Horse is to be the subject preferred, and next to that the nature, causes and treatment of Glanders, and the diseases of the Eye in horses: And if there should be no successful dissertation at the end of seven years, then the amount of the said accumulations shall be disposed of by the said Governors in such manner as they in their discretion may think proper, so as they are applied for the promotion of Veterinary Science'.

The will was proved at London on 21 August 1839. Nothing about the medal seems to have happened until a meeting of the governors on 2 August 1848. They resolved that, if the money was now obtainable, it should be applied to assist the funds of the journal designated at that time the *Veterinary Record* (not connected with the present journal of that name) which was edited by professors of the College. This seems somewhat cool behaviour, considering that the governors appear to have done nothing to put the medal up for competition. Then, on 9 July 1859 (11 years later) Professor Spooner was asked to report to the governors on the state of the fund, and to ascertain who were the current trustees. On the following 18 October, he was asked to consult with his staff colleagues and such other veterinarians as he might think fit, 'with regard to the terms upon which the funds bequeathed by the late Professor Coleman for the advancement of Veterinary Science can be best appropriated . . .'

On 17 January 1860 Spooner was asked to transfer the legacy from the bank into the names of the treasurer (J.W. Bosanquet), M.B. Behrens and Spooner. It was resolved to purchase silver and bronze medals, and an embossed certificate of merit. Notice was to be given to the pupils that prizes would be awarded for the best essay on the eye of the horse, embracing its anatomy and physiology, and also the laws of light applicable to vision, the chemical composition of the humour, and the pathology, treatment and results of the disease known as constitutional ophthalmia. It was agreed that the face of the medal should show the head of Coleman, and the first awards were made that year. In 1861, the subject was the anatomy and physiology of the skin in domesticated animals, including the pathology and treatment of the disease termed mange or scab.

In the course of time, the Coleman prize became awarded as a result of examinations posing pathological and practical subjects relating to the foot of the horse, the principles and practice of shoeing, the diseases of the horse's eye, and the disease known as glanders. More recently the prize, a silver medal, is awarded on the result of a written examination on some aspect of veterinary science relating to the horse in health and disease.

Coleman published little in his long life — all his works came out within nine years of his appointment as Professor. They did, however, include the first number of *Veterinary*

Transactions, containing observations on the effect of treatment of wounds of joints and other circumscribed cavities. Published by order of the general meeting of subscribers to the College, London, 1801, Smith described it as '. . . a very poor product for seven years' work: it was the first and the last'.

The College has been much criticised for failing to produce more than one volume of the *Transactions* that were required annually by the original constitution. Two factors may be pleaded in mitigation. The College was woefully under-staffed; the preparation of a worthy volume of transactions would require not only staff to do the work that would be reported, but also staff to write up the material. Secondly, Coleman may have been one of the numerous band of teachers, at present out of fashion, who put their main energies into what after all may be considered the prime function of a teaching institution — teaching. (A university school must be a place of research, but it should not be overbalanced by this, and it ought to have plenty of room for scholarship too.) A countervailing factor was the great tendency at that time to preserve secrecy over the College's lectures and practice, lest practitioners 'steal' knowledge to their advantage and to the College's detriment.

The criticisms that have been levelled at Coleman on educational and other matters have included assertions that he admitted unsuitable pupils; unduly shortened the course of instruction; concentrated that instruction solely on diseases of the horse; allowed undue medical interference in the development of the profession, particularly in respect of the examining committee, solely composed of medical men; barred veterinary surgeons from becoming subscribers to the College, and thwarted attempts by the profession to obtain a charter.

Those who formulated the rules for admission to the College, who were afraid they might deter men from coming forward to train for membership of a still infant profession, limited the requirement for admission to an ability to read and write well — quite a severe restriction at the time — plus personal recommendation. The original regulations of the College stated that candidates for entry must not be under 15 nor over 22 years of age, and that preference would be given to those youths who had received the elements of a good education. Early pupils were mainly youths who had just completed general schooling, and medical students, who may have served some years of apprenticeship to a surgeon, and to whom the contrast between an overcrowded surgical profession, and the developing veterinary profession, favoured the latter. Other entrants had been apprenticed to farriers, druggists, and so on, or were following their fathers in practice.

It was a constant complaint that Coleman lowered the standing of the young profession because of the unsuitable pupils he admitted. It is however impossible to believe that among these — bearing in mind that each applicant had to be sponsored by some reputable person — there were, as some claimed, barbers, man-milliners, tailors, shoemakers, mercers, mutton pie men, rat catchers, razor-strop makers, razor grinders, a druggist's porter, insolvent debtors, and in general, the out-at-elbow fraternity. That blacksmiths and the sons of blacksmiths and grooms were admitted is indisputable — perhaps the most famous example was William Dick, founder of the Edinburgh veterinary school.

Smith claimed that, although Coleman invited medical men to attend the College with the promise of an early diploma, these educated people were not looked on with favour, for they were able to see through Coleman's 'shallow and fatuous system'. Apart from the absence of any selection board, and any other substantial barrier to student entry, Coleman had some sense on his side. He constantly proclaimed that the sons of blacksmiths and grooms made the best veterinary surgeons — a general proposition supported by Percivall in 1842 — although he denied that he ever said surgeons made the worst. A remark by Behrens suggests a modification of the statement that is extremely significant: 'The late Professor Coleman used to observe that where talent was united with an early knowledge of the horse, the sons of these men (namely farriers and grooms) proved the best veterinarians'. The farrier's son would recognise spavin, splint and stringhalt in the living horse although he did not know their nature. Such students, it was said, would listen with mingled pleasure and wonder to the professor's lectures and would perform their task with the greatest cheerfulness. On the other hand, the student with previous medical training might grasp the rationale of these conditions, but he could not recognise them, and might well soon find his task a dirty drudgery.

Coleman was blamed for reducing the period of three years as originally fixed for the course of instruction in Vial's time, to as little as three or four months, so that some men were sent out into practice at 19, 18, or even 17 years of age (as a contrary example, Coleman's nephew, E.C. Dray, was a student for nine years).

The durations prescribed by the Royal College when it became responsible for the curriculum and examination have steadily increased. The two-year course was introduced in 1844 and endured for 32 years. From 1876-1885 there was a three-year course. The four-year course, started in 1885, was replaced in 1932 by the five-year course which has lasted into the university degree era, with occasional variations.

We have no evidence that Vial provided, or indeed could have provided, a three-year course (apart from that, he was at one point rebuked by the governors for not paying enough attention to his teaching duties).

Even at the then much praised Alfort school, their four-year course was found to be too long. It was held that about half this time would serve except in cases of great idleness or stupidity. Moorcroft spent only one year on the Lyons course, planned to occupy four years. Students at that time could apparently choose when they wished to be examined (after the continental custom) as there was no fixed examination schedule as we know it. The examination committee records in London show that the majority of students were examined after nine or 18 months' instruction, and even then they stood a chance of being referred back for a further period of study. The student could leave at any time he wished and take up unqualified practice, usually permanently, but sometimes temporarily. It was further agreed that a three-year course would be too expensive, especially as entrants might have served a part or the whole of a long apprenticeship beforehand.

The first College certificate was granted on 22 April 1794 to Edmund Bond, after 18 months' instruction while a resident pupil. Bond was examined at 8.00pm on the Tuesday evening in the Crown & Anchor tavern in the Strand by Cline (in the chair), Baillie, Abernethy, Home, Houlston and Cooper, with Coleman in attendance and W. Mounsher as secretary. He received his certificate which stated: 'These are to Certify that Mr Edmund Bond has attended the Veterinary College as a resident pupil for 18 months and having been examined by us, we consider him as qualified to practise the Veterinary Art'. Henry Cline was surgeon at St Thomas's Hospital and teacher of anatomy. Dr Baillie was lately teacher of anatomy, and physician to St George's Hospital. John Abernethy was surgeon to St Bartholomew's Hospital, and teacher of anatomy and surgery. Houlston was a surgeon in Chancery Lane. Everard Home was surgeon at St George's Hospital, and Astley Cooper was surgeon to Guy's hospital and teacher of anatomy and surgery. The certificate was signed by Coleman a mere 18 days after Moorcroft's resignation. On 5 July certificates were granted to Richard Lawrence, John Mills, Richard Thompson, John Field, Bracy Clark and William Stockley. On 12 March 1795 certificates were granted to F.J. Nash, William Wilkinson, J. Atfield and James Jones.

It is recorded somewhat ruefully that, after years of struggle, when the *Veterinarian* had won its fight to get the course lengthened, students who had previously been apprenticed for three

58

or four years to a practitioner claimed they at least ought to be able to leave the College after 12 months, and not have to stay the same period — two years — as the non-apprenticed.

We would need to know far more about the actual course of study students had been following, albeit briefly, under Vial, before we could accept that Coleman maliciously reduced it, and that his motive, as claimed by Smith, was mercenary self-interest (the 20 guineas student's fee going into his pocket). In 1844, after Coleman's time, the course at the Edinburgh 'Dick' School was apparently a mere five or six months' duration. Pugh pointed out that the greater the output of veterinary surgeons, the swifter the development of the new profession. Perhaps in the light of the demand for veterinary surgeons in the Revolutionary and Napoleonic wars, we could interpret Coleman's efforts favourably as a 'crash programme', already anticipated by Vial. In five years from 1796, Coleman furnished 44 veterinary surgeons to the army.

Another criticism levelled at Coleman was that his teaching neglected animals other than the horse, contrary to the original constitution of the College. A further charge was that practical and theoretical instruction, even on diseases of the horse, was limited and in some cases erroneous. When he came to the College, Coleman was presumably almost totally ignorant of veterinary matters (although he may have been studying the subject during the 'interregnum'). The restricted range of animals he saw at the College, and the limited nature of their diseases, inevitably meant that his experience was narrowly based. This arose from the unsatisfactory location of the College, which was on the edge of a rapidly expanding urban area increasingly remote from any true farm practice.

There is a vigorous defence of Coleman by Mayer: 'The energies of Coleman's mind were more exclusively devoted to anything bearing upon the horse: and no wonder, for the College, constructed as it was and is, can only be adapted for the reception of that animal. Consequently, it alone, of all our domesticated animals, has absorbed the whole attention, until very lately, of the professors of that establishment. In Mr Coleman's early career, and even until within a very few years, the veterinary art, so far as regards its application to cattle, sheep, swine, dogs, etc., was in the lowest state of barbarism and degradation. We cannot, therefore, feel surprised that Professor Coleman, beset by so many obstacles in that particular branch of our art, and having arrived at an advanced period of life, could not fling himself into its pursuit; nor was it reasonable to expect it from him'. An observer noted that 'the day is happily gone by, the dark age has passed over, when the village farrier had a clyster-pipe and bladder in one pocket, and a roll of tow emerging from another, and brandishing his twitch as a weapon of offence and defence, is the only person to whom our domestic animals are entrusted'.

It is not particularly surprising that Coleman, a redoubtable big fish in a very small pond, although giving great attention to his early cases, later assumed a sometimes unjustified confidence, and came to believe, or at least teach, that the diseases of the horse were few as compared to those of man, and that he could carry all the drugs necessary for veterinary practice in his waistcoat pocket. Smith says Coleman's opinions were final and never underwent revision. This hardly tallies with the sentiments expressed in a letter in the possession of the College in which Coleman, writing on 24 February 1813, gracefully declined an invitation to become President of the London Veterinary Society:

'Gentlemen,

I received your letter, and it gives me great pleasure to see so much zeal for the improvement of the veterinary art in Gentlemen, whom any & every Teacher might well be proud to call his Pupils — I shall most willingly grant the use of the College Theatre for the examination and discussion of such points as may be considered by you most important for the advancement of the Veterinary Science . . . you rightly observe that a number of minds concentrated on one object cannot fail to improve any art far beyond the reach of any individual and I have no doubt that the Public will ultimately derive great benefits from your united exertions. You do me great honor in proposing me as your President, & if I did not feel that my acceptance of this favour would tend much to defeat the laudable object of your pursuit I should most certainly gratify my own ambition, & have the pleasure to preside at your meetings. But Gentlemen for your deliberations to be useful they must be free — your opinions must not be shackled by authorities; & I know that were I present your candor and delicacy towards me would be such, as to prevent that freedom of discussion and investigation, which is absolutely necessary to obtain a knowledge of facts. Many opinions I formerly entertained are now given up & probably many of my present opinions will share the same fate — I wish them to be closely and fully (as I know they will fairly) examined without any regard to the author & therefore I cannot by my presence aid your cause. Be assured however that if I can in any manner contribute to the success of your efforts, either by the proposal of questions for discussion, or subjects for Papers or giving my opinions on any part of the Veterinary Art which you may think proper to investigate I shall at all times feel myself honored by the request, & I am persuaded that Mr Sewell will be most happy to (?add) his exertions in any way congenial to your wishes.

I have the honor to be Gentn.
   With great esteem
     Yr most faithful & Obdt.Sert.
      Edw. Coleman'

Practice was largely limited to horses by the peculiar constitution of the College, whereby subscribers of the richer sort sent their animals in for free treatment and received drugs at half-price. No coach- or cart-horses, subject to hard work and gross negligence and ignorance were likely to be presented. Further, no instruction was possible on racehorses, hunters or hackneys, or on stud practice. The Royal Agricultural Society of England later made great, continuous, and finally successful efforts to remedy this undoubted narrowness in the syllabus.

The College was underfinanced. Subscriptions and students' fees were not adequate to provide a properly staffed establishment, and the choice made of this method of financing the College, in preference to direct government funding (which would have had to be much greater than the government grants received from 1795 to 1813) was to hamper the growth of the College well into the present century. Almost as soon as it was begun, the College became virtually bankrupt, and it had to be taken firmly under control, notably by Lord Kinnaird, Byron's banker friend. So bad was the situation that on one or two occasions half-hearted explorations of the possibility of selling off the College land and buildings were made. In 1828, for example, when Coleman was sadly in need of an operating theatre, the various builders' estimates were so high that the project was abandoned 'for the time being'.

Lack of finance inevitably meant that the College was understaffed. Astley Cooper claimed (incorrectly) that the constitution of the College would not allow more professors to be appointed, although it is difficult to imagine that a course, ideally lasting three years and covering the health and diseases of all species of domesticated animals, could have been undertaken by a professor, an assistant professor and a demonstrator. The content of the Coleman course is shown by near-verbatim notes taken at different times by students, and preserved in the College and at the Royal College. However absurd these may seem in some respects, we have to read them in the light of the knowledge then available. Large areas of science we take for granted were unknown, and even unsuspected. T.W. Mayer Jr was to write in 1837: 'Pathology . . . exhibits considerable progress, though it has not yet attained that perfection which is desirable'. In 1839, Pritchard referred to 'colourless globules in pus like those observed in the blood'.

Coleman's lectures can be read even today with pleasure as well as interest. His thoughts often centred on the foot of the horse, and he wasted no time in his introductory lecture before remarking on the correlation of structure and function that was exhibited by the frog of the foot. His next interest was comparative anatomy, and he soon referred to the 'celebrated Dr Hunter'. He addressed his students as 'Gentlemen', and drew them into his subject by the use of 'we' and 'you' (a contrast with McFadyean's 'one' that fits in well with the relationships between these two different teachers and their classes.) He had the good lecturer's habit of referring back to the previous lecture, and looking forward to the next, so that the course flowed smoothly on. He used homely but thought-stimulating examples. In his discourse on indigestion in the horse, he posed the question, why did ploughmen seldom suffer from indigestion, while members of the higher classes were prone to this? He was an advocate of warm water as a means of reducing inflammation. He was not slow in pointing out that some facts had to be taught, and learnt, for which there was not, nor sometimes was there ever likely to be, a satisfactory explanation. Coleman's lecturing skills were not confined to his College students. Apart from his lectures at Woolwich, he delivered a course of lectures on the horse at Guy's Hospital in 1817.

In Europe the veterinary schools, which were state-funded, had four or even six professional men as teachers, but even there criticism was not lacking. At Alfort, for instance, the professors were constrained to reply to the same charge as was levelled at Coleman — that of neglecting animals other than the horse. They pointed out that near large towns horses were, in any case, more numerous than cattle, and that diseased cattle would be sent to slaughter rather than to the veterinarian. Farm animals could not be led to the school, and their illnesses were often too rapid in course to permit of their transport. However, Alfort tried to some extent to offset the disadvantages of its location. A considerable number of cattle were kept in pastures belonging to the school, along with sheep and pigs. In the late 1830s, the idea of buying a farm as a field station for the London College was mooted but not pursued — again for lack of funds.

Even allowing for the restricted staff, there appears to have been some lack of organization of the lecturing programme in Coleman's later years. Teachers were constantly late or even absent, without proper provision for a deputy. There was a lack of instruction in shoeing, and operations classes were poorly organised. Coleman seems to have been rather silently supported by Sewell as assistant professor. Cherry noted, as a most extraordinary circumstance, that Sewell had given a demonstration which actually lasted nearly 10 minutes 'which might be short and sweet: if it was intelligible, it was the first time'.

Coleman's introductory lecture began late in November, and students had to stay in London in the heat of the following summer, when in those pre-formalin days they cut up carcasses at some hazard to their health. The students dissected donkeys rather than horses and even Coleman used donkey material to demonstrate horse muscles. Donkeys were the typical animals of costermongers, and were cheaper than horses. Any horses that died in College went to 'old Cross' for salvage to reduce the charge to clients, and it was pleaded that a proper post-mortem examination ought to be made of all these animals. Richard Cross was a knacker in Camden Town. He supplied dead horses and asses for dissection, and also dealt in dead cows. (Someone suggested that 'old Cross' even lectured on morbid anatomy from these carcasses.)

There has possibly been some exaggeration in this matter of concentration on the horse. Coleman's view was that a sound basis of training in diseases of the horse would enable the veterinarian to acquire equal skill in the diseases of other species. If he failed at first, he would know better next time. Coleman once referred to 'heartbreaking' letters which he heard had been written by practitioners who had gone unprepared into country practice, but he said 'I have no compunctious visitings in the matter'.

Coleman's first class numbered 14, but later classes sometimes exceeded 70 students. By the 1830s, some 50 students yearly were awarded a diploma. At that time the animal population of the country was around 1½ million horses, five million cattle, four million pigs, 30 million sheep and two million dogs. The students were examined, before being awarded their diploma, by a committee consisting of prominent medical men (plus Coleman and Sewell, the latter serving as treasurer and secretary). The examination, held at the Freemasons' tavern, was entirely *viva voce* and the complaint was made that the candidates did not even have to cast a horse, or operate on a dead one, still less on a live one which might have benefitted.

The arrangement of having medical men only as examiners, which grew to be a prime cause of discontent in the profession, started as a reasonable plan. When the College was in its early years, certain outstanding medical men signed the diploma awarded to successful candidates. Although the diploma was called 'a scrap of paper' by Baron Vaughan it was a guarantee that students had received a superior education, raising them far above the status of the farrier. The diploma (at an examining fee of three guineas) was, Coleman claimed, signed by people known to all Europe, and this would undoubtedly carry great weight in the country town in which the qualifying student might go to practise; local medical men would see that the certificate must refer to men with whom they might safely associate.

Unfortunately the arrangement, however justified originally, went on too long. Coleman tried to obtain veterinary representation on the examining committee, but all efforts failed until after his death. The medical examining committee met at the Crown & Anchor tavern up to 31 July 1809 and thereafter at the Freemasons' tavern until at least 1821. At first the students achieved a certificate on qualifying, but this was called a diploma from 24 June 1808. Certificates were mentioned again on 29 April 1819, but diplomas appeared on 7 July 1819.

Coleman always claimed that the examination conducted by the medical committee was not a farce, but that unambiguous questions were fairly put, and no student was ever failed because he dissented from his teacher's views. It is recorded in 1810 that two 'six months pupils were advised to study a little longer'. On 29 December 1812 Thomas Mayer, a seven months resident pupil, received his certificate. Some students felt they had been rather hard pressed in relation to their knowledge of chemistry, but Coleman rightly said that a properly educated gentleman could be expected to understand the general principles and applications of chemical science. He adopted the same line in his lectures on the foetal circulation — this was a subject of little practical importance, but it was one of which a properly educated man should have some appreciation.

The College in Coleman's reign took a long time to recover from the difficulties of its early days. It was built in an unsuitable situation and given an inadequate constitution. It was severely under-funded, and it quickly became a horse infirmary primarily, and a teaching body secondarily. Meeting the demand for veterinary surgeons for the army, while raising the social status of the young profession, did nothing to support the needs of agriculture. Coleman, when he was appointed, was uninformed on veterinary matters but, as Moorcroft's resignation was not followed by the appointment of a veterinary successor, he was left inadequately supported. His staff was much too small to give a reasonable teaching course, and the absence of serious opposition that might have been provided by another English veterinary school meant there was no great stimulus to change. Further, Coleman was appointed without time limit and, since his friends held the key positions in the councils of the College, due reform was delayed.

On the whole, it can be said that Coleman, in the circumstances, served the College, the profession and the country, well and that a balanced assessment, tending neither to adulation nor to denigration, is indicated. Smith's unfavourable opinion, which does not seem justified in respect of Coleman's professional career, is expressed in what seems to be is an inexplicably biassed manner. In Mayer's fine words: 'I hope we shall no longer hear Mr Coleman reflected upon for not accomplishing impossibilities. I shall ever esteem the man and revere his memory: and although I feel myself incapable to do full justice to his merits, yet posterity will'.

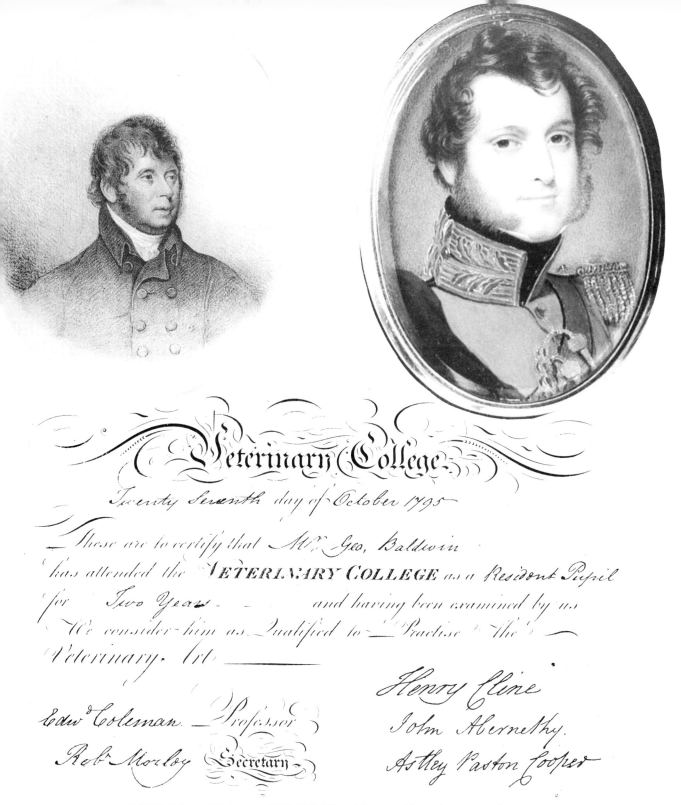

Veterinary College

Twenty Seventh day of October 1795

These are to certify that Mr. Geo. Baldwin has attended the **VETERINARY COLLEGE** as a Resident Pupil for Two Years and having been examined by us We consider him as Qualified to Practise the Veterinary Art

Edwd Coleman — *Professor*

Robt Morley *Secretary*

Henry Cline

John Abernethy

Astley Paston Cooper

LEFT: Edward Coleman. BELOW: The oldest certificate known to the College, issued to George Baldwin, a resident pupil for two years, on 27 October 1795. RIGHT: William Percivall, who founded the *Veterinarian* in 1828.

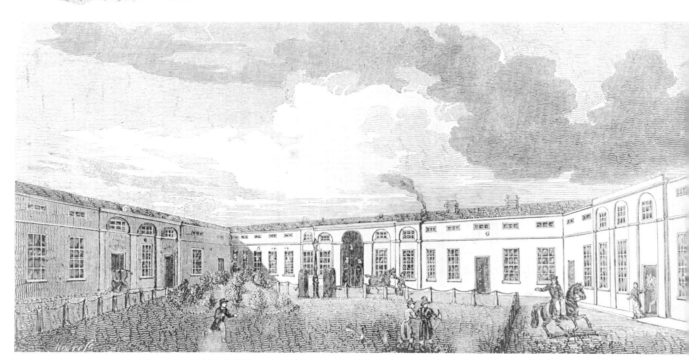

ABOVE: William Dick's notes on 'Mr Coleman's Introductory Lecture', made while a student at the College. BELOW: The College quadrangle, as pictured in *The Farrier and Naturalist*, January 1828.

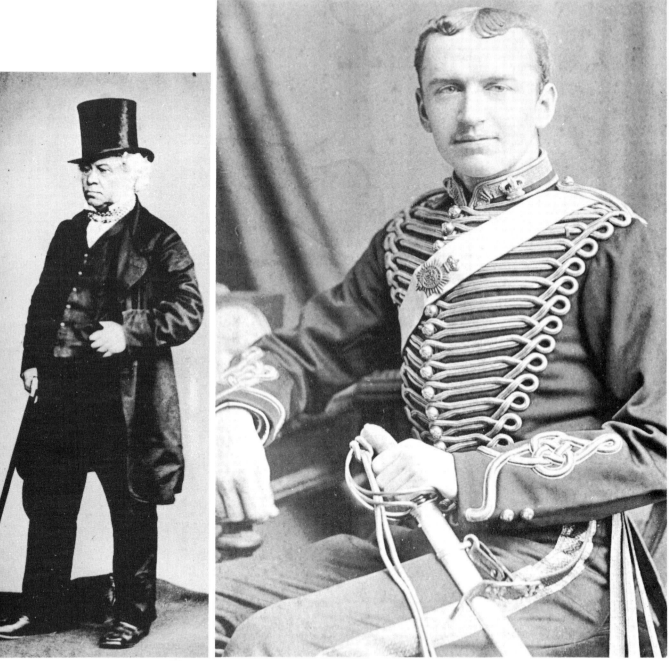

LEFT: William Dick, who qualified at the College in 1817 and founded his own school in Edinburgh in 1823. RIGHT: Major-General Sir Frederick Smith (1857-1929), a student at the College from 1873-1876, later director general of the Army Veterinary Corps. (RCVS)

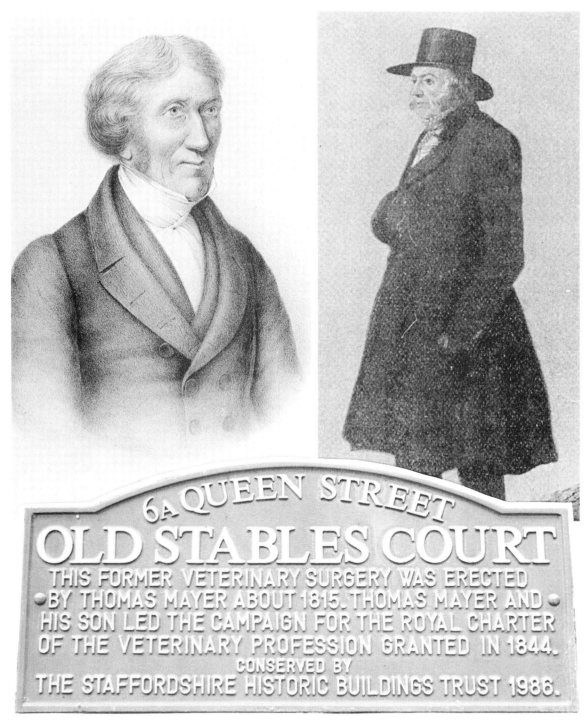

LEFT: William Sewell. RIGHT: William Youatt, who frequently quoted the advice given to students at the College by Sir William Blizard in 1828: 'Remember, gentlemen, that your reputation and success must be founded on the union of science and humanity'. BELOW: Plaque donated by the Veterinary History Society, marking Thomas Mayer's surgery in Newcastle-under-Lyme. (JC)

PART II

Birth of the Profession

WILLIAM SEWELL

Professor 1839-1853

The death of Coleman was the end of an era. He had held sway at the College for 45 years, for 40 of which he had been assisted by his faithful subordinate William Sewell who now, at the age of 58, was to succeed his master as Professor. No doubt Sewell would have maintained the old order but there were forces outside the College working for change.

In 1828 William Percivall had founded the *Veterinarian* as a journal for the emerging profession. It included scientific and clinical articles, abstracts from foreign journals, news items and editorials. One of its objectives was the reform of the London College, which it pursued in a generally persuasive and constructive way. The *Farrier and Naturalist* had also been founded in 1828 and it too was critical of the College, but its style was one of personal attack on Coleman.

Another important event during Coleman's long reign was the opening of a veterinary school in Edinburgh by William Dick in 1823. Dick had qualified from London in 1817 but his new school was too remote from London to affect Coleman's autocracy and there developed two monopolies, the old one in London and a new one in Edinburgh. An incredible example of the attitude in London can be seen in the response to a request from practitioners that they, like anybody else in the land, should become subscribing members of the College. The governors adamantly excluded veterinary surgeons from becoming subscribers because they 'might learn some of the secrets of the College' thus 'becoming more skilful and successful' and 'might interfere with the interests and lessen the profits of the College'. By the time Coleman died it was said that the number of veterinary surgeons practising in the three kingdoms fell little short of 1,000. It was a critical mass.

With Coleman gone, the practitioners lost no time in taking the initiative. Thomas Mayer and his son, Thomas Walton Mayer of Newcastle-under-Lyme, sent to every veterinary surgeon in the United Kingdom the draft of a memorial addressed to the governors of the London College, with the ultimate objective of gaining a Charter of Incorporation 'to protect us from illiterate and uneducated men, and to afford us the same privileges and exemptions which other professional bodies possess'. This was followed up by a deputation to the governors on 10 June 1840, led by Thomas Turner. The reply from the governors, dated 3 July 1840, was addressed to Messrs Mayer and Son. It said that the governors 'do not see the immediate necessity for applying to the Crown for a Royal Charter to be granted to this Institution' but that 'every facility' would be given to the veterinary surgeons 'for procuring an Act of Parliament to prevent certain grievances complained of by the Memorial, which could not be relieved by a Charter'.

Thomas Walton Mayer was undeterred. He became the secretary of a standing committee of veterinary surgeons dedicated to petitioning the Privy Council for a Royal Charter 'conferring upon the graduates of the Royal Veterinary College and the College of Edinburgh the title of the Royal College of Veterinary Surgeons, upon the same plan and constitution as the present Royal College of Surgeons'. On 22 March 1841 Thomas Turner, chairman of the committee, sent a memorial and petition to the Marquis of Normanby, Secretary of State for the Home Department. The memorial read:

'Feeling the necessity that exists for a better regulation in the management of our profession and for a more organised system of educating and examining its practitioners, we have condensed in the annexed Petition the principal substance of our wants and to which we most humbly but most anxiously solicit your Lordship's kind attention'.

The petition was not successful but a deputation to Sir James Graham, Home Secretary, in April 1842 received some encouragement and an amended petition and a draft of a Charter of Incorporation was submitted to him on 24 March 1843. In a letter to Sir James Graham on 23 March 1843 Thomas Turner wrote: 'During the period that has now elapsed [since the deputation was received "some months since"] favourable circumstances have arisen and resulted in a complete union between the heads of the Veterinary Colleges of London and Edinburgh and the profession at large and I am enabled to state that the accompanying petition and draft Charter have received the signatures of the several Professors of the said College. . . .'

On 27 July 1843 Her Majesty was 'pleased to refer this Petition together with Draft of Charter thereunto annexed to Mr Attorney and Mr Solicitor General. . . .' On 24 November the lawyers replied 'respectfully to state our opinion that Your Majesty may properly grant a Royal Charter', but it was not until 14 February 1844 that Thomas Turner was able to report to the standing committee of veterinary surgeons that their determined efforts had been rewarded and that the Royal College of Veterinary Surgeons had been incorporated.

The success of the second petition had turned on the fact that it included the signatures of the professors of the two schools — Sewell, Spooner and Simonds for London and Dick for Edinburgh — but no sooner had the Charter been granted than the two schools were in dispute with the Royal College. The contention continued for four years and the underlying reason for it was pique. The schools had never imagined that the practitioners would be successful and, when they were, the schools were annoyed to realise that they had lost their monopoly powers. The details of the antagonism were complex, devious and not always consistent. There is an account of them in Pattison's history, *The British Veterinary Profession 1791-1948*.

The governors of the London school were incensed. They lost no time in petitioning the Home Secretary 'complaining that their privileges had been infringed upon by the Charter granted to the Royal College of Veterinary Surgeons and praying for relief'. The petition was signed by 'W. Sewell. On the part of the Governors'; Sewell was doing the governors' bidding. A copy of the petition was sent to the Royal College and in the reply to Sir James Graham, dated 27 July 1844, Thomas Turner, the President, felt confident that he was able to 'prove the aspersions made in the two petitions to be entirely groundless'. The petition did not succeed, but the governors did not give up.

On 28 May 1845 Joseph Berent, chairman of the committee of governors, sent the Home Secretary a draft of a proposed charter for the veterinary school. As before, a copy was sent to the Royal College with a suggestion that the 1844 Charter should be amended because Sir James Graham was 'disposed to attach weight to the representations'. The Royal College resisted the compromise and the Home Office did nothing. The governors were still waiting for action one year later. On 11 May 1846 W.M. Wilkinson, their lawyer, wrote to the Home Office to ask what was happening:

'The Governors of the Veterinary College at Camden Town are anxious that the Charter for which they have petitioned Her Majesty or such modification thereof as you may approve

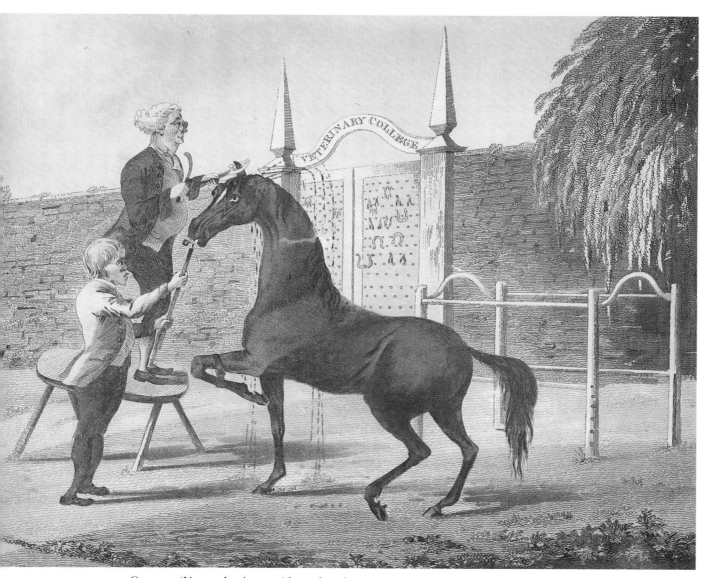

Cartoon 'Upon the improv'd mode of cropping' — one of a series
published in 1792 as part of a campaign by farriers to ridicule the
Veterinary College.

should be granted without further delay, as great inconvenience and loss to the Institution is arising from the want of such Charter.

'It is now clearly ascertained that the present chartered body will not accept the terms which is is understood have been proposed to them and for the information of the Governors of the Royal Veterinary College I shall feel much obliged by your informing me whether or not a Charter will be granted to them.'

Professor Dick in Edinburgh was also much displeased with the Charter and in 1848, after four years of recrimination, the sponsors of his school, the Highland and Agricultural Society, joined with the governors of the London school to petition yet again for another charter. Thinking this would be successful, Dick then declared independence from the Royal College of Veterinary Surgeons. He was not acting illegally, as no Act of Parliament gave statutory force to the terms of the Charter of 1844.

The London governors were by now contemplating extreme measures but they could not persuade the Royal Agricultural Society of England to provide support of the kind Dick was getting in Scotland and their veiled threats in the petition were likewise unsuccessful. The official report said:

'The petitioners remark that "the Royal Veterinary College of London is the private property of the subscribers thereto who may continue or close the same at their discretion; that it is only from their desire to advance the veterinary art that they have allowed their institution to be employed as a College of instruction; and that thereby the veterinary profession in this country owes even its existence to their establishment".

'I scarcely know whether these remarks are intended as the mere superfluous assertion of an abstract right, or whether they are intended to imply a covert threat, that if the petitioners are dissatisfied with the answer to their application, they may resort to the extreme course of closing that useful place of veterinary education. Many reasons occur why it is improbable that they would take such a step which both students and professor would have cause to regret. . . .'

Again, the petition was rejected. Harsh words and animosity persisted for a year or so but by 1851 there was a thaw in relations between the London school and the Royal College. In 1852 the breach was healed by the election of Professor William Sewell as president RCVS.

William Sewell was born into a Quaker family in Essex in 1781. He was apprenticed to Professor Coleman in 1796 when aged 15, and received his certificate from the College on 30 March 1799 (for some unknown reason, this certificate disappeared for good that very same evening). He became assistant to the Professor and demonstrator of anatomy, at £25 per annum, plus coals for his sitting room. On 1 January 1803 he was appointed assistant professor at 100 guineas per annum. After Coleman's death, Sewell was appointed Principal and Professor on 23 July 1839. He suffered from ill health in 1840, and again in 1842 and 1844. In 1852 he relinquished his teaching duties on grounds of poor health and was appointed to the sinecure posts of director of the College, secretary and resident governor. Late in life he married a member of the Wilkinson family (whose firm had for many years been solicitors to the College). His wife predeceased him in 1841, leaving no children. In a black-edged letter to the College Veterinary Medical Association, Sewell declined an invitation to their dinner. 'Between the cup and the lip it has pleased the Great Disposer of events to visit him with the greatest of all afflictions in the bereavement of his most affectionate wife. Her heart was full of benevolence to our own species, and most sensitively alive to suffering animals, and might in truth be called as a member of the society to which she belonged, the Animals' Friend.'

William Sewell died in the College of pneumonia on 8 June 1853, aged 72, and was buried at Highgate cemetery.

As a young man, Sewell appeared to some observers to be eccentric and reserved, but at the same time he was looked upon as a steady, attentive and exemplary apprentice. He was tall, slim and dignified, and showed no anger even when provoked. He was not scholastically talented, and was said by some of his students to be a poor lecturer: 'Never was there a more irregular course of lectures, so that we scarcely knew what he was talking about'. He was also said to be unpopular with some members of the profession, although he was elected president of the London Veterinary Medical Society. Sewell was free in his criticisms of others, including his fellow teachers, but he generally failed to state his own experience and opinions clearly. On one occasion he even offered 'money back' to anyone dissatisfied with his lectures.

Sewell was a dedicated surgical operator, although he was sometimes greatly inconvenienced by the disorderly conduct of students crowding and jostling each other for even a glimpse of what was going on. He successfully performed vesical lithotomy in the horse, and also amputated the equine penis. He practised subcutaneous periosteotomy for the relief of pain due to exostoses, and he was well aware of the value of post-mortem examinations as a check on his surgical successes and failures. In his 57 years at the College, he undoubtedly gained a great deal of clinical knowledge, which he unfortunately carried with him to the grave. He is one of the select band of teachers (including Dick and Macqueen) of whom it was said that they could tell if a horse was lame, merely by listening.

Sewell made one significant anatomical discovery. In 1803 he demonstrated the presence of the central canal of the spinal cord, studying it in the horse, ox, sheep, pig and dog. In the *Veterinarian* of 1831 we read 'A letter on a canal in the medulla spinalis of some quadrupeds. In a letter from Mr William Sewell to Everard Home, Esq., F.R.S. (Copied from the *Philosophical Transactions of the Royal Society*, A.D. 1808): Sir, According to your request, I send you an account of the facts I have ascertained, respecting a canal I discovered in the year 1803, in the medulla spinalis of the horse, bullock, sheep, hog and dog: and should it appear to you deserving of being laid before the Royal Society, I shall feel myself particularly obliged by having so great an honour conferred upon me. Upon tracing the sixth ventricle of the brain, which corresponds to the fourth in the human subject, to its apparent termination, the calamus scriptorius, I perceived the appearance of a canal, continuing by a direct course into the centre of the spinal marrow. To ascertain with accuracy whether such structure existed throughout its whole length, I made sections of the spinal marrow at different distances from the brain, and found that each divided portion exhibited an orifice with a diameter sufficient to admit a large sized pin; from which a small quantity of transparent colourless fluid issued, like that contained in the ventricles of the brain. The canal is lined by a membrane resembling the tunica arachnoidea, and is situated above the fissure of the medulla, being separated by a medullary layer: it is most easily distinguished where the large nerves are given off in the bend of the neck and sacrum, imperceptibly terminating in the cauda equina. Having satisfactorily ascertained its existence through the whole length of the spinal marrow, my next object was to discover whether it was a continued tube from one extremity to the other: this was most decidedly proved, by dividing the spinal marrow through the middle, and pouring mercury into the orifice where the canal was cut across: it passed in a small stream with equal facility towards the brain (into which it entered), or in a contrary direction to where the spinal marrow terminates. By many similar experiments, I have since proved that a free communication of the limpid fluid, which the canal contains, is kept up between the brain and the whole extent of spinal marrow. I have consulted the most celebrated authors on comparative anatomy, but do not find any such structures of those parts described; and as it is not known to you, I may presume that it has not been before taken notice of. I have the honour to be, sir, your obedient, faithful servant, Wm. Sewell'.

Sewell also described the trachealis muscle of the horse. Another discovery he claimed was that of a cure for glanders: one horse had remained 'cured' for four years after treatment with what was popularly known as 'Sewell's Blue Broth' — three ounces of copper sulphate in a quart of water. More significantly, he showed that glanders was a disease of the lungs, and that lung nodule material would produce glanders in another horse.

Sewell had been made responsible to Coleman for maintaining discipline among the students. A particular problem in and after his time were the 'meat fights' in the dissecting room. Sewell lived in a house in College, and it is pleasing to note that in 1807, £50 was set aside by the College for furnishing two ground floor rooms in his house, and for applying oil paint to floor, architrave, dado and skirting, in white, and to the walls in a light French gray. Like other teachers, he was allowed to keep a horse in the stables.

Sewell was not completely College-bound. He visited certain continental veterinary schools in 1815 and 1816, but did not submit his report on these visits to the governors until June 1818. The report, which was subsequently sent out to subscribers, has been compared to an auctioneer's catalogue, and dismissed as uninformative and useless. However, considering that Sewell characteristically was uncommunicative and that the College's general policy was not to give away information helpful to others, the report does have some interest.

The defeat of Napoleon at Waterloo on 18 June 1815 had opened up travel on the Continent, and Sewell, fully realising that his visits were cursory, seems nevertheless to have enjoyed them. In November 1815 he was in Lyons, carrying a letter of introduction from Sir Thomas Webbe (a College subscriber) to the mayor of that city. He was introduced to M Bredin, the director of the veterinary school, and made repeated visits, noting the museum, infirmary, forge and botanical garden. Lectures were given on botany and chemistry (subjects not covered in the London College at that time). The anatomy theatre, in which lectures on medicine and surgery were also delivered, held about 100 pupils, and adjacent to it were a dissecting room, yard and paddock. Here and elsewhere, Sewell was keen to note details of flooring and ventilation, and he took care to collect horseshoes, books and instruments.

Next, Sewell carried letters of introduction from M Bredin to Alfort where M Huzard was inspector-general of the French veterinary schools. Alfort was described at that time as four miles from Paris, and Sewell spent a whole day at the veterinary school. The buildings and arrangements were generally superior to those at Lyons, and special mention is made of the museum and the library — there was even a resident librarian. Lectures were given on agriculture, rural economy, and medical jurisprudence; Sewell considered the latter subjects worth adopting in London. He obtained the usual samples of horseshoes, some novel instruments, and books on subjects relevant to the veterinary art.

In July 1816 Sewell set off for Vienna, Berlin and Hanover. He arrived in Berlin in late August and spent some hours inspecting the College. The detached building housing the anatomy theatre, museum and dissecting room was praised, and the theatre's similarity to the one in the London Veterinary College and that in St Thomas's hospital (which Sewell had visited when it was still in Southwark) is noted. A riding-house was attached to the school for use of government-financed pupils intended for the army. Special mention is made of 'the most powerful Electrical apparatus that, probably, was ever constructed', which was said to have been employed successfully in various diseases, such as 'paralytic attacks, tetanus or lock-jaw, cataract & gutta serena (paralysis of the optic nerves)'. Visits were also made to the royal stables and barracks. Sewell received some 'useful instruments for relieving sheep and cattle when afflicted with an over-distension of the stomach, from gas being evolved called Hoven'.

In Hanover, Sewell was introduced to Professor Havemann, whose plans to visit England in 1777 and in 1796 unfortunately came to nothing (the missing link, possibly, in a chain that might have set the Hanover veterinary school, founded in 1788, rather than Lyons or Alfort as an immediate model for the London Veterinary College). The infirmary and stables had become dilapidated during the wars, having been occupied by enemy cavalry, and were empty. The royal stables near the school could hold 2-300 horses. Sewell obtained more horseshoes in Holland, which had no veterinary school, and praised the royal stables at The Hague. In Brussels, the method used to drain one large stable housing about 200 horses was also noted favourably.

It is hard to know why this report has been so severely criticised by Smith and others. Sewell at least must have benefited by the visits, and the varied material he brought home, including books as well as horseshoes, would surely have been put to use in the Veterinary College. Joseph Gamgee recorded that on his return from the Continent, Sewell said 'I have seen more lame horses while posting from Harwich to London than I have met with in all my journeys and during my inspection of veterinary schools and public places in France, Switzerland, Germany and Belgium'. (Gamgee himself found that 42% of 2,664 horses in this country were lame, but only 9% of 286 horses in Paris.) For his journeys abroad, and his neurectomy study, Sewell received a gratuity in 1819 of £300, plus a salary increase of £50 per annum. Later, the College permitted him to be the veterinary examiner for the East India Company.

As befits a Quaker, Sewell was a humane man. He thought the firing of horses should be prohibited by Act of Parliament, and he condemned the practice of nicking horses' tails. From 1818 he popularised the practice of neurectomy for alleviating foot lameness, performing the operation several hundreds of times. Naturally, he took a great interest in horse-shoeing, and horseshoes seem to have been a main interest in his continental journeys. He had a great fondness for the application of setons, particularly in cases of lameness — a curious lapse for such a humane man.

After the death of Coleman, one of the main problems was how to widen the scope of instruction at the College, until then restricted to horses, and embrace the diseases of other animal species, particularly cattle and sheep. (It is surprising to read in the *Veterinarian* of 1841 an article on the diseases of cats, and still more surprising to see the statement in the issue of 1850 that many practitioners were restricting themselves to dog practice).

In 1827 Sewell, in his introductory lecture, said he would not, in his lectures on surgery, confine himself to the horse. This in effect meant the delivery of only a handful of other lectures: circumstances ensured that no teacher at the College could expect to become knowledgeable on the diseases of farm animals, which practically never came into the College infirmary for attention. Although some practitioners advocated the purchase of a farm, where students could learn about the practicalities of management and disease, nothing came of it. The members of the Royal Agricultural Society of England (founded 1838) were invited to submit diseased animals to the College, but this met with an almost complete lack of response.

Sewell tried in 1841 to establish a cattle infirmary at Thomas Flight's famous dairy (formerly Laycock's) in Islington, housing some 600 or 700 cows (there were thousands of cows in London until the railways facilitated milk supplies from the country). This plan did little to provide clinical material. The most students could hope to see were cases of diseased udders, feet and skin; there were few parturitions. It is questionable whether the spaying of cows was widely practised at that time, but it is well known that London dairymen were only interested in a continuous milk supply. Cows were spayed in full milk and when eventually the supply was uneconomic, the animal was fat and ready for the butcher. Approaches to other institutions were peremptorily rejected by their proprietors. It was proposed that the College should attempt systematically to buy in diseased animals, perhaps appointing a special member of staff for that purpose, but nothing came of this, nor of a linked suggestion that students' fees should be increased to allow relevant staff increases.

73

It is no exaggeration to say that the task of providing classes of students with adequate and representative material to illustrate a course on the diseases of farm animals is still one of the most intractable problems veterinary colleges face today; few have solved it satisfactorily.

Although Sewell claimed in 1840 that the governors were fully satisfied with his ability to teach cattle pathology, his inadequacy was so patent that drastic measures were needed. Fortunately, the Royal Agricultural Society of England, prompted no doubt by William Youatt, a member of its veterinary sub-committee, eventually proposed the creation of a chair of cattle pathology at the College, to be funded by the Society.

William Youatt (1776-1847) was born in Exeter, the son of a surgeon. In 1811 he was a pupil of Delabere Blaine in Nassau Street, becoming Blaine's partner in 1813. In 1828, he was editor of the *Veterinarian*. Youatt became owner of the Nassau Street infirmary, where he lectured on diseases of the dog; he also gave lectures at University College. He was veterinary surgeon to the London Zoological Society, and made a loan of his magnificent library of over 400 volumes to the Veterinary Medical Association library at the College.

On 6 October 1840 Sewell reported an annual grant of £200 from the Royal Agricultural Society of England to finance lectures on the anatomy and treatment of the various disorders of cattle, sheep and other domestic animals. Society members were to get free treatment of their animals, but would pay for their keep. The plan aroused much interest and in 1842 James Beart Simonds was selected as lecturer from half a dozen candidates. This appointment was apparently predeterimined, and it caused some offence in the profession. A Mr E. Friend complained (as did Mr Tombs) that he had not been informed that his application was unsuccessful. Simonds, who was to give three to five lectures a week, admitted that, coming from practice in Twickenham, he was not an experienced teacher, and had never lectured to such an audience as attended his inaugural discourse.

In 1843 Mr Read of Crediton suggested attaching a farm to the College, where every kind of stock-farming, manuring, buying and selling, could occasionally be left to the judgment of the senior students.

Although Sewell failed to secure appointment as Principal Army Veterinary Surgeon on Coleman's death, he was veterinary surgeon to the London and Westminster Light Horse Volunteers from July 1805 and was presented as such at one of Prince Albert's levées in 1850. With the death of Coleman, the way was cleared for Edinburgh-qualified veterinary surgeons to receive regimental appointments.

In Sewell's time the course of instruction, lasting generally for two sessions of nine months each, was given in the cooler months of the year, the brief *viva voce* examinations qualifying for entry to the Royal College's diploma examinations being held in the unsuitable surroundings of the Freemasons' tavern. The students were given three lectures a day (Simonds was strongly against any more lecturing than this) and it was estimated that 50 to 60 horses were available for examination each day.

In 1846 Edward Mayhew resigned as anatomical teacher at the College. He had been appointed demonstrator in anatomy in his second year as a student, a remarkable achievement. He left after a dispute with the deputy professor, Charles Spooner, who may have been jealous of Mayhew's popularity with the students. Indeed, when he left, the students presented Mayhew with a microscope so that he could carry on 'with his investigations of structures, a subject of vast importance, but hitherto untaught and little known in the Veterinary College'. Mayhew continued to give private lessons, and set up in practice near Paddington Station. He subsequently published several works on the treatment of dogs, as well as the popular *Illustrated Horse Doctor* and *The Horse's Mouth: Shewing the Age by the Teeth* which he illustrated himself.

In 1844 it was reported that College graduates had gone to South Africa, South America, Egypt and Australia. At that time, more veterinary surgeons held commissioned rank in the East India Company than in the Queen's service.

From 1844 to 1873, the Royal College curriculum consisted of two sessions, followed by a single oral examination, in (i) chemistry, *materia medica* and pharmacy; (ii) anatomy and physiology of the horse; (iii) pathology and treatment of the horse; (iv) anatomy and physiology of the ox and other domesticated animals. Prior to 1884, the various veterinary schools imposed their own preliminary examination in general education.

When the Charter was granted in 1844, graduates of the London and Edinburgh schools became members of the Royal College of Veterinary Surgeons, although they did not obtain exclusive right to the title 'Veterinary surgeon'. W.J.T. Morton was the first to receive the diploma of membership, on 15 May. Sewell, Spooner and Simonds became members of the council of the Royal College. There was at first some confused skirmishing over the actual terms of the Charter — the College's solicitor, Mr France, had apparently not seen some amendments and had agreed to others from the practitioners' side without fully informing either the College professors or William Dick. More trouble arose over the decision by Dick to submit his students to examination, not by the Royal College, but by the Highland and Agricultural Society. Eventually, matters were resolved, and Sewell, after a 3-11 defeat in an 1850-1851 election, was unanimously appointed president of the Royal College in 1852-1853.

Sewell has been overshadowed by Coleman, in death as in life. He was a devoted and loyal colleague who was too old and set in his ways when he became Professor to introduce major developments, but signs of change were seen, coming to fruition in his successor's reign.

As a tailpiece, the author's study window overlooks a link with the history of the College — the home of Joseph Green, one of the medical men forming the examination committee.

Joseph Henry Green FRS (1792-1864), twice president of the Royal College of Surgeons, died at The Mount (now St Martha's Convent school) at Hadley Green, Barnet, 13 January 1864. His mother was a sister of Henry Cline. In 1818 he joined Astley Cooper as joint lecturer on anatomy and physiology at St Thomas's Hospital. In May 1819 he was unanimously chosen as a member of the board of examiners of the Veterinary College, succeeding Cline. In 1840 he delivered the annual oration in memory of 'the immortal Hunter'. When the Royal College of Veterinary Surgeons received its Charter in 1844 Green, along with other members of the board (Paris, Stanley, Liston, Richard Bright and Bransby Cooper, Astley's nephew) sent in his resignation with every wish for the future success of the Royal College. These members, with the exception of John Ayrton Paris, recently elected president of the Royal College of Physicians, agreed to serve on a temporary mixed board of medical and veterinary examiners. Green's memorial tablet is in the church of St Mary the Virgin at Monken Hadley, only a few miles from the College's Hawkshead campus.

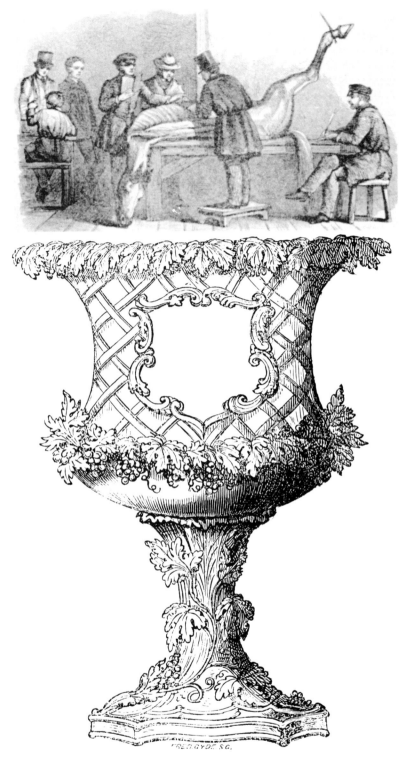

ABOVE: Students dissecting at the Royal Veterinary College, London, drawn by Edward Mayhew for his *Illustrated Horse Management*, published 1864. BELOW: One of numerous gifts he received, this silver vase was 'presented to Professor W. J. T. Morton by his private class pupils, session 1846-7, in admiration of his talents; as a token of their gratitude for his unwearied assiduity; and as a mark of their unqualified esteem and respect'.

CHARLES SPOONER

Professor 1853-1871

Important additions to the College buildings were made during Spooner's term as Professor. A dissecting room, a covered enclosure for post-mortems, a chemistry laboratory and a new theatre helped improve the scope of instruction courses, while a student's room, a professor's room and a boardroom were welcome amenities. To answer criticisms that the educational standards of incoming students were too low, the College instituted its own matriculation entrance examination.

Spooner was one of the first leading veterinary surgeons of his day to condemn vivisection, both in the form of unnecessary demonstrations at medical schools, and in experiments being carried out in France. Like Sewell, Spooner came from Essex. He was born on 19 October 1806, the third and youngest son of William Spooner, a dairy farmer at Mistley Park, Manningtree. After being apprenticed to G. Jervis, a chemist in Westbar, Sheffield, he entered the College in November 1828, at the same time attending Youatt's classes in Nassau Street. He and James Beart Simonds, who succeeded him as Principal, were fellow students. Spooner graduated on 21 July 1829 and then, mainly through the influence of his friend Sewell, was appointed to succeed Youatt as veterinary surgeon to the London Zoological Society, serving until 1833. On 3 November 1834 he began lecturing in his newly opened private school of veterinary anatomy, dealing almost entirely with the horse. This school was some 200 yards up College Street, on the opposite side of the road from the College, and comprised a yard, stable and dissecting room. The classes had the approval of Coleman as useful, indeed essential, supplements to the instruction in the College.

Following the retirement of Vines, Spooner, at the express invitation of Coleman, was appointed demonstrator in anatomy in October 1838. He became assistant professor on 20 June 1839 just before Coleman died, and in 1842 (when Simonds was installed in the chair of cattle pathology funded by the Royal Agricultural Society of England) Spooner was appointed deputy professor. Eventually, on the death of Sewell, he was appointed Professor and secretary of the College on 23 June 1853 at the age of 47. Early in 1840, Spooner had married Mary Anne Boulton (1817-1858) of Manchester, and had moved from No 5 to No 1 Great College Street. They had five sons and three daughters. One son, Percy Boulton Spooner, graduated MRCVS in January 1877 and died in May 1914, aged 57. For many years he had a large horse practice in Florence Street, Islington. Another son, veterinary major Walter Boulton Spooner, died in 1902 aged 48. He qualified from the College in December 1873, entering the Army Veterinary Department in 1874. He served in three campaigns: Afghan War of 1879-1880; Egyptian Expedition of 1882; Nile Expedition of 1884-1885. In the Afghan War, he took part in the defence of Kandahar, and was mentioned in despatches.

Professor Spooner died in the College on the morning of 24 November 1871 after a short illness. Classes were suspended for the day. He was buried in Highgate cemetery; the mourners included 160 students, walking four abreast and wearing crêpe bands. Some of them bore the coffin from the hearse to the chapel, and thence to the grave. In December 1871 the governors granted Mrs Spooner £500 and, when her son Percy entered the College, fees due to the College were remitted to her.

Spooner was a good-looking man, with whiskers and sometimes a beard. He was presented with a marble bust of himself, sculpted by a young Suffolk man known to Simonds, by the College students in the 1834-5 session. This bust was donated to the College by Spooner's son Frank, on 14 October 1913. Simonds said it was a good likeness, and some of Spooner's descendants have commented on the strong likeness of the bust to the current male generation in the family.

As a man, Spooner has been described as wilful, headstrong and quick-tempered, but also as extremely astute. His temper apparently worsened as he grew older, and by 1844 some observers thought he was suffering from megalomania. He often complained of not feeling well, and he tended to grow unduly excited over events of little intrinsic importance.

Spooner was a man of high moral principles. He spoke out strongly against drunkenness, which he thought had been one of the greatest failings of the veterinary profession since its inception (an opinion which remained widespread to well within living memory). He protested against vivisection, in the shape of unnecessary demonstrations to medical students, and he eventually urged the chloroforming of animals before they were subjected to experimentation. He picked out for criticism, among others, French experimental physiologists, including the celebrated Magendie. Spooner also supported the Society for the Prevention of Cruelty to Animals, and was a member of its council. In 1852 he was served with a summons for eightpence; his servant had called cab, but Spooner had refused to use it, as the horse was severely lame. The case was dismissed.

Spooner was held to be an able anatomist, and most students considered him an exceptionally fine teacher. He had a great fluency of speech, but some students complained that he failed to impart practical instruction, causing discontent in the class and involving additonal work for his colleagues. He had a habit of taking snuff while lecturing, and in April 1849 the students presented him with a handsome silver snuff box.

A vivid description of the College in the early days of Spooner's term as Principal was given by Pritchard (who qualified in 1860) in his opening address in 1890. In his time as a student 'the institution of a matriculation examination had not taken place; then, more frequently than one cares to recollect, the embryo veterinary surgeon's education was painfully meagre, and he was but very ill-fitted for the teaching dealt out to him — a disadvantage, the enormity of which I need not dwell upon. The teaching staff consisted of three professors, an assistant professor, and a demonstrator in anatomy; all men well selected for their appointments, gifted with rare abilities, with an ardent love for their calling, and an amount of zest for their duties which commanded much admiration and every respect; men who live well in the memories of their numerous pupils, and the fruits of whose labours will live long after them. But when we think of the amount of matter embraced in the different items of the curriculum with which they had to deal, one conclusion only can be arrived at — that, however good and great the ability, the energy, the labour, and the desire of these men to fully and completely accomplish the task to which they were devoted, it must of necessity have been beyond them.

'A passing thought on the class room or theatre, for there was only one: it was so small that extra movable seats had to be placed around the lecture table, encroaching inconveniently on the lecturer; and even with this arrangement it was overcrowded, and consequently very ill-fitted for an audience whose attention should be undivided. The dissecting room, which should be one of the best appointed parts of the school, was a long, narrow, low-roofed, badly floored, miserable-looking place; fitted with a few rough tables and forms, the general appearance of the whole arrangement of which was exceedingly well calculated to rob the aspirant to anatomical honours of at least half of his good intention to have an afternoon's instructive dissertation immediately upon his entrance.

'There was no chemical laboratory, either for the use of the professor of chemistry or for the pupils to carry on practical work in. The pharmacy was a small room set aside for containing the drugs needed for the treatment of patients in the infirmary and was only entered occasionally by a pupil, whose visit was more out of curiosity than anything else. Indeed, there was only one other room, a small one, set aside for the use of students, which was designated the pupils' room, and which was intended to serve for reading and writing in, but for which purposes afforded little (or no) accommodation, and which was more frequently used as a retreat by the lazy, or for depositing coats, parcels, and the like in. The teaching in the theatre consisted of three lectures daily, Saturday excepted, when there was only one; and an examination on chemistry. The professor on duty usually made a daily visit around the well-filled infirmary, when those who chose to attend him had an opportunity of hearing something of the nature of the cases and the instruction given as to the treatment of them, varied occasionally by a horse being seen out with a view to determine the seat of lameness, or whether treatment adopted was having the desired effect. Be it said to the credit of the students, such [a] professor was usually numerously attended. But this constituted the whole of the [clinical] teaching.

'There were very good opportunities for seeing horses examined as to soundness, as large numbers were sent to the College for that purpose; but very frequently such examinations took place without the students, who happened to be present, learning the opinion of the professor who carried out the examination. All operations were performed by members of the staff, clinical clerks were selected from the class weekly, but the casting and securing of the animals to be operated upon was always performed by the grooms, and all medicines were administered by the head groom. A student was never so much as requested to put a bandage on a horse's leg, consequently few of them knew how to do it. Each student was expected to dissect a certain number of subjects during the session, which dissections, considering the facilities provided, were on the whole well carried out. No practical instruction in shoeing was given. With the exception of the Coleman prizes, none were offered for competition to the general class; and no books were provided for the students, excepting those who had joined the Veterinary Medical Association.'

Spooner was a member of the London Veterinary Medical Society (he and Morton, having voted for Vines' exclusion in 1831, both resigned in 1836). He became president of its successor Veterinary Medical Association, re-elected annually until his death. His clinical and pathological demonstrations at the association's weekly meetings were felt by many to be more instructive than his formal lectures. He was conscious of the need (and of the difficulty) of securing animals other than horses for demonstration purposes. He tried to buy sick animals, and nothing came of yet another suggestion that the College should acquire a farm.

He was a noted surgical operator. His first operation — a successful one — was on a horse with a vesicle calculus. He later removed a calculus from a horse's bladder while the animal was under the influence of chloroform. In another case, again with the help of chloroform, he successfully divided a horse's metacarpal nerves. Unfortunately he failed to put his clinical experience on record for future generations.

During Spooner's regime, numerous additions were made to College House, and separate rooms for students and professors, with a boardroom for the governors, were provided in the main buildings. A new dissecting room was built in 1863, and a covered enclosure was erected for the slaughter and dissection of animals and for the post-mortem examination of patients dying or being destroyed in the infirmary (although too many of these were apparently sent, unproductively from the teaching point of view, to the knacker's yard). Several loose boxes and outbuildings were provided, and also a chemistry laboratory. There followed in 1867 a commodious theatre, and a new museum.

In 1859 John Hunter's remains were transferred from St Martin-in-the-Fields to Westminster Abbey. In the same year, a proposal was made that a College monument to Coleman should be erected. This, like the suggestion of an annual Coleman memorial lecture to be delivered at the Royal College, came to naught. However, in the 1860s, Coleman prizes were offered for the first time. Prizewinners from then on generally proved to be outstanding members of the profession. In 1866, for example, J. Wortley Axe of Tuxford, who qualified on 26 April, won the silver medal (and the Veterinary Medical Association prize); four years later he was appointed assistant professor to succeed the unfortunate O.W. Gordon-Brown, who had followed Pritchard as demonstrator and curator of anatomy. On 24 March 1868, Gordon-Brown had visited Hampstead on a horse borrowed from a friend; coming home the horse bolted, slipped on the pavement and fell on its side. Gordon-Brown was thrown against a wall and died of his injuries a few hours later. In 1875 Axe was appointed professor of histology and morbid anatomy. He instructed students in the daily practice of the College, and became a great teacher. Axe published a number of books and papers, including an interesting treatise on *actinomycosis bovis* (including *actinobacillosis*) 'with drawings by himself'.

In July 1866 the Midland Counties Extension Railway offered to buy the College an alternative site near Chelsea Bridge, and erect new buildings thereon, in exchange for the College site. The offer, most unfortunately, lapsed when the railway was eventually laid further east.

The long saga of the Brown Bequest had started in 1852, when Thomas Brown of Dublin bequeathed £20,000 to found 'an Animal Sanatory Institution' for 'investigating, studying and . . . endeavouring to cure maladies, distempers, and injuries among Quadripeds or Birds useful to man may be found subject to.' The tangled subsequent history of the bequest is set out in fascinating detail by Sir Graham Wilson in the *Journal of Hygiene* (Cambridge) 1979. The terms of the will were complex and proved difficult to meet. The institute had to be within a mile of Westminster, Southwark or Dublin and, if the University of London had not established it within 19 years from the date of Brown's death, the bequest would go to Trinity College, Dublin to establish professorships in certain ancient, eastern languages. There were legal wrangles and by 1865 the Senate of the University of London, fearful that they would lose the money, formed a committee to see what could be done.

John Gamgee, who had just transferred his New Edinburgh Veterinary College to London as the Albert Veterinary College in Queens Road, Bayswater, suggested the Brown Institute could be established on land leased by his college. The Royal Veterinary College also put in a proposal but it, like Gamgee's, was rejected because the site was not within a mile of Westminster or Southwark, and because the university did not want to surrender its independence in the matter.

Instead, the committee proposed a scheme for the higher education of veterinary practitioners, whose professional qualifications they considered inferior to those in France or Germany. The Senate took this advice and suggested that the Committee on Examinations in Medicine should draw up a curriculum of study and a scheme of examinations for conferring certificates of proficiency in veterinary medicine and surgery. So much for the Royal College of Veterinary Surgeons and the three veterinary schools! The Brown Institute was eventually established in Wandsworth in 1871. There were two departments, one for the treatment of sick and injured animals (both in-patients and out-patients) and one for scientific research. In the first 20 years, nearly 50,000 animals, mainly horses and dogs, were treated. The institute, which remained under the control of the Senate, was damaged and subsequently destroyed by bombs in the Second World War. It was never rebuilt and, after legal proceedings that dragged on for 25 years, the assets were divided between the universities of London and Dublin. The London share was used to endow the Thomas Brown research fellowship in veterinary pathology at the College.

For some time, concern had been freely expressed that the educational standard of pupils entering the College was too low. Spooner referred to this in his introductory address in 1864, when the College decided to institute its own matriculation examination. He reminded the new entry that in lectures they would tend to be passive, and would usually be observers in the clinic. In the dissecting room, however, they had to do things for themselves: only students of weak character and industry might regard it as an area for gossip and irregular amusement. He also reminded students that they would be required to act as clinical clerks in the second session, and if they were diligent in this they would receive a certificate from the professors.

A matriculation examination was accordingly introduced, and by the time of Spooner's death this was being conducted by the College of Preceptors — exemption being granted for holders of recognised certificates and diplomas. The candidate had to be capable of writing from dictation, parsing a simple sentence, reading aloud, and understanding the first four rules of arithmetic and the simple rule of three. It is interesting to note the background of entrants in Spooner's time. They included medical students, stud grooms, assistants to chemists and druggists, farriers, farmers, surgeons, and often of course, youths from veterinary families. Students came great distances to College, and were recorded as having lived in Dublin, Belfast, Australia, New Zealand, Calcutta, United States (Boston, New York), St Kitts, Paris, Toronto, and Russia.

The quality of veterinary teachers also became a matter of concern. Fleming, in a slightly later presidential address to the Central Veterinary Society, said he thought it essential that teachers should be highly educated scientific men. To achieve this, the veterinary schools should be aided financially by the government, and should in consequence be subject to periodical inspection. Teachers should have no pecuniary interest in the number of students who entered or left the schools.

Students' standards of behaviour did at times seem rather low. In 1857 George Scott admitted in writing that he had stolen something from one of his fellow students on more than one occasion: the College showed the mailed fist in the velvet glove, for Spooner was instructed to suggest to Mr Scott that it would be advisable that he should withdraw himself from the College. In 1864 a Mr Hinge was suspended, being in the habit of disturbing lectures by 'very indecent behaviour' (the imagination boggles). In 1871 Mr Condon's name was struck off the list of pupils; he had used College notepaper in offering betting information for £5. In contrast, some of the students gave a weekly collection for the Lord Mayor's Fund to help distressed Lancashire operatives. Other students revealed interesting degrees of enterprise after qualifying. Thus Henry Corby, graduating in 1854, became demonstrator of anatomy in 1857 but then went to America in May 1859 and practised in St Louis. He joined the federal volunteers at the outbreak of the Civil War and was present at the battle of Springfield on 10 August: wounded four times, he died on the 14th. Another former student, Thomas K. Quickfall, was appointed veterinary surgeon to the New Jersey cavalry in 1863.

Spooner travelled extensively in England on consultations, and attended the Vienna veterinary congress on 21-26 August 1865. One of the original petitioners for a Charter for the veterinary profession, he became president of the Royal College in 1858, his period of office marred by his brief resignation over some imagined slight, fortunately followed by rapid reconciliation. On 22 April 1844 he was a member of the small party (Spooner, Mayer

Jr and Gabriel, Royal College secretary) who attended the examinations at Dick's school in Edinburgh and which generally condemned the examination, the clinical instruction, and Dick's attitude to the examiners, thus further widening the rift between the Royal College and the Edinburgh School.

The list of subscribers in the second half of the century includes a number of brewers (Allsop, Bass, Buxton, Charington, Meux). Others, such as Pickfords and the South Eastern Railway Company, also have an obvious interest, but why did the warden of Dulwich College subscribe?

Four of the College teachers in Spooner's time require special mention: Morton, Tuson, Varnell and Pritchard.

William John Thomas Morton (1800-1868) was born in London, but was brought up in Devonshire, where he became apprenticed to a druggist in Tiverton. He came back to London in 1819 and joined a firm of retail chemists, remaining there until 1822. He was then appointed clerk and dispenser at the College, succeeding Mr Cupiss (later known as the 'constitutional ball' celebrity of Diss) who quitted this post on qualifying in 1822. Morton began giving private classes in *materia medica* and pharmacy in his own house in 1826, with Coleman's approval. In 1829 he arranged to give his classes in the evening in Spooner's private school of anatomy, and later he also lectured on chemistry. Prior to this, a student might have to walk to St George's Hospital to attend chemistry and *materia medica* classes, return to College for Coleman's lectures, go three times a week to Bart's for physiology lectures, and in the evenings go to one of the borough schools for surgical instruction (if he was one of the few lucky enough to have a ticket). In 1836 Morton's class gave him the first of a long series of presentations, finally numbering over a score.

Morton was appointed professor of chemistry in the College in 1839. He moved to Coleman's house, with Mrs Facer as housekeeper and manager, her daughter being house and parlour servant. He was the first to take the Royal College diploma examination in 1844, after a *pro forma* identification, and it was he who suggested the professional motto of the Royal College — *Vis unita fortior* — (in unity lies strength). This was the motto of the Earls of Mountcashell in Ireland, and is today used by many others, including the City and County Borough of Stoke-on-Trent. It had been the motto of the Veterinary Medical Association. Morton was a driving force of this association, being secretary from 1836-1850, and editor of its proceedings and transactions.

Morton far-sightedly urged the formation of a professional benevolent fund. He was elected a member of Royal College council in 1850, becoming treasurer in 1854; he was examiner in chemistry at the Royal College from 1864 until his death. Elected president of the Royal College in 1867, he declined the office on grounds of advanced age and ill-health.

A prolific writer, Morton published some notable monographs on chemistry and *materia medica*. He frequently wrote editorials in the *Veterinarian*, and was particularly effective, in the manner of his times, as an obituarist. He was the first to urge the need for a summer session at College, and he supported Percivall's request for a good practical test in the Royal College's diploma examinations.

On his retirement in 1860 students and members of the profession made a magnificent presentation to Morton (the 21st he had received) at the London Coffee House on Ludgate Hill. He had been given a silver tea and coffee service in 1844; the salver he now received was worth £85, comprising 146 ounces of silver, and was meant to accommodate this service. With the salver, Morton received a purse containing 135 guineas (further money was handed to him later) — an unprecedented sum.

Morton was at his best as a teacher. Griffith Evans, who qualified at the College in 1855, said in 1935 that Morton was naturally a poet, who sometimes gave a poetical twist to his lectures. One of his lectures dealt with the action of acids and alkalis on each other; the attraction, or repulsion, he said resembled love. 'His method of teaching, the choice selection of soul-stirring passages from the immortal works of Britain's noblest bards . . . renders the otherwise somewhat tedious and difficult subject of chemistry at once agreeable and instructive'. Perhaps there was a touch of personal reminiscence in his condemnation of students indulging in boisterous mirth before the beginning of lectures. However, students (although not perhaps some of his colleagues) may have felt he was speaking for them in suggesting that too much attention was given to the course in anatomy. He was obviously widely read in the classics, and an admirer of Lord Bacon: 'knowledge is power' was a much-used tag, and he quoted Bacon in urging students not to pursue wealth immoderately nor, like Atalanta, to be deflected from professional probity by chasing the golden ball of personal riches. He was the first College professor to retire into private life. He died in Dawlish on 2 April 1868 and was buried in Honiton old churchyard.

Morton was followed in the chair of chemistry and *materia medica* by Professor Tuson FCS, appointed on 18 September 1860 (at the same time, William Pritchard was appointed anatomical demonstrator). In 1872 Tuson was given the use of the College laboratory for his voluntary private classes in practical chemistry. He made his reputation by discovering the active principle of the castor oil bean. He wrote often in the *Veterinarian*, which he co-edited for some years, and his *Veterinary Pharmacopoeia* passed through several editions. An officer of the College for 28 years, he was kind-hearted, and made many friends. Tuson advocated the formation of a training college, where prospective students could learn the basic sciences before coming to College. He also proposed establishing a hall of residence for College students. He thought his veterinary students were a better group than his medical students: his class reciprocated by presenting him with a microscope. Tuson died in November 1888 aged 56, from 'structural disease of the valves of the heart', leaving a wife and six children.

George William Varnell (1806-1879) was the son of a Suffolk farmer. He took up the fattening of cattle, and then emigrated to America in about 1827. He started a veterinary practice in New York (there was no veterinary school in America at that time) and wrote to his father asking for the best books on veterinary practice. Simonds was consulted, as a neighbour of Varnell's father, and Blaine's works were sent out. After practising for about 10 years, Varnell returned to Britain and qualified in London in 1846. He showed a special aptitude for anatomy and took over as demonstrator when Mayhew resigned in 1846, becoming assistant professor in June 1853. Three years later he proffered, and then withdrew, his resignation on grounds of an inadequate salary. In 1862 he became professor of anatomy and clinic, retiring through ill-health in May 1867 and taking a farm at Beech House, Belton, in Norfolk. There he received a testimonial from the students — £100 and a silver tea urn, which had been chosen by his wife to match a previous gift of a silver tea and coffee service.

Varnell was a thorough master of his subject. In clinical classes he reportedly had an affable and comprehensible way of explaining and simplifying complex symptoms. He tested many horses for soundness, pointing out that by the aid of anatomy the patient was 'as it were, rendered transparent'. Varnell, like most anatomists, was a clever draughtsman (as was, for example, McCunn in this century). He was an untiring worker, and especially noted for his careful post-mortem examinations. He was a prolific writer and stressed the importance of putting matters on record for the benefit of future enquirers, for 'an academic life that leaves no record is indeed partly wasted'. The pages of the *Veterinarian* contain many 'Remarks by Professor Varnell', forming excellent accounts of autopsy findings and specimen examinations that show pathology was a well-taught subject before the advent of McFadyean. He was a forward-looking teacher, who (unsuccessfully) urged the College governors to institute a systematic course in morbid anatomy, and pressed for the greater use of the microscope. He was one of the first veterinary surgeons to stress the importance of urine examination in the diagnosis of disease. He devised the famous Varnell's gag for horses. He was a well-read man, and quoted Virchow's *Cellular Pathology* with approval.

One of Varnell's great interests was the pathology of parasitism, although he is said to have overlooked in 1864 the presence of parasites in haemorrhagic mucosal nodules in a colt's intestines, correcting this error when his attention was drawn to them by the submitting veterinary surgeon, Mr Littler.

In his introductory address in 1865, Varnell referred to the current lecture timetable. Every day, except Saturday, there was an anatomy lecture at 9.15. At 11 o'clock, chemistry and cattle pathology alternated, and at 1pm, four days a week, lectures were given on the physiology and pathology of the horse. As to students' leisure, Varnell told them to avoid reading novels, and not to go to plays or concerts.

In the professional field, Varnell urged the formation of a legal defence society. He proposed a series of postgraduate lectures every year at the Royal College, of which he was president in 1865. He was an ardent worker in the cause of prevention of cruelty to animals.

Like Morton, Varnell was the recipient of a number of student testimonials to his skill as a teacher. In 1848 he was given a gold watch, and in 1850 a microscope. In 1855 he received a silver tea and coffee set, and in 1859 a silver salver, cruet stand and an elaborately-chased cakebasket. On that occasion, he unexpectedly confessed that he found the monotony of his occupation sometimes rather trying, and referred to the not always congenial companionship he had experienced in discharging his College duties — yet, to read his life, he seems to have been a man of many parts and numerous rewarding activities.

Varnell was succeeded by Assistant Professor Pritchard. William Pritchard (1838-1906) qualified at the College in 1860 and shortly afterwards was appointed demonstrator in anatomy, one of his tasks being to preserve order and gentlemanly conduct in the dissecting room. He became teacher of anatomy on Varnell's retirement in May 1867 and professor in February 1872, after Spooner's death. He spent 20 years in College, and undertook a large part of the clinical work. His students respected and admired him, and gave him the usual quota of testimonials including a silver claret jug and inkstand, a 'superior' microscope, silver plate, a portrait in oils, and a silver cup.

Pritchard was sometimes stern, and even cross, but his students knew he meant what he said. They must have liked him because, on his wedding day (he married Spooner's daughter, Emily), he left the class without telling them where he was going, so that they could not be tempted to follow him and neglect their classes.

Pritchard was accused in 1880 by the general purposes committee of having broken Bye-law No8 by examining two horses at Cricklewood, for four guineas, at which he resigned.

After his resignation Pritchard remained in London, building up a large town practice and a vast consultative practice. He was said to be an unsurpassed clinical observer and a skilled operator, and was much sought after as a professional expert witness. He was appointed to the Royal College's board of examiners, and became a member of Royal College council, serving as president in 1888-1889.

Two great men qualified from the College in Spooner's reign — the sculptor, Adrian Jones, and the scientist Griffith Evans.

Adrian Jones was born in Ludlow, Shropshire, on 9 February 1845, the fourth son of James Brookhandling Jones, a veterinary surgeon in comfortable circumstances. He qualified MRCVS on 25 April 1865 aged 21, and saw 23 years' service as an army veterinary surgeon. His *Memoirs of a Soldier Artist* were published in 1933. He died on 24 January 1938 and had one son, the etcher Adrian Jones.

There is a memorial tablet to Adrian Jones senior on the outside of the south wall of the nave of Ludlow Parish Church (near a tablet commemorating A.E. Housman) which disappointingly does not state his veterinary qualification. On 11 January 1867 he was gazetted and went to India to join a battery of Royal Horse Artillery. Later that year England declared war on Abyssinia; Adrian Jones was veterinary surgeon to the advance brigade in the 400-mile push fron Annesley Bay to Magdala. He gave the *Times* correspondent a detailed account of the glanders-like disease which affected their horses, mules and camels. Jones was one of the officers to find the body of King Theodore, who shot himself when Magdala was stormed.

After the Abyssinian campaign, Jones returned to India to rejoin the Royal Horse Artillery. In 1869 he was gazetted to the Queen's Bays in Brighton and went with the regiment to spend 10 years in Ireland. He accompanied the 7th Hussars to Africa in the First Boer War in 1881 and was attached to the Eniskillen Dragoons when peace was declared.

On his return from Africa, and while still in the army, he began his first opus, a study of one of his own hunters in the form of a statuette called 'One of the right sort', which was shown at the Royal Academy exhibition in 1884. His experience in the Camel Corps in the Nile Campaign of 1884-1885 led to the statuette 'The Camel Corps Scout'. At the same time, his statuette 'Gone Away' — a mounted huntsman and two hounds — won the Goldsmiths Company's first prize. Initially, Adrian Jones had problems with the artistic establishment, who found it difficult to accept someone who had not been formally trained as a sculptor. However, his knowledge of equine anatomy and experience with horses proved invaluable in the equine subjects which dominated his works, and he became a well-known and respected artist, attracting royal patronage.

Among the highlights of his impressive output are a model of Persimmon, King Edward VIIth's favourite racehorse: the memorial to the Duke of Cambridge in Whitehall; the equestrian statue of Sir Redvers Buller VC, in Exeter, and the cavalry memorial at the Stanhope Gate in Hyde Park.

Undoubtedly his two most famous works are 'The Quadriga of Peace' on top of the Decimus Burton Arch on Constitution Hill, and 'Duncan's Horses', now at Hawkshead. Both masterpieces suffered a series of disappointments and delays before being installed in their present sites. It appears that a prototype of the Peace Quadriga in the Royal Academy exhibition of 1891 attracted the attention of the Prince of Wales (later King Eward VII) who proposed to the sculptor that such a Quadriga could be placed on the Arch on Constitution Hill. Over a period of 16 years, drawings were submitted to the Office of Works, who said they had no funds to implement the plan. Eventually, in 1907 Lord Mickleham, a noted philanthropist, agreed to meet the costs. Edward VII thus initiated the development of the Quadriga, but died before it was completed in 1912. Adrian Jones produced Duncan's Horses in 1892, the year after he left the Army.

Griffith Evans was born at Ty Mawr, near Towyn, Merionethshire, on 7 August 1835 (when Coleman still had four more years to live). His father was a farmer. He qualified from the College on 24 May 1855. He was commissioned in the Royal Artillery in January 1860, and stationed in Montreal in 1861. Evans graduated from McGill University as MD, CM in 1864, following the medical course, and worked as a postgraduate there for a year. His experiences in the American Civil War were described at length in the *Veterinary Record* of 3 August 1935, and make fascinating reading. Evans returned with the troops to England in 1870 and was stationed at Ipswich, where he continued his medical studies at the infirmary. He transferred from the Royal Artillery to the Army Service Corps in 1871, and was stationed at Woolwich for a number of years. He further studied medicine at King's College, the Royal Ophthalmic Hospital and the London Hospital. In 1877 he was ordered to India to investigate what turned out to be anthrax in horses. In 1880 he was asked to study a fatal disease of horses and camels in the Punjab known as 'surra'. He demonstrated 'microbes, swarming in the first drop of surra blood examined', and transmitted the disease by subcutaneous injection and by feeding the blood of an affected horse. The organism is now called *Trypanosoma evansi*, which he also demonstrated in the blood of camels. Evans thus discovered the first pathogenic trypanosome.

Evans retired from the army in 1890 and settled in Bangor, giving lectures on veterinary hygiene at its university for 20 years, finally retiring at the age of 75. He was awarded, among other honours, the John Henry Steel medal of the Royal College in 1918. He died in December 1935, shortly after the 100th anniversary of his birth had been commemorated by the College, the Royal College, the profession and the community he had served for so long.

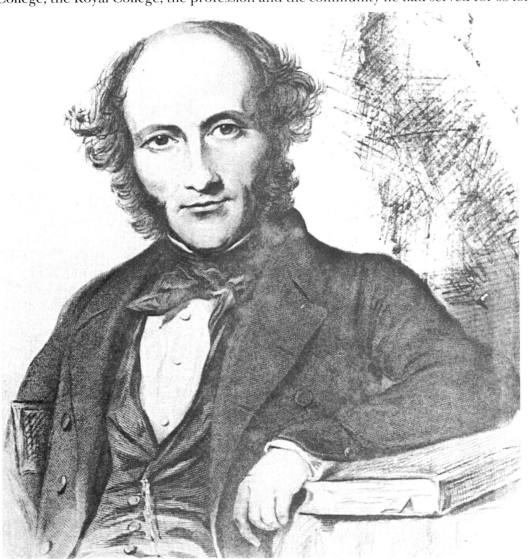

Charles Spooner in his prime.

NOTICE!

Mr. FOSTER, *COWLEECH*, issued handbills last week in this market, stating that he had removed from Double-street to Pinchbeck-street, soliciting also a continuance of favors, and designating himself *a Veterinary Surgeon !* Now the term "Veterinary Surgeon" was **a FORGERY**—an appellation to which *he has not the slightest claim.*

To constitute a Veterinary Surgeon, it is essential to be in possession of a **Diploma,** granted by the Court of Examiners of the Royal College of Veterinary Surgeons, London. That, at the said College, Candidates for the said Diploma are taught Anatomy, Physiology, Dissections, and the Nature and Proper Treatment of all Diseases incident to Domesticated Animals, as also Chemistry and Materia Medica; and unless such Candidates are found Proficient in each of these Branches of Veterinary Science on their examination, they are rejected, being considered unqualified to practice.

Mr. FOSTER, like many other **Blacksmiths, Bell-hangers, &c.,** professing a knowledge of the **Healing Art,** has not acquired the above essential branches, and consequently will, ere long **be compelled** to represent himself in proper terms, by adopting the words **"FARRIER"** or **"COW-LEECH"** *instead of Veterinary Surgeon.*

The Veterinary Body, under their Royal Charter of Incorporation, have the power of compelling Empirics *to erase from their Door-plates, Sign-boards, &c., the words "Veterinary Surgeon,"* it being an Imposition and a Forgery ! and is not allowed by other Professions.

R. METHERELL,

Veterinary Surgeon, and Fellow of the Veterinary Medical Society.

Veterinary Infirmary, Pinchbeck-street, Spalding,
  October 18th, 1852.

R. Metherell, who qualified at the College in December 1838, having enrolled in October 1837, attacks a cow-leech for misrepresentation.
(RCVS)

87

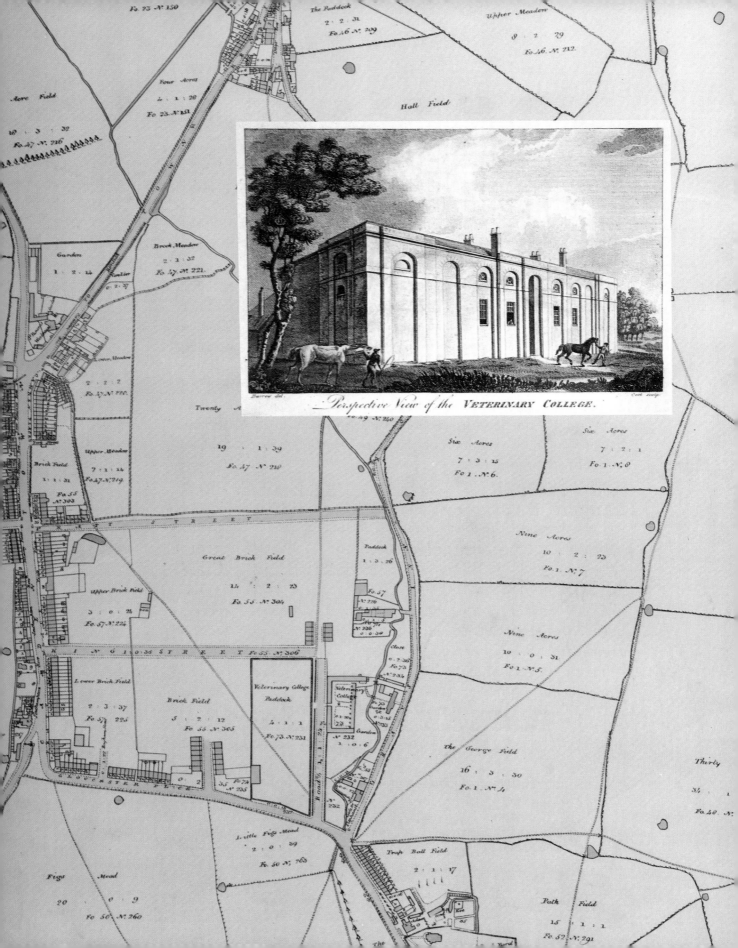

Perspective View of the VETERINARY COLLEGE.

OPPOSITE: Tompson's map, 1801, showing the Veterinary College with the Fleet River running behind the building. (LBC) INSET: 'Perspective view' of the west front of the College in about 1793. The height is greatly exaggerated in this engraving, which shows the round-headed arcades visible on the Great College Street facade until it was demolished in the 1930s. BELOW: Charles Spooner (seated left) R. V. Tuson, C. W. Varnell and (seated right) James Beart Simonds, photographed in about 1860.

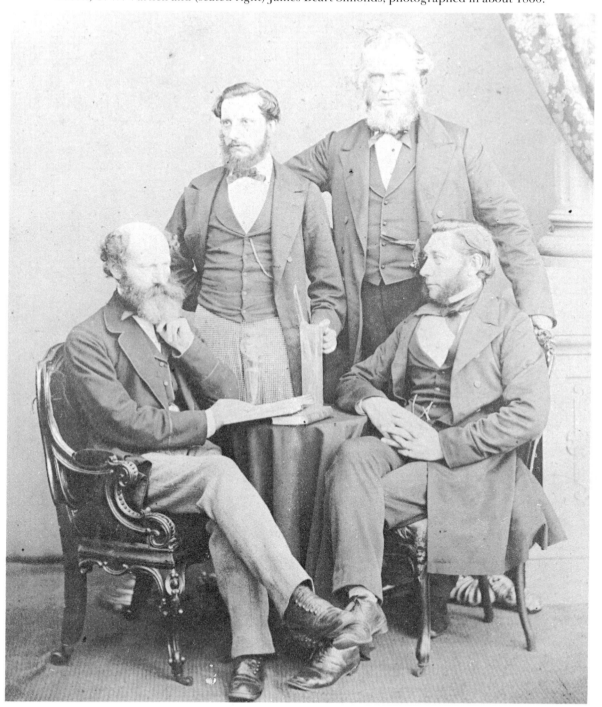

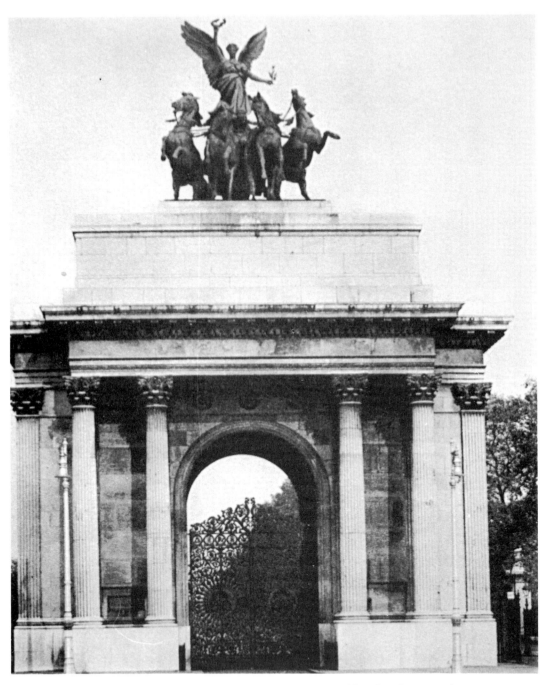

The Quadriga of Peace, 'one of the most superbly placed statues in London', on the Decimus Burton arch, Constitution Hill. The sculptor was Adrian Jones, who qualified at the College in 1865.

THE SHEEP:

ITS HISTORY, STRUCTURE, ECONOMY, AND DISEASES.

IN THREE PARTS.

Illustrated with fine Engravings from Drawings

By W. HARVEY, Esq.

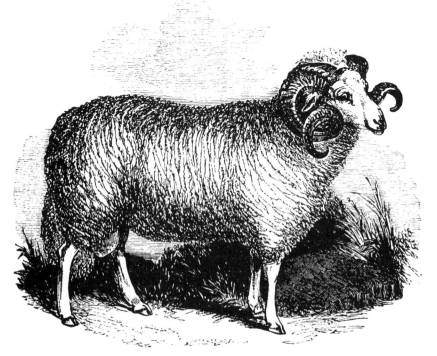

By W. C. SPOONER, V. S.

MEMBER OF THE COUNSEL OF THE ROYAL COLLEGE OF VETERINARY SURGEONS,
HONORARY ASSOCIATE OF THE VETERINARY MEDICAL ASSOCIATION,
AUTHOR OF DISEASES OF THE HORSE'S FOOT, EDITOR OF
THE NEW EDITION OF 'YOUATT ON THE HORSE,' AND
OF 'WHITE'S CATTLE MEDICINE,' &c.

SECOND EDITION.

LONDON:
CRADOCK AND CO., 48, PATERNOSTER ROW.

William Charles Spooner (1809-1885) who became an expert on sheep
and horses, was not related to Professor Charles Spooner. They studied
together at the College, where W. C. Spooner qualified in 1829.

ROYAL VETERINARY COLLEGE,
GREAT COLLEGE STREET, CAMDEN TOWN.

FOUNDED 1791.—INCORPORATED 1875.

PATRON—HER MAJESTY THE QUEEN.

PRESIDENT:

FIELD-MARSHAL H.R.H. THE DUKE OF CAMBRIDGE, K.G., &c. &c.

Annual Subscription, Two Guineas. Life Subscription, Twenty Guineas. Annual Subscribers for two consecutive years may become Life Subscribers by payment of Sixteen Guineas.

JAS. B. SIMONDS,

ADMISSION AND DISCHARGE OF PATIENTS.

Ordinary Cases are admitted or discharged daily, Sunday excepted, from 9 o'clock until 6 in the Summer, and 5 in the Winter.

Accidents and Urgent Cases are admitted on Sundays as well as on other days and at any hour.

Admitted *July 26* 1876

Animal *Roan Gelding*

Owner *Messrs Bailey*

W Pelling Clerk.

This Card must be produced on the removal of the Animal from the College. Communications are to be addressed to the Principal.

LEFT: Admission ticket dated 1876, for a roan gelding. The ludicrously low subscription fees, fixed soon after the College was founded, remained in force until the middle of this century. In 1876 charges for keep were: horse, 3s 6d per day; ox 1s 6d; dog 5s per week; sheep and pig 3s 6d. Shoes were charged 5s a set to subscribers and 6s to non-subscribers. RIGHT: James Beart Simonds.

92

JAMES BEART SIMONDS

Principal 1872-1881

The College grew in size, scope and stature with Simonds as Principal. During his regime, in 1875 the College was incorporated by Royal Charter, thus giving it an entirely new status. Almost before his appointment was confirmed, Simonds set about reorganising the daily life of the College. He brought method and organisation into the hospital routine, with increased involvement for the students in all forms of practical work. With Professor Brown, he submitted a detailed review of the educational system, with recommendations for its improvement. A summer teaching session was introduced. The 'cheap practice' (later known as the Out Patients' Department) was opened. In addition, Simonds's own contributions to veterinary science added lustre to the reputation of the College.

James Beart Simonds rather touchingly (if unconvincingly) claimed descent from Simon, Lord of St Sever in Gascony, who fought at the Battle of Hastings and was granted land in East Anglia by William the Conqueror. Simonds was born in Lowestoft on 18 February 1810 into an agricultural family. Two uncles — Samuel and John — were veterinary surgeons. Simonds was orphaned when his father, James, died at the age of 25, and he was educated, while under the care of his paternal grandfather, first at a commercial school, and then at Bungay Grammar school. He entered the College on 7 January 1828 and qualified after 14 months' study, on 7 March 1829. As a student he had also attended, with some half-dozen others, Youatt's private school in Nassau Street where the main interest was in canine pathology. He also attended *materia medica* classes given by Morton. He took a course of human anatomy at Tyrell's school in Aldersgate Street, and classes on chemistry at Dr Agar's private residence. Simond's qualifying examination was conducted at Astley Cooper's house in Conduit Street, Hanover Square, by Cooper, Babington, Bell, Brodie, Joseph Henry Green, Coleman and Sewell. Cooper remarked on the fact that he himself had been born at Brooke, six miles north of Bungay, and he encouragingly invited Simonds to breakfast with him the next morning.

Simonds's veterinary uncles, Samuel and John, married two sisters, the daughters of James Beart, a farmer and breeder of Suffolk horses, living near Diss. Simonds's paternal grandfather and guardian, Samuel, was also an agriculturalist. Simonds himself was to continue his farming interest at Oakington Farm near Wembley, some 2-300 acres in extent.

In April 1881, when he had been Principal for nearly 10 years Simonds, who was reported to have been ill for six weeks, wrote to the governors: 'Painful as it may be to speak of oneself, I feel that the time is fully come for me to seek relief from some portion of my work, more especially that of delivering lectures day by day to the Class. At the close of the Summer Session I shall enter on the fortieth year of my official service under the Governors, which, with my advanced age and I fear diminishing physical powers, clearly point to the improbability of my being able to fulfil all the duties of my office, especially during the Winter Session, in a manner satisfactory to the Governors or myself'. A little later, in his report of 1 July, Simonds wrote for the information of non-executive governors, and subscribers: 'It has seemed to me that the time has arrived when I should give place to a younger and more energetic man. Great as my desire ever has been to continue to serve the Governors until the end of my career in the position I have had the honour to occupy so long, I feel that this will have to yield to circumstances over which I have no control. It can scarcely be hoped that even with diminished work I should be enabled for any lengthy period to perform the duties which would still evolve on me'. Nevertheless, the kindness which he always had at the hands of the governors led him to leave the matter entirely to their decision.

Simonds appears to have meant nothing more than what he had asked for — relief from some of his duties, particularly lecturing — but the governors read his remarks otherwise, for Simonds was taken aback when the governors suggested it would be conducive to his comfort and health if he retired. However, he dutifully resigned, moving to St Helens, some three miles south of Ryde on the Isle of Wight, having been granted a reasonable annuity by the College. He was given a testimonial signed 'George' (the Duke of Cambridge, president of the College) and was made an Honorary Associate of the Royal College. His health was restored in six months but the Veterinary College doors remained closed to him. He continued to be an active member of the Royal Agricultural Society and in 1894 he was present at the jubilee meeting of the Royal College (of which he had been president in 1862). He was then the sole surviving petitioner for the 1844 Charter.

Smith knew Simonds, and described him as follows: 'In appearance he somewhat resembled the statesman, Mr Gladstone: the writer remembers him as a little above the middle height, with a slight stoop, probably due to age, jet black hair without a bald patch, side whiskers, otherwise clean-shaven, large mobile features which always bore a solemn expression. Perhaps no one ever saw him laugh' (a phrase applied also, understandably enough, to some subsequent College principals). Smith further said that Simonds deserved all credit for being the first real organiser of the College. He had gained considerable official and worldly experience, and moved in different circles from Spooner. Smith praised Simonds as the first Principal to come to power with clear ideas of improving the College: in fact, Smith considered, he reconstructed the College materially and morally.

To take up the story of what followed Spooner's death in 1871, in Simonds's own words: '. . . in November 1871 . . . I was therefore requested to act as Director of the School and Hospital until the appointment of a Principal in succession to Professor Spooner was determined on at the Annual meeting of the Governors. As Director, however, I was empowered to make such changes as were deemed to be pressing. In addition, therefore, to the daily Hospital visits, special clinical demonstrations were held twice a week, and a day set apart for operations. Clinical Clerks and Dressers were likewise appointed from the Second Session Students to attend week by week to the patients, under the direction of the acting Professor. Monitors, having the oversight of the dissecting-room duties, were selected to act under the direction of the Assistant Professor of Anatomy. The Professor of Chemistry had also power given for carrying out practical analytical work. These and some other changes of minor importance being approved, the Governors at their meeting on 20th February, 1872, conferred on me the honour of Principal of the College. At an adjourned meeting, it was determined to add a summer session to the existing winter one. The instruction to include Botany, Practical Pharmacy, the principles and practice of Shoeing and the performance of operations on the dead subject.' (Helminthology was later added to botany, and Dr Cobbold was appointed teacher of both subjects.)

'In order to carry out these additions to the curriculum, the strength of the teaching power had necessarily to be increased. The consideration of these important matters relating to the

Infirmary was, however, postponed for the decision of a general meeting of the Governors. At that meeting, Professor Brown was appointed Lecturer on Physiology, Therapeutics and Pharmacy. The Education Staff of the Institution being completed, consisted of — J. B. Simonds, Professor and Principal of the College, Lecturer on Pathology. Professor R. V. Tuson FCS, Lecturer on Chemistry, Materia Medica and Toxicology. Professor G. T. Brown, Lecturer on Physiology, Therapeutics and Pharmacy. Professor T. S. Cobbold FRS, Lecturer on Botany, Parasites and Parasitic Diseases. Assistant Professor J. W. Axe, Demonstrator of Anatomy of Domesticated Animals. In addition, Hospital Surgeons — pupils of the Institution who had obtained the Diploma of the RCVS — were appointed annually; to act under the Professors. It was also arranged that monitors, Clinical Clerks, Dressers and Prosectors, be periodically selected from the Class.'

Among the students entering the College in 1872 was John Henry Steel, after whom the medal of the Royal College is named 'to perpetuate the memory of an earnest worker, so that his example may incite others, and to benefit the profession by encouraging and rewarding merit'. John Henry Steel (1855-1891), son of Charles Steel, an army veterinarian in the 12th Lancers, qualified in 1875, taking the first Fitzwygram prize (50 guineas) as well as the Spooner gold medal and the Coleman silver medal. He spent nine months in the army, and was then appointed assistant demonstrator at the College. He contributed many translations to the *Veterinarian*, especially of articles from French journals and, with Cobbold, visited Alfort in 1879. Steel resigned as lecturer in anatomy in 1881, instancing pecuniary considerations and his not achieving an anticipated promotion to professor — the College plan was to abolish the post of professor of anatomy — and he hinted at other causes he would not disclose. On leaving the College, he was presented on 25 March, in the lecture theatre, with a handsome gold lever keyless watch. He stated then his view that the students should have more direct access to the governors of the College, and he urged the governors in turn to make themselves more acquainted with the working of the College. Steel rejoined the Army Veterinary Department in 1881 and was later appointed professor of veterinary science at the Bombay Veterinary College, which he started. He died — much lamented, according to Simonds — on 20 January 1891 at the early age of 35.

Steel's publications included books on equine anatomy, diseases of the ox, and diseases of the camel. He investigated surra in mules in Burma. With Banham, he developed a veterinary congress from which the National Veterinary Association, precursor of the present British Veterinary Association, evolved.

Only one application for Steel's post was received — from William Hastie Kennedy of Wrexham, Shave having declined to be a candidate. Kennedy resigned due to ill health in 1881, and Shave was appointed lecturer in anatomy.

In 1872 the Principal had been empowered to appoint two newly qualified students as hospital surgeons by examination, with an honorarium of £10; this was raised to £50 in 1874 as there were few or no takers at the lower rate. In 1873 two examinations of one hour each were instituted — the first after winter and summer sessions, the second after the next winter session. By 1876 the course was nearly three years, with three Royal College examinations, still all *viva voce*. In 1876 proposals were considered which might have led to the appointment of associate professors, for the recognition of veterinary surgeons in practice who gave vacation instruction to College students. Although a College library was available from October 1878, only one student out of 200 was a subscriber, yet many students joined the Veterinary Medical Association, at two guineas, to use its much superior library.

The year 1879 saw the introduction of a 'cheap practice' for poor owners. This practice was carried on by students under the direction of one of the professors. The cheap practice, later known as the Out Patients' Department and more colloquially as the 'back gate' or 'back bed', mostly concerned horses with persistent lameness. The defence by the College, against complaints of undercutting made by members of the profession, was that those attending the cheap practice would not be able to afford normal veterinary fees.

In 1878 considerable insubordination was noted among students of Class A. In 1881 a student was suspended for using bad language (which was overheard by the head groom) at the College gate while ladies were passing. In the same year a Mr Burghope got two months' hard labour for worrying cats and assaulting a policeman; surprisingly, he was allowed back into College. In 1883 the preliminary examination taken in College to determine whether students should go forward for the Royal College diploma examinations was dropped.

The non-teaching staff had its troubles too. In 1874 the head groom broke his right leg while walking on Hampstead Heath; he was lucky, for his full wages were to be continued at the Principal's discretion. The next year, a groom suffered three broken ribs from the kick of a horse. On a more cheerful note, in 1874 the gate porter was provided with an official uniform — blue coat, blue waistcoat, black or dark-mixed trousers, a hat, and white buttons stamped 'RVC' in raised letters.

Changes in staffing were accompanied by a building programme as reported by Simonds in his autobiography: 'At subsequent meetings of the Governors, decisions were come to with reference to the erection of New buildings and the conversion of existing ones to the increasing requirements both of the School and the Infirmary. Those most needed were begun forthwith. Thus by the opening of the Educational year 1872-3 a Pharmaceutical Laboratory, a Class room specially arranged for Histological Investigations and the study of Morbid Anatomy [20 years, be it noted, before McFadyean came to London] as well as a new Lecture and Dissecting room were sufficiently advanced for occupation. Much of the work of adding to and improving the Infirmary was in a sufficiently forward condition to meet the evidently increasing practice. Old sheds had, however, to be pulled down, and new loose-boxes and an entire new Ward erected for the reception of Horses, Cattle and Sheep and other animals. Hot, cold, douche, vapour and foot baths, with an operating room &c., were in due course also added. Ultimately a new and more imposing front to the College was also erected.' In 1873 the Principal was given the right of disposal among staff of all rooms and stables. In 1875 a brick wall replaced the dilapidated wooden fence at the back entrance from College Grove. The following year, the College decided to give up land it had sub-let west of Great College Street; it was presumably long before then that the tunnel under the street, leading from the College to the pasture, was closed.

Two outstanding developments affecting the College took place during Simonds's regime — the incorporation of the College in 1875 by Royal Charter and a detailed review of the College educational system. These are the main features of the Charter of 1875:

Paragraph 1 sets out briefly the history of the College, and names the petitioners — the Duke of Cambridge (President), Viscount Bridport, Charles Newdigate Newdegate CB, MP, Sir James Tyler and James Whatman Bosanquet. It states (without supporting evidence) that the site of the College in Camden Town was selected as being both healthful and convenient. The College comprised an ample infirmary for sick animals, a museum, a lecture theatre, dissecting rooms, operative theatre, chemical laboratory, library, board and committee rooms, an official residence for the Principal, etc. Paragraph 2 states that there had been some early Parliamentary financial assistance for the College, but for upwards of 50 years, the main resources, from subscribers' fees, students' fees, plus legacies and donations, had proved sufficient for its support. Veterinary surgeons had been appointed to the forces by commission. The Royal Agricultural Society provided £200 per annum towards the teaching of diseases of animals other than the horse and for investigating them and their treatment. Paragraph 3 notes that a matriculation examination was conducted by the College of Preceptors, and students had to pass two examinations of the Royal College.

Subsequent paragraphs list powers granted to appoint from time to time a Principal, professors, assistant professors, and other officers, to remove them, and to appoint successors. Exhibitions, scholarships, medals and other prizes and certificates would be conferred, to conduce to the proficiency of the students and the maintenance of a high standard of education. The governors would be able to create fellows of the College.

The College would be incorporated, to give it permanence as a public body, and the current form of government (president, vice-presidents, governors, treasurer, and general purposes committee) would continue.

The officers and subscribers were to form 'The Royal Veterinary College', and the Charter lists the new president and governors and others who were to form the College.

The government of the College was to be vested in president, vice-presidents, governors and treasurer, who would have power to appoint trustees, secretary, fellows, licentiates, honorary and foreign associates, Principal, professors, assistant professors, demonstrators, hospital surgeons and other officers. An annual general meeting was to be held.

Power was given to enact bye-laws, which must not prejudice or interfere with the rights and privileges of the Royal College of Veterinary Surgeons under its charter. Executive management was vested in a general purposes committee.

As an addendum, there is a note on the arms of the College which came into use with the charter of 1875.

The education committee of the College made reports in 1876 and 1878 which led to a scheme for running the business of the College being put forward by Professors Simonds and Brown. Their recommendations, which by inference show the extent of current deficiencies, were:

1. All incoming letters relating to College business should go through the secretary's office, and be open to inspection by the Principal. (Had Hobday observed this recommendation he might not have been forcibly retired on 'age limit'.)
2. The entry and exit of all animals should be recorded in a book to be kept by the porter, who should not be allowed to leave his post during College hours.
3. Regulations 12 to 18, and 21, should be strictly enforced. These were: '12 — The Principal, in addition to his other duties, shall exercises a general supervision over the whole of the daily practice of the College, and shall have the medical care of all the animals in the Infirmary, receiving such assistance as he may require from the other Professors and Officers whose duties are connected with the ordinary daily business of the College.

   '13 — The Officers who shall be in attendance day by day during College hours shall be the Principal, the Professor of Anatomy, and the Professor of Histology, or any other Officer or Officers who may be appointed for the purpose by the Governing Body or the General Purposes Committee; and on occasions requiring the temporary absence of any of the Officers, such arrangement shall be made by the Principal as will secure the constant attendance of not less than two of the other Officers during such absence.

   'In order to ensure the uninterrupted attendance of the Principal and other Officers to the business of the College, each of them shall, as far as possible, avoid giving opinions in cases in which litigation is pending, or likely to arise on the question of a breach of warranty, or of soundness of horses or other animals.

   '15 — The Assisting Infirmary or Hospital Surgeon and Dispenser shall reside within the College, and shall give his entire services to the duties of his office, under the immediate direction and supervision of the Principal, or in his absence, of one of the other Professors or Officers in attendance. He shall dispense all medicine under the direction of the Principal, to whom he shall be responsible for the safe custody of all drugs, chemicals, instruments, utensils, and pharmacy fittings: and shall see that all rules and regulations respecting the attendance of the Students in the Infirmary and in the Pharmacy shall be strictly carried out. He shall not order any drugs, chemicals, or medicinal agents of any kind, but when such are required he shall report the same to the Principal.

'16 — None of the Professors or Teachers whose duties, besides those of instructing the Students, are connected with the Infirmary department of the College, shall engage in private practice; but with the special permission of the Principal they may investigate cases of extensive or serious outbreaks of disease, and visit individual animals with the object of their removal to the Infirmary for treatment.

'17 — The Principal shall see that a complete record is kept daily of every animal brought to the College for admission as a patient, or for treatment as an out-patient, or for examination for soundness, or for opinion on disease. This record shall be so kept under the direction of the Principal that it can be referred to by any of the Professors or Officers in attendance as a guide to the opinions that have been given.

'18 — All documents and correspondence relating to the business of the College shall be considered official, and shall be kept for reference by the Secretary.

'21 — Besides the Annual General Report to be presented to the Annual General Meeting, which shall contain an account of the state of the College as a whole, quarterly reports and returns of the infirmary, and Chemical departments and School, together with a report of all the work done by the Professors in their several departments for non-subscribers, agricultural societies, and their members, shall be presented by the Principal to the Governing Body or the General Purposes Committee, who shall take notice of any irregularities which may have occurred on the part of any of the Officers in carrying out their respective duties'.

4. It was recommended that operations should be performed at fixed hours, to be arranged by the professors and notified so that students would be able to attend. A record should be kept by the demonstrator of all morbid specimens sent to the College, and this record should be signed by the Principal.

5. 'College business admittedly often interfered with Classwork, but as far as possible, the Students should be kept to their duties under the inspection of a teacher. If a teacher is unable to take a class, he should let the Principal know, so that a substitute may be provided. The Principal should arrange the subjects for Classwork, and he should report to the Governors or the General Purposes Committee every instance of non-compliance with his directions or of any infringement of any Regulation relating to the educational or general routine work of the College.'

This final recommendation of Professors Simonds and Brown is surely a *cri de coeur* that other principals have echoed: 'Lastly we are of the opinion that, unless several members of the College staff actively and heartily co-operate with the Principal, it will be difficult, if not impossible, to carry out the reforms we have suggested'.

Although Simonds had been appointed secretary as well as Principal, the posts were separated in 1876. The advertisement in *The Times* of 19 June 1876 showed the salary of the secretary to the £200 per annum. No veterinarian would be eligible. Over 600 applications were received, including one from a woman — Susan Ferrer, dated 23 June, who offered to accept a lower salary than a man would receive. A short list of five was hastily prepared, and interviews were held at Arlington House on 30 June. One of the five, Mr Pennell, was recommended for appointment but he declined, and the post went to R.A.N. Powys, who proved to be a great success.

Richard Atherton Norman Powys was College secretary for 37 years. It was noted that hundreds of students and parents met him, mostly during the awesome period of a first interview at their *Alma Mater*, and that his clear, bold handwriting was generally the first thing that started candidates on their way to a career as a veterinary surgeon. To the students, he was always courteous and to his colleagues at the College he was a warm-hearted friend. He established a methodical way of working, arriving and departing so regularly each day that students might set their watches by him.

Powys died suddenly from heart disease at East Sheen, Surrey, on 10 July 1913 in his 70th year. He had been obliged by failing health to resign his appointment some two months before but, until his successor, Thomas C. Wight, clerk to the Edinburgh and East of Scotland College of Agriculture, was able to take up his duties, Powys had carried on working to 7 July.

Subsequent College secretaries were T. C. Wight, 1913-1935; J. F. P. Maclaren, 1935-1938; C. G. Freke, 1938-1946; H. W. J. Adams, 1946-1974, and Derek W. Gordon-Brown, the present incumbent, who was appointed in 1974.

Simonds contributed in two major ways to the advancement of veterinary science: firstly by the investigation of diseases, especially of infectious diseases, largely at the instigation of the Royal Agricultural Society, and secondly by the use of the editorial columns of the *Veterinarian*, which he and Morton co-edited after Percivall's death in 1854, to bring current advances to the notice of the profession.

Particularly noteworthy was his work in respect of foot-and-mouth disease, sheep-pox, cattle plague and contagious bovine pleuro-pneumonia (details of this and other work may be found in Smith). Simonds states that England appeared to have been free of foot-and-mouth disease until the autumn of 1839, when almost simultaneously it was detected in Smithfield Market, and near Norwich. From London the disease spread quickly, particularly into Middlesex. It appeared in Simonds's practice on a farm about five miles from Twickenham. Experimentally, Simonds placed some hay in the mouth of a diseased cow, for saturation with saliva and with the contents of ruptured vesicles. On his return home, one of his own cows was made to chew the hay, and she became infected in three days. His next experiment was to test her milk. Having at that time a litter of pigs old enough to be weaned, some of them were isolated and given warm milk from the infected cow. They also contracted the disease, but by strict isolation, neither the piglets left with the sow, nor either of two other cows, became infected.

Simonds found sheep-pox in Mr Statham's flock at Datchet, near Windsor, on 4 September 1847 and is said to have handled the situation with considerable understanding and skill. Erasmus Wilson, a noted medical dermatologist with a strong interest in animal disease, agreed with Simonds that the lesions resembled those of human smallpox. The disease spread all over the country, and Simonds pressed for a controlling Act of Parliament. This was passed in 1848, giving authority for the destruction of affected animals and flocks entering this country. The experiments he made showed the disease could be spread by inoculation and by contact. Vaccination with human vaccine lymph was shown to be useless, but the method of 'ovination', using 'lymph' from affected sheep, reduced the mortality from 50% to 3%. Simonds set out his experiences at length in his 1848 textbook. When sheep-pox was re-introduced in 1862, in a self-contained flock in Wiltshire, it was diagnosed by Simonds. The disease was eradicated from the United Kingdom in 1866.

In April 1854 Thomas Mayer junior resigned from the council of the Royal College and gave up the family practice in Newcastle-under-Lyme, to join the army and serve in the Crimean War. He heard in the late summer of a plague that was destroying immense numbers of cattle in Asiatic Turkey, and which shortly afterwards appeared in his camp. Following consular reports, Simonds was invited to visit the Continent to see control measures in force on the eastern frontiers with Russia. The expenses of the visit, made in company with William Ernes, a polyglot Belgian MRCVS, were borne by the Royal Agricultural Society of England, the Highland and Agricultural Society of Scotland, and the Royal Agricultural Improvement Society of Ireland. On 9 April 1857 the two men set off on an extensive tour, during which they saw cases of the disease at a quarantine station in Galicia. Simonds submitted a report published in 10 issues of the *Veterinarian*, with the following conclusions:

'1. That all the countries of Northern and Western Europe from which cattle are exported to England are perfectly free from the Rinderpest; and that the only disease of an epizootic or destructive nature which prevails therein is the one known to us as Pleuro-pneumonia, which disease has existed here since 1841.

'2. That in the greater part of the official despatches and reports which have been forwarded to the Government, and by them transmitted to the Royal Agricultural Society of England, the Rinderpest has been confounded with Pleuro-pneumonia, 'Milzbrand', and other destructive maladies to which cattle are liable.

'3. That the Rinderpest is a disease which specially belongs to the Steppes of Russia, from which it frequently extends, in the ordinary course of the cattle trade, into Hungary, Austria, Galicia, Poland, &c.

'4. That whenever circumstances have arisen which called for the movements of troops, and consequently the transit of large numbers of cattle, in Southern and Eastern Europe, and particularly when Russian troops have crossed the frontier of their territory, the disease has been spread over a far greater extent of country.

'5. That the disease which has recently prevailed in Galicia — where it was specially investigated by ourselves — as well as in Poland, Austria, Hungary, the Danubian Provinces, Bessarabia, Turkey, &c., is the true Rinderpest, or Steppe Murrain of Russia.

'6. That with the exception of a few places in the kingdom of Prussia and others in Moravia, near to the frontier of Galicia and Poland, the disease in its outbreaks of 1855-56, and -57, did not extend to any country lying westward of a line drawn from Memel on the Baltic to Trieste on the Gulf of Venice.

'7. That, speaking in general terms, Rinderpest has not existed in Central and Western Europe for a period of forty-two years; its great prevalence at that time being due to the war which was being then carried on between the different Continental kingdoms and states.

'8. That all the facts connected with the history of its several outbreaks concur in proving that the malady does not spread from country to country as an ordinary epizootic. And that, if it were a disease exclusively belonging to this class, the sanitary measures which are had recourse to throughout Europe would be inefficient in preventing its extension; and consequently that in all probability we should long since have been both painfully and practically familiar with it in this country, as hundreds of our cattle would have succumbed to its destructive effects.

'9. That it is one of the most infectious maladies of which we have any experience, and that it is capable of being conveyed from animal to animal by persons and various articles of clothing, &c., which have come in contact with the diseased cattle.

'10. That the ox tribe is alone susceptible to the disease; and that the morbific matter on which it depends lies dormant in the system for a period of not less than seven days, and occasionally, according to some Continental authorities, as long as twenty days, before the symptoms declare themselves.

'11. That an attack of the disease which has terminated favourably renders the animal insusceptible to a second action of the *materies morbi* which gives origin to the pest.

'12. That the deaths often amount to 90 per cent.

'13. That the malady is one in which the blood is early, if not primarily, affected; and that subsequently the mucous membranes throughout the entire body become the principal seat of the morbid changes.

'14. That the symptoms are in general well marked and quite characteristic of the affection.

'15. That all varieties of medical treatment which have as yet been tried have failed in curing the disease; the recoveries which take place having for the most part depended on the *vis medicatrix naturae*.

'16. That no fear need be entertained that this destructive pest will reach our shores. Its present great distance from us would, of itself, afford a fair amount of security; but when we add to this that no cattle find their way from thence, directly or indirectly, to the English market; and also that in the event of the disease spreading from Galicia, it would have to break through hundreds of military *cordons*, one after the other, before it could possibly reach the *western side* of the German states; and, moreover, that for years past commerce has been unrestricted with regard to the importation of skins, hides, bones &c., of cattle from Russia and elsewhere, all alarm, we believe, may cease with reference to its introduction into the British Isles.'

Pattison observed that the clear conclusion was that because of the remoteness of the affected areas, and of the draconian measures that were taken to control the disease on the Continent, 'no fear need be entertained that this destructive pest will reach our shores'. That this conclusion referred only to that particular time and to the circumstances then prevailing is made clear in a Morton editorial praising the report: '. . . since the time may come — although there is no fear at present — when this formidable malady will reach our shores through the introduction of foreign cattle'.

In a letter to *The Times* of 10 November 1863 Gamgee warned that cattle plague would find its way into this country with a cargo from a Baltic port. In fact, cattle plague from Russia appeared in the London market on 14 June 1865, having entered by the port of Hull. On 4 July, Simonds was asked to see some affected cows at an Islington dairy. On 10 July he reported the matter to the Privy Council. The Order in Council of 11 August described the disease as 'a contagious and infectious disorder, of which the nature was uncertain [on 24 July] but which has since been ascertained to be of a typhoid nature, and is generally designated as cattle plague'. Smith claimed that Simonds failed to recognise the disease when he first saw it, and did not make up his mind on the nature of the disease until early August. Pattison considers that an examination of the literature, official reports, and minutes of the Privy Council's proceedings failed to reveal the basis for Smith's strictures on Simonds and for his support for Gamgee in the cattle plague affair. In particular, no explanation had been found for Smith's contention that Simonds believed that cattle plague could arise spontaneously. The use of the description 'a disease of malignant character', instead of 'cattle plague' has been held against Simonds, suggesting that he did not recognise the disease. This, Pattison considers, is unjust. Simonds was a cautious man, and it was far better to be cautious at first, and correct in the end. When the disease had been stamped out, a Veterinary Department of the Privy Council was formed, of which Simonds was created chief officer.

Contagious bovine pleuro-pnemonia reached London in the winter of 1841-42; Simonds believed it originated 'spontaneously' in Ireland. He infected a healthy cow at the College by placing it in contact with a diseased animal.

Simonds recognised swine fever as a specific disease in 1862 in Berkshire.

Pattison — who is not, be it noted, a London graduate — has written 'There is extensive documentary evidence that Simonds' personal contributions to the profession have not been surpassed by any other individual. First a rural practitioner, then Professor of Cattle Pathology at the London school. Member of the Charter Committee and signatory to the Charter. Field investigator of diseases of sheep and cattle, notably sheep-pox, foot-and-mouth disease, pleuro-pneumonia, cattle plague and parasitic diseases. First veterinary adviser to the Royal Agricultural Society and to the Privy Council, veterinary adviser to the Privy Council in the successful control of cattle plague, and first veterinary surgeon in the Government

101

being scarce. Probably the first treatise exclusively devoted to the subject which was published in the English language.

Jas. B. Simonds

department in consequence established. For many years editor-in-chief of the *Veterinarian*. Author of numerous scientific papers. RCVS Councillor for over twenty years, and President in 1862. Principal of the London school for ten years, and architect of its incorporating Charter of 1875. In retirement, historian and biographer. Because he thought deliberately and spoke quietly, Simonds has been overshadowed by more flamboyant but less worthy men.'

A
DECLARATION
OF SVCH GREIVOVS
accidents as commonly follow

the biting of mad Dogges,

together with the cure
thereof,

BY
THOMAS SPACKMAN
Doctor *of* Physick.

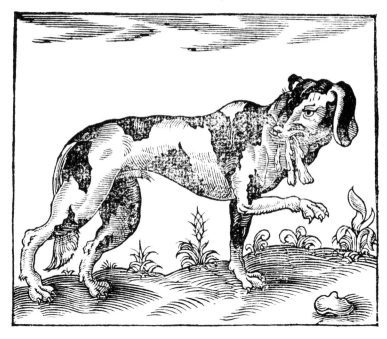

LONDON
Printed for *Iohn Bill* 1613.

Frontispiece of one of the many books donated by James Beart Simonds
to the College library. His note on the flyleaf reads 'Very scarce. Probably
the first treatise exclusively devoted to the subject which was published
in the English language'.

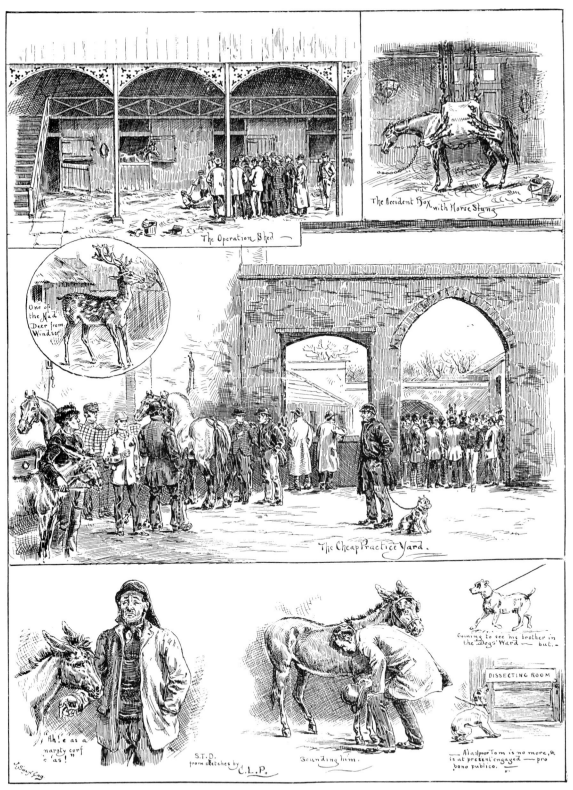

Sketches published in *The Illustrated Sporting and Dramatic News*, January
1888, which described the College as 'one of the most important
institutions in the country'.

WILLIAM ROBERTSON

Principal 1881-1887

Robertson is the least written about of the College principals. He was born in Kelso in 1830 and was brought up in the ways of a Scottish country practice. He was thus 'familiar with the hard drudgery of forge and of saddle practice'. Educated at Selkirk Grammar School, he was at one time intended for the Church. He studied Greek and Latin and at the age of 17 was awarded the gold medal for mathematics by the University of Edinburgh. Despite this promise of a brilliant academic career, Robertson was led by his early experience of practice, and by his love for animals, to train for the veterinary profession. He went to the 'Dick' school, where his chief teacher, William Dick (whom, it was said, he resembled in more ways than one) was a great stimulus to him.

Robertson obtained the certificate of the Highland and Agricultural Society of Scotland in 1852, and began to practise in Kelso, greatly impressing people by his skill and endurance. His diagnosis was said to be rapid and accurate, and his treatment prompt. On 9 May 1860 he became MRCVS and was elected to the Royal College's examining board for Scotland, remaining a member for nearly 20 years, specialising in cattle pathology. He served as a member of Royal College council from 1879, having become FRCVS in 1877.

When Dick died in 1866, Robertson was offered the chief professorship at the 'Dick' school, but this he declined. In 1880 a vacancy occurred in the staff of the College when Professor Pritchard resigned, and a committee was set up to find a successor. On 24 February the post was ordered to be advertised, and on 16 March nine applications were considered. The committee reported that they believed Robertson to be eminently qualified for the appointment, both by his practice and by his theoretical skill in his profession. Mr Robertson, they said, had gained a great reputation for his knowledge of the diseases of cattle as well as of horses, and his testimonials were eminently satisfactory. So Robertson was appointed professor of hippopathology from 12 July 1880, at £800 per annum. His terms of appointment allowed him to leave the College (presumably for private consultations) at 2 pm every day, unless his services were required in the College. On Simonds's resignation in 1881, Robertson was elected Principal on 19 July. He was to occupy the Principal's residence, and get coals, gas, water, the keep of a horse, the services of a man, and taxes.

Robertson was a man whose general physique and healthy looks were thought to presage a ripe old age, but this proved to be wrong. On the morning of Thursday 15 December 1887, the day Royal College examinations began, Robertson complained to Professors Axe and Brown of not feeling well, and said that for the first time in his life he had been reminded that he had a heart. At about 2.30 pm that day John Doyle, a College messenger, entering Robertson's office, found him lying on the floor. He called for help from Powys, the College secretary, who hurried to the room. There he loosened Robertson's tie, but it seemed that the Principal was drawing his last breath. He was buried on 19 December at Highgate Cemetery.

In 1888 a letter from Robertson's son (one of his four children) elicited from the governors a grant of £312 10s to the widow. On 14 March 1888 it was decided to appoint G. T. Brown as Principal (despite the availability of J. Wortley Axe, professor of pathology and morbid anatomy, who had been connected with the College for 20 years).

Robertson was a good teacher and a prolific writer. He had the faculty of using every odd fragment of time that might be available. He developed the free clinic, took students on sick rounds and conducted examinations for soundness. He contributed papers to the *Veterinarian* (his copies of this journal were neatly bound) and to the *Journal of the Royal Agricultural Society*. His major work, *Equine Medicine*, was published in 1883 — he presented a copy to the College library on 15 October. He was correcting proofs of a proposed companion volume on equine surgery at the time of his death.

A number of staff changes were made in 1881. G. T. Brown was transferred to the chair of cattle pathology vacated by Simonds. Henry Power FRCS was appointed lecturer in physiology — a Mr Collins thought it should not be lost sight of that this office should at some future date be held by a veterinarian, who could if wanted assist in the general work of the College. E. Simpson Shave was appointed lecturer in anatomy, succeeding Kennedy, who had resigned due to ill-health. (In 1883 Shave was granted permission to practise outside the College, and in 1886 he was awarded the title of professor.) John Penberthy, Coleman bronze medallist, was appointed hospital surgeon. T. Spencer Cobbold MD FRS resigned as lecturer in helminthology in 1885, and Dr Thomas B. Lowne became lecturer in helminthology and botany (the teaching of the latter being transferred from Shave). Lowne appears not to have been a successful teacher; in 1886, for example, it was noted that there had been somewhat unruly behaviour of a section of the botany class during the first winter term. He resigned in 1888 in protest at the abolition of his course in helminthology.

In Robertson's early years as Principal, the financial situation led to a committee under Sir Frederick Fitzwygram to consider ways of reducing annual expenditure. The committee proposed to do this in the classical way, by reducing the salary of some of the staff and increasing the work-load of others. This proposal naturally upset the staff concerned, but it is not clear how rigidly they adhered to the committee's recommendations. Brown was required to reduce his lectures from three to two per week, his £300 salary being reduced accordingly.

In 1885 Penberthy, entering the controversy over whether experience of veterinary work by a student before entering the College was helpful, observed that, of the last 150 students admitted to the College, 90 had previously been with a veterinary surgeon, and others had gone to one after passing the first or second Royal College examinations (the course was then three years). Of the last 50 students who failed to satisfy the diploma examiners, more than four-fifths had been apprenticed to veterinary surgeons. For example, Trevor Spencer left school at the age of 15½ years and was articled in 1886 to a veterinary surgeon in a large mixed practice in Berkshire. He remained there until he came to College in October 1887, continuing his pupillage in Berkshire during each College vacation. He qualified as a member of the Royal College in 1890, but he had to wait for his diploma until he reached the required age of 21. Spencer was in practice in Northamptonshire from 1893, and during the First World War had been responsible for the veterinary care of some 36,000 remount horses and mules. He also, for a short time, had the veterinary responsibility for about 500 horses at the artillery training school.

Penberthy also gave some figures for the College's clinical work. In the three years 1882-1884, 3,268 horses had been examined for soundness and 4,129 were examined for lameness or other diseases. There had been 2,387 horses as in-patients in the infirmary, besides a number of dogs and other animals (it was noted that cases of rabies were regularly admitted). Over 6,000 animals had been seen in the cheap practice, one-tenth being submitted to surgical operations, while one half were lame. All medicines were dispensed and administered by students, who also performed operations under professional supervision in the cheap practice.

The annual reports of the time make interesting reading. In 1883 the falling number of student admissions and subscribers were matters for concern. To make the teaching at the College more generally known, besides using the regular veterinary journals, advertisements were put in 32 different papers, including the *Field, Land and Water*, and *Bell's Life*, shortly before the opening of the winter session. Also in 1883, a practitioner said that owners of animals attending the cheap practice should have a certificate from a veterinary surgeon saying they were too poor to pay the fee. In 1884 a new lease was being negotiated with the Ecclesiastical Commissioners — the old lease would expire in 1889, and £750 per annum for 99 years was on offer.

In 1886 the long connection of the Angerstein family with the College was broken when William ceased to be a governor, having failed to attend meetings for over two years. In that year, too, the Principal and a house surgeon visited Pasteur's laboratory in Paris, with financial support from the Royal Agricultural Society. In 1887 the Society's grant to the College was renewed, having been discontinued in 1876. Also in 1887, Nigel Kingscote was elected chairman of the governors, succeeding Newdigate, who had been a governor since 1838 and who was chairman under the 1875 Charter of incorporation. It appears that rugby matches between the London and Edinburgh veterinary schools were instituted in 1886.

Some insight into Robertson's mind can be obtained by reading his address at the opening of the session on 1 October 1886. It is a model of its kind, and could, with little alteration, be delivered acceptably today. Robertson comes through as an intelligent and humane man, and his relatively early death must have curtailed what could have been an outstanding contribution to the development of the College.

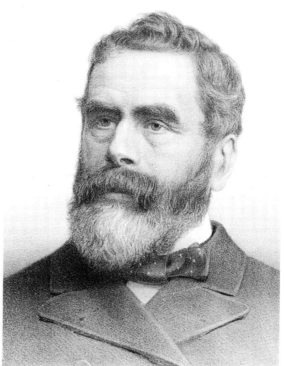

William Robertson.

107

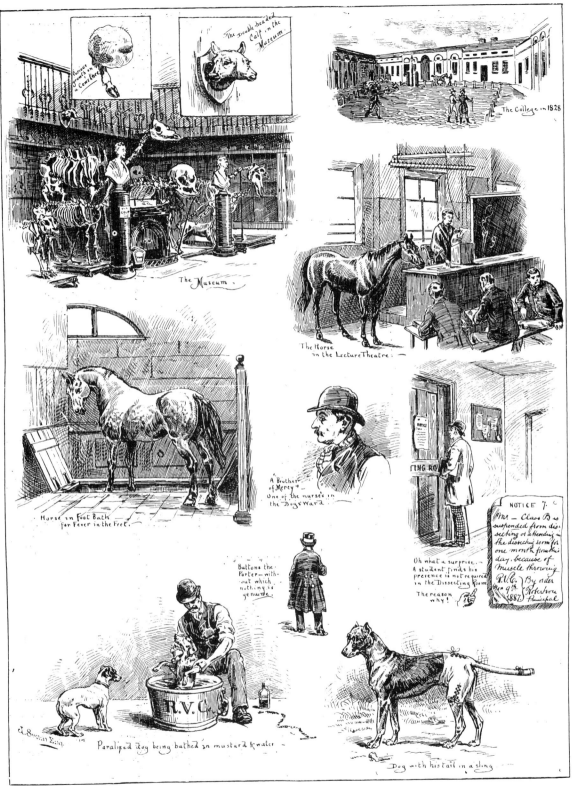

Sketches published in *The Illustrated Sporting and Dramatic News*, January 1888.

George Thomas Brown

Principal 1888-1894

The centenary of the College was celebrated in 1891 when the Prince of Wales opened a new lecture room, library, museum, reading room and bacteriology laboratory. There were then some 300 students on the roll but, throughout Brown's term as Principal, women were still refused admission.

George Thomas Brown was born in 1827. He entered the College in 1846 at the age of 19, took his MRCVS diploma in 1847, and went into practice in London. In 1850 he was appointed professor of veterinary science at the Royal Agricultural College, Cirencester, whose secretary had approached the College for someone to fill the appointment. There he taught classes of 60 to 80 agricultural students for 13 years, and learned the skill of presenting veterinary science interestingly to non-specialist audiences. He built up a museum there, and conducted an agricultural consultative practice, chiefly dealing with cattle, sheep and pigs. He made a particular study of the dentition of farm animals, and in his spare time studied agriculture and geology. His students expressed their appreciation of his qualities by giving him a silver tankard, and later, a timepiece and a purse of sovereigns towards the purchase of a microscope — he wrote a notable account of microscopy in veterinary medicine in 1867. He designed a pocket microscope in 1872, and a pocket clinical thermometer the following year.

In 1863, when a new principal was installed at Cirencester, Brown, along with senior colleagues, resigned (no precise reason emerged) although he remained an honorary associate of the Royal Agricultural College, delivering a lecture there annually. He went back into practice in London but, in June 1865 on the outbreak of cattle plague, he was appointed under Simonds to the veterinary department formed by the Privy Council. Here he was to demonstrate to the full his administrative ability and infinite commonsense. The State Veterinary Service, founded on 14 October 1865, is virtually Brown's creation.

In 1868 Brown succeeded Morton as Royal College examiner in *materia medica*. He was elected a member of Royal College council in 1864, 1876 and 1884. In 1868 he became vice-president of the Royal College, an honour repeated seven times. He was president in 1874-75, and was elected an honorary associate in 1881.

The president, with two other members of the council of the Royal College (Harpley and Field) were co-opted on a committee set up by the governors of the College to investigate its curriculum. This committee recommended, and the governors agreed, that the College's power to appoint licentiates and fellows should be removed from the 1875 Charter and the only honour conferred by the College should be an honorary associateship (which Fitzwygram, Harpley and Field accepted). The College has since revived its power to elect fellows; current fellows include the Queen Mother and the Princess Royal, chancellor of London University.

Brown was appointed lecturer in physiology, therapeutics and *materia medica* at the College in 1872, the latter two subjects forming the course of the newly instituted summer session. In 1872 he succeeded Simonds as chief adviser to the State Veterinary Service, becoming head of that department in 1877 and serving until 1893. His claim to fame is that he freed the country from cattle plague, foot-and-mouth disease and contagious bovine pleuro-pneumonia.

In 1881 Brown took the chair of cattle pathology, under Principal Robertson. After Robertson's death in 1887, the general purposes committee asked Brown if he would undertake the duties of Principal without being required to live in College, but to be responsible for general management and discipline. This was clearly looked upon as a part-time and interim arrangement to which Brown agreed, saying he could not undertake any duties which would interfere with his official work for the agricultural department of the Privy Council. The *Veterinary Record* asked whether Brown could discharge two posts satisfactorily, but Lord Cranbrook, Lord President of the Council, saw no grounds for objecting, and Brown was appointed Principal on 5 July 1888. Professor Axe went into residence in the Principal's house, and shared the infirmary practice with Professor Penberthy. Axe was to represent the Principal in his absence, and to share with the Principal lectures on the diseases of farm animals (a few years before, it was estimated that there were in the United Kingdom two million horses, 10 million cattle, 30 million sheep and four million pigs).

Professor Shave, who was admitted FRCVS by examination on 21 October 1890, in addition to teaching anatomy, was to take on board histology and morbid anatomy, and was to assist in the infirmary and in clinical instruction. Professor Lowne was to discontinue lectures on helminthology, that subject being adequately covered by the lectures on animal diseases, but he was to provide botany lectures at a fee of £100 per annum. It was made clear to the staff that no pension was attached to any appointment.

In 1890 Brown presented a report on the course of study at the College. He considered that the patched-up course then current had resulted from intermittent and haphazard responses to changes introduced from time to time by the Royal College, additional duties having been taken on by staff not properly prepared for them. The course of study introduced in 1876 now occupied three years, and there were three Royal College examinations (still *viva voce*; the first written examination was not held until 1892). Anatomy was taught by three members of staff, one of whom also taught histology (a subject which Brown thought properly belonged to physiologists); one taught bacteriology (a division of pathology) and one, botany. These subjects required special attention, but a major thrust of Brown's report was in regard to pathology, a subject taught by a staff member who was not a recognised pathologist. Brown said that pathology (including morbid anatomy and bacteriology) should be taught by a scientist who had given special attention to this subject, and he looked forward to a chair about to be established, with Royal Agricultural Society funding, supported by a College grant. (In July 1891 there was speculation in the *Veterinary Record* on the possibility of forming a faculty of veterinary science in the University of London.)

Brown also thought that improvements in the system might, with advantage, be associated with corresponding improvements in the College buildings, and he urged that the scheme submitted to the general purposes committee a few months previously, for the construction of lecture rooms and other offices over the ride, deserved more serious consideration. If the plans of Mr Vernon, the architect, were accepted at once, the new buildings might be ready for occupation in time for the celebration of the centenary of the College, and no more fitting memorial could be suggested. The estimated cost was £4,500 (though the actual expenditure proved to be £8,000).

The foundation stone of the new buildings was laid by the president, the Duke of Cambridge, on 7 June 1890. The stimulus was the £500 grant from the Royal Agricultural Society for the establishment of a department of scientific research, with special reference to diseases of farm animals.

The stone-laying ceremony was performed in a marquee in the main quadrangle. Among those present were Simonds, the former Principal, and a large number of ladies. The Duke stood in the centre of the marquee, facing the stone, which was suspended by ropes, and around which were gathered the staff of the College and the visitors. Colonel Sir Nigel Kingscote, chairman of the Board of Governors, reviewed the history of the College, pointing out that the Duke's father had been the second president. The current lease of 99 years, granted by the Ecclesiastical Commissioners in 1887, had encouraged the erection of new buildings, including a lecture theatre which could seat some 350 persons, a library, a museum, a reading room and a bacteriology laboratory.

The outside iron staircase, a striking feature of the new buildings, would give more room inside by avoiding the need for corridors.

The secretary commented that, in a cavity in the stone, there were copies of four London newspapers of that day's date, the current copy of the *Veterinarian*, two copies of the regulations of the College (one of which contained a list of subscribers) and a programme of the day's proceedings. Then, with a silver trowel, the Duke spread the mortar, applied the level, tapped the stone three times on each end with a mallet, and in time-honoured phrase, said 'I declare this stone to be well and truly laid'. On the stone, which does not appear to have survived the re-building of the 1930s, the inscription read: 'This stone was laid by Field Marshal His Royal Highness the Duke of Cambridge KG, President of the College, on Saturday, June 7th, 1890. Col Sir Nigel Kingscote GCB, Chairman of the Governors. Professor G. T. Brown CB, Principal of the College. Richard Benyon Berens, Chairman of the General Purposes Committee. Richard A. N. Powys, Secretary. Arthur Vernon, Architect; G. H. and A. Bywaters, Builders'.

In his opening address in 1890, Pritchard described some of the improvements achieved in the College since his student days 30 years before: 'Such a standard of matriculation examinations has been established as enables the pupil to easily grasp all that is taught, and possesses him with other immense advantages. The period of study has been much extended, and instead of the same subjects being dealt with each session, as heretofore, every term has its work, the pupils divided into classes "A", "B" and "C" having to make themselves efficient in one set of subjects before passing on to cope with others. The teaching staff has been increased no less than threefold, and the appliances wherewith to carry out their work of instruction very considerably improved and added to. The theatre, lecture- and class-rooms have been increased in size and trebled in number, and at the present time even these are being magnificently added to . . . The dissecting-room, which for some years past was in every respect a vast improvement on the original one, has been considerably extended, and is now equal, if not superior, to anything of the kind in this country. A room is being fitted up for bacteriological research; a new row of buildings is in course of erection over the site of the ride, in which is a large lecture-theatre capable of accommodating comfortably over 300 students; a museum of much larger dimensions than the present one, and an extensive reading-room and library with other rooms; besides which one of the quadrangles has been covered in with glass to afford facilities for surgical and other practical teaching. A professor's chemical laboratory, with one for the students, and a large pharmacy have also been erected . . . The examination of horses as to soundness, and the cases of disease in the infirmary, which now are not only those affecting horses and dogs as heretofore, but include those which oxen, sheep and swine are the subjects of, are well utilised as means of instruction. The art of shoeing is practically as well as theoretically taught. You are permitted to cast and secure horses for operation, to compound and administer medicine to patients. You are practically taught to bandage, dress and otherwise treat wounds; and, more valuable than all, you are, by an arrangement made by the governing body, which allows of the animals of the needy being treated at low rates, given the golden opportunity of being trusted with, and made responsible for, the treatment of the subject, than which nothing teaches better . . . a further inducement held out for your encouragement are certificates of distinction, medals, scholarships, exhibitions, and other awards, the like of which my confrères had no opportunity to compete for . . .'

When Pritchard resigned in 1880 the College gave him a large silver teapot, milk jug and sugar basin, with 500 guineas in the teapot. It is said that Pritchard once sewed back a torn flap of skin of a horse falling in a race, using string as a suture, and a nail from the foot to sew with. Pritchard was president of the Savage Club, and was in attendance on the horses of many leading members of society.

In October 1890 Henry Chaplin (president of the Board of Agriculture) offered the College the skeleton of the horse Hermit. He was bred by Mr Blenkiron in 1864, and in the following year was purchased by Mr Chaplin at the Middle Park sale for 1,000 guineas. As a three-year-old he won four races out of nine, including the Derby at Epsom. In 1870 he was put to stud at Blankney, where he remained until he died. His reputed skeleton is now in the museum of the College. He sired two Derby winners, Shotover and St Blaise, besides many other good horses. Before he died, his progeny had won over £340,000.

Various ideas were mooted for celebrating the College centenary in 1891 — Woodroffe Hill FRCVS proposed an international conference, followed by a banquet and soirée. The College set up a centenary committee, comprising Berens, Marjoribanks, Gilbey and Brown. In July, this committee recommended that a substantial cold collation be given to the students (who numbered some 300) and about 100 guests, at a cost of not more than ten shillings per head. Each student was to receive a centenary silver medal, with the College arms on one side and a suitable inscription on the other; Gilbey negotiated with Mappin & Webb to supply 300 medals for £162 10s. It was further proposed that an annual centenary scholarship of £21 be awarded to the candidate obtaining the highest marks in the matriculation examination.

The firm of E. G. Moore of Eversholt Street, who had for several years provided refreshments at the opening of College sessions, estimated to feed 400 persons at three shillings per head, with table requisites and attendance. They would also supply Moet and Chandon champagne — one bottle per two guests at 6s 6d per bottle, with sherry (3s) and claret (2s) respectively, per each six guests, which would amount to about £80, raising the total cost of the luncheon to 9s per head.

A marquee, floored, carpeted and lined throughout with scarlet and white bunting, and lit by gas (the College did not have electric light until the 1900s) and a supply of chairs and tables for 400 people, plus two small supplementary marquees for the convenience of the caterer, would cost £74.

The centenary was observed (a little late) on Monday 19 October 1891. The Prince of Wales was present, and his first task was formally to declare the new buildings open. Luncheon was then taken in the marquee in the quadrangle, tastefully decorated with ferns and autumn flowers. Moore's cold collation was indeed substantial — it consisted of roast joints, raised pies, dish pies, galantines, tongues, hams, roast fowl, salads, jellies, creams, patisserie and cheese — as promised, everything was 'of the best description and in abundance'.

The Duke of Cambridge, as chairman, proposed the toasts to the Queen, the Prince and Princess of Wales, and other members of the Royal Family. The Prince toasted 'success and continued prosperity to the Institution, coupled with the name of your Principal'. Sir Nigel proposed a toast to the Duke of Cambridge as president of the College. In his reply, the Duke called on the public to increase its financial support for the College (the subscription rate was still what it had been 100 years before). The architect of the new buildings, Arthur Vernon, of Great George Street, Westminster, was presented to the Prince after luncheon.

With a part-time Principal, a full-time officer was necessary for the day-to-day functioning of the College. Professor Crookshank, who gave lectures on bacteriology to College students, thought a dean, on the lines of the one in his own college — King's in the Strand — would serve. The Principal thought it might be necessary to go to Germany to find an occupant for the new chair in pathology, and an approach by Fleming to German scientists was suggested. However, with the approval of Brown (but not, it appears from a letter of Fleming's, by unanimous vote in the general purposes committee) John McFadyean was appointed dean and professor of pathology and bacteriology in 1892. When Brown resigned in September 1894, McFadyean succeeded him as Principal.

Although Brown was first-class as an administrator, as a lecturer he was reputedly dull and uninspiring, and even at his best not exhilarating. Curiously, as a public speaker he was said to be 'gifted beyond measure' — impressive, severely logical and with a wide choice of language. He was apparently not popular with students, owing to his reserved manner, his somewhat melancholy expression, and the extreme rarity of his smile. Indeed, some of the students called him 'miserable Jimmy', because he invariably looked as though about to weep (although in private life he was said to show an unexpected sense of humour). Despite this, like Simonds, he never ceased to command respect. He received public recognition for his work under the Privy Council, was appointed CB in 1887, and received a knighthood in 1898 (some would have liked Simonds to be similarly honoured). In 1881 he received the rare honour of associateship of the Royal College. Brown was for many years veterinary editor of *The Field*, veterinary adviser to the Royal Agricultural Society, and to the Bath & West of England Agricultural Society. He retired from active State service in 1893 on reaching the age limit, but was kept on as a consultant for three years. He died on 20 June 1906.

During Brown's term as Principal, Walter Gilbey was appointed a governor in 1886. Gilbey thought the previous system of having a clinician as Principal was unsatisfactory, because principals had not always been good administrators. At about that time Powys, the College secretary, commented to an enquirer that several students obtained the diploma of the Royal College without seeing practice with a veterinary surgeon 'though to do so is no doubt advantageous when practicable'.

In 1889 a deputation, led by W. J. Mulvey, complained that the College was undercutting practitioners' prices — a perennial complaint. In April, it was noted that the students used the waiting-room as a smoking-room — the room would be converted into a library and reading room. Most students lived in 'digs' near the College, although some professors (Macqueen, Penberthy, Shave) boarded a few by private arrangement. The fee for the three-year course of lectures was £45. A number of students were suspended for poor attendance.

Axe and Penberthy shared the infirmary practice in 1893. Axe, who had been appointed demonstrator in anatomy, was liked by his pupils. He apparently conducted flourishing private classes, for in 1874 his private pupils presented him, on 4 March in the Crowndale Hall, with a 'beautiful marble timepiece, inlaid with Egyptian figures, and surmounted by a sphinx in bronze'. Four months later, on 14 July, Axe was called upon to make a full apology for his behaviour to the dean. This he did, and then resigned; apparently he had told McFadyean to keep out of his office.

In 1894 Powys twice wrote to ladies applying for admission as students, saying that the regulations of the College did not admit them to the course of instruction. This was somewhat disingenuous, as the regulations did not categorically exclude them.

A Students' Union was formed at the College in 1891, described in the first issue of *The Student* in November as 'the year in which we suddenly woke up to the necessity of protecting our own interests'. By the following month, the name of the periodical had been changed to *The Students' Record* because it had been found that 'there are several "Students" now in circulation at the different medical schools'. The committee had grandiose plans for the new organisation. The existing football, swimming, boxing and musical clubs were made sections of the students' union, and it was envisaged that 'new sections will inevitably arise from year to year, such as dramatic, debating, athletic, cycling, shooting, terpsichorean and research clubs'.

The sports and athletics clubs continued to flourish, but interest in the other activities dwindled over the years, so much so that in February 1921 the *Veterinary Record* reported that a provisional council had been formed at the College 'with the object of forming a Students' Union'. The report of the first meeting promised that every effort would be made 'to promote the social welfare of the students by the provision of organised recreation, apart from the athletic clubs already established, concerts, dances, lectures and debates on general subjects being included within its scope'.

It was this 'new' organisation which laid the foundations for the students' union which has come to play such a vital part in the life of the College. An Association of Veterinary Students (AVS) from all the British schools was formed in 1942, and held its first conference at Streatley the following year. Students from the College now (in 1990) participate fully in the AVS, in the International Veterinary Students' Association, and have formed close links with the veterinary school in the University of Munich.

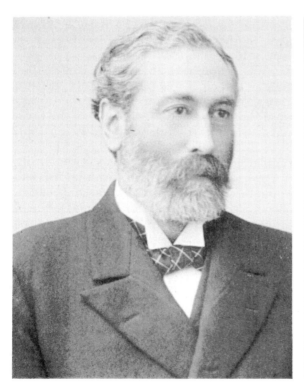 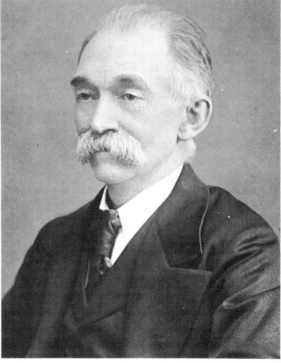

LEFT: William Hunting, who founded the *Veterinary Record* in 1888 and edited it until 1907. (RCVS) RIGHT: George Thomas Brown.

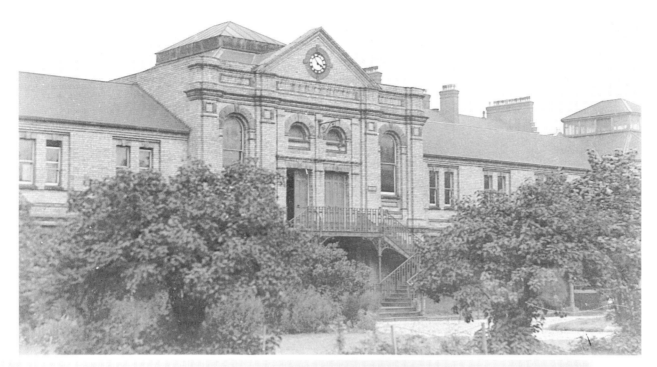

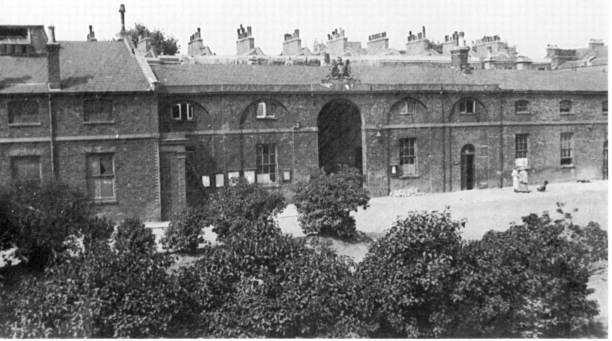

ABOVE: The lecture theatre and 'new buildings' of 1890 seen across the College quadrangle. BELOW: Inner side of the quadrangle of the old College, looking towards the entrance arch which, with the bays on either side, was obviously part of the original building.

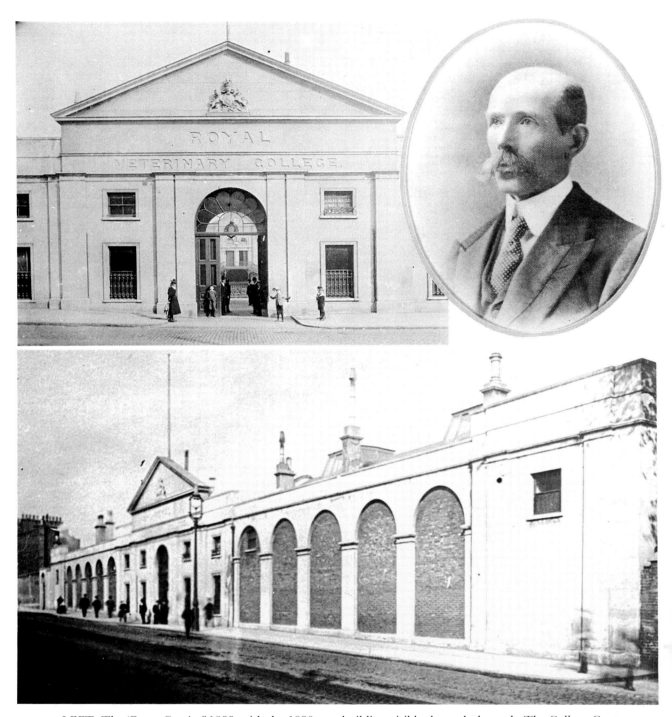

LEFT: The 'Front Gate' of 1895, with the 1890 new building visible through the arch. The College Coat of Arms above the entrance is now at Boltons Park. RIGHT: Sir John McFadyean. BELOW: The College facade in the early 1900s, showing the road surfaced with granite blocks, inlaid with tramlines. The Principal's private gate is on the right.

116

PART III

A New Era of Scientific Progress

JOHN MCFADYEAN

Principal 1894-1927

Looking back over the first 100 years of the College one can see how the course of veterinary medicine was shaped by the momentous changes — social, economic and scientific — that characterised the 19th century.

When the College was founded, the horse was of supreme importance for both civil and military purposes. It was the need to improve veterinary care in the army that persuaded Parliament to grant-aid the College so that it could produce more qualified men, who in 1796 became known as veterinary surgeons. The East India Company, too, was in urgent need of advice. It was critically short of cavalry horses following Cornwallis's second war against Mysore in 1791-2 and was unable to import the right sort of stallions from England, because the Napoleonic wars were making enormous demands on a dwindling supply.

The civil requirements for horse-power were also expanding. The Industrial Revolution was gaining momentum; products and people had to be transported on the canals and turnpikes and, until steam could be harnessed, the horse was the prime mover. Infectious equine diseases were commonplace and lameness, much of which was due to poor standards of shoeing, was a cause of suffering for the horse and loss for his master. The needs and opportunities were there for the veterinary profession to improve matters.

At the time of the census in 1801 the population of England and Wales was 8.8 million. Fifty years later it was 17.9 million. Not only had it doubled but there had been a shift in its distribution. By 1851 over half the people living in the big towns had moved there from the country and they had to be fed. The new railways could bring produce from the country and the ports, but there was no refrigeration for perishables such as meat and milk. To a large extent that problem was solved by keeping the cows in buildings in towns. There they provided a ready supply of fresh milk and, when they went dry, they became a source of meat. The town dairies were not self-sustaining as they depended on a supply of freshly-calved cows, sent up from the country. They were also hotbeds of disease.

For many years there had been no importation of cattle into Britain, but in 1839 the founding of the Anti-Corn Law League marked the renewal of the drive for free trade. But free trade in animals meant free trade in animal diseases and in September of that year an unusual disease was reported among the cows in dairies close to London: it was foot-and-mouth disease. In 1842 the 'new disease', contagious bovine pleuropneumonia, appeared and in 1847 sheep pox broke out near Windsor. But the worst was yet to come — rinderpest in 1865. Imported, contagious diseases of cattle and sheep were a new challenge to the profession, but there were few veterinarians with any experience or knowledge of them. James Beart Simonds had been appointed professor of cattle pathology at the College when the Royal Agricultural Society sponsored the post in 1842. It was he who went on a tour of Europe in 1857 to determine the risk of Britain importing rinderpest and it was he who became the chief veterinary adviser to the government on the epidemic diseases.

117

It was a difficult time for a veterinary adviser. The political climate was firmly resistant to any controls on the legitimate importation and movement of livestock, and there was by no means full agreement on what caused epidemics. Simonds, for instance, believed that, although foot-and-mouth disease and pleuropneumonia were diseases that could be spread by contagion, they arose, in the first place in the 'epizootic form', by which term he implied spontaneous generation. These were the days before Pasteur and Koch provided the experimental evidence that micro-organisms were the specific cause of infectious disease.

In 1876 Koch demonstrated that anthrax was caused by a bacterium which he was able to isolate from cases of the disease and grow in the laboratory. Pasteur confirmed the finding and went on to isolate the organism causing fowl cholera. Thereafter, 'new discoveries were being announced like corn popping in the pan' and many of the discoveries related to animal disease. The new science of bacteriology was a triumph for the Germans and the French and the crowning achievement was the isolation of the tuberculosis bacillus by Koch in 1882. The first bacteriological laboratory in Britain was at King's College London, founded by Edgar Crookshank, who studied under Koch in Berlin. The London veterinary students had lectures from Crookshank.

The importance of the new science was recognised by the Royal Agricultural Society of England when, once again, they funded the appointment of a professor at the College. This time it was for the chair of pathology and bacteriology, for which they made an annual grant of £500. In 1891 the governors confirmed the appointment of Professor John McFadyean from Edinburgh. He took up office the following year and became Principal in 1894. A new era of scientific veterinary research had begun.

In 1890 there were rumours of problems at the Royal Veterinary College. At the opening of the session Sir Frederick Fitzwygram, the chairman, commented that the educational standards, as in other veterinary schools, appeared to be falling, as evidenced by the rising number of students failing the examinations of the Royal College, and an increasing rejection of unsuitable candidates for army commissions.

The problems facing the College were considered at a meeting on 9 December 1891. Professor Crookshank spoke of the advantages of a resident dean and Fitzwygram proposed that a chair of pathology and bacteriology should be instituted, to be supported by a grant of £500 from the Royal Agricultural Society. At first, despite his son Andrew's unsupported and probably erroneous statement that the chair was founded for John McFadyean himself, it seems the College was uncertain how to fill it.

John McFadyean was awarded the Royal College diploma at the 'Dick' School in April 1876 and had by 1891 gained a wide reputation, both as an anatomy lecturer in Edinburgh, and as the author of *The Anatomy of the Horse*, and other publications.

The College decided to write to McFadyean to discover under what terms he would accept both the chair and the deanship. The salary proposed by McFadyean was £800, but the College offered £600; this McFadyean declined, so the original £800 was agreed.

The Edinburgh school gave its farewell presentation to McFadyean on 2 May 1892, and he delivered the inaugural address to the College later that year on 5 October.

While the general view is that McFadyean was the natural and inevitable successor to Brown, when the latter decided to resign from the principalship in 1894, there were alternatives who were considered by some as equally if not more worthy of consideration. Two particularly mentioned were J. Wortley Axe and J. A. W. Dollar.

Axe began his career as a pharmaceutical chemist, but became a College student and joined the teaching staff in 1869. In 1893, after a brush with McFadyean, he resigned the professorship of medicine and built up a large consulting practice. He was active in Royal Agricultural Society affairs. At College he had been a good teacher, and made many studies of medicine, surgery and pathology. He was a noted surgeon, one of his specialisations being equine vesical lithotomy, operating with perfect sang-froid, unhurried and deliberate. He is permanently remembered for discovering *T. axei*, a non-pathogenic strongyle of the horse. He traced anthrax to imported hides and wool, and its distribution in the neighbourhood of manufacturing towns through the carting of waste with town refuse and its ultimate employment on the land. In the famous Hendon scarlatina outbreak, he clearly traced the disease to the water employed in washing milk utensils, thus exonerating the cow of suspicion. He wrote and spoke often on veterinary matters, but his best-known work is *The Horse*, in nine volumes, the manuscript of which was just completed when he fell terminally ill. The final volumes were edited by Harold Leeney MRCVS, who wrote a graceful obituary in the *Veterinary Record* after Axe's death in 1909. Axe was active on the council of the Royal College, and president in 1889-1890.

The early career of John A. W. Dollar, son of T. A. Dollar MRCVS suggested to some observers that he was being groomed for eventual principalship of the College. John Archibald Watt Dollar (1866-1947) was born in Lewisham. After leaving school he worked for a time in his father's practice, keeping the books and helping in the dispensary. He entered the College in 1884 as student assistant in chemistry, and qualified in 1887 as a member of the Royal College.

Dollar attended Crookshank's pioneering bacteriology course at King's College. In 1889 he visited Lyons, where his brother, W. W. Dollar, was trained, and in 1892-1893 he attended classes at the Berlin Veterinary College and in Koch's laboratory in Berlin. In the winter vacation he toured Lower Germany, Austria, Hungary and Czechoslovakia. In 1893 he attended courses in Alfort and at the Pasteur Institute, and again travelled extensively in Europe. In 1894 he went to the international congress of hygiene and demography in Budapest. For some unrecorded reason, Dollar did not offer himself as a candidate, but supported McFadyean's appointment to the chair. On the matter of the transfer of McFadyean from Edinburgh, Dollar claims to have recommended McFadyean personally to Fitzwygram. J. A. W. Dollar recalled that 'My deeply loved principal, Professor Robertson, died at his desk in Camden Town early in the summer session of 1887. At the opening of the College next autumn not a word was mentioned of the man who had given his life for the College. His successor's career was not long, its principal feature appeared to be extravagance. Very soon the College was virtually bankrupt . . . The governors met, the successor resigned, a new Atlas had to be sought. None of the "old gang" were to be thought of. Sir Frederick Fitzwygram, who as an "externe" student about 1849 or 1850 had known my father and never relinquished the friendship, came to consult my father and obtain his advice. By bad luck, my father was out. Sir Frederick, who knew that I had been a student at Great College Street, and was acquainted with affairs behind the scenes, mentioned the governors' dilemma and actually asked me whom I thought the most likely man. I unhesitatingly said McFadyean. I had already a knowledge of his genius as an anatomist, his interest as a student, working for the Edinburgh MB between his own lectures and demonstrations, his courage in defending his students against unjust action by the Colossus (Fleming) of those days — and I was strongly drawn to him. "But", said Fitzwygram, "he has a very dangerous temper" (this was the reputation given forth by Fleming). I explained the situation to Sir Frederick and he departed *more suo*, whistling all out of tune and inscrutable. The next thing I knew was when Professor McFadyean arrived at our house, 56 New Bond Street, to announce he was to meet the governors of the RVC the following day over the question of his appointment. The position was anxious, as I assured him, the College nearly bankrupt, its resources nil, the "old gang" bitterly hostile, and the College's reputation with the public at a very low ebb. Even its own students were against its policy. Professor McFadyean came, saw, and was accepted. What he has done is plain to all.'

Dollar was over 70 years old when this was published. It is not clear whether he is referring to McFadyean's appointment as dean or to his later appointment as Principal. The 'successor' (G. T. Brown) did not resign when McFadyean was appointed dean, and it was Brown himself who recommended McFadyean for the principalship two years later.

What was McFadyean like as a man? He has been described as relatively tall and spare, with broad and slightly-rounded shoulders. He walked with an easy stride, his fair-haired head carried at a slight tilt backwards. McFadyean was probably the last professor to wear the traditional top hat (eventually discarded in favour of a bowler) and he maintained his aplomb even when a piece of thrown flesh struck his hat when he unexpectedly entered the dissecting room.

Most observers of McFadyean have noted his air of austere dignity and extreme reserve. Few students spoke to him in a personal way, looking on him sometimes with veneration, always with respect and often with awe. To be interviewed by him was something of an ordeal. There was a certain lack of geniality, reinforced by his air of always being absorbed in some problem.

McFadyean did have some relaxations, leaving the College at 7.30 am for a daily ride in the park. Consternation reigned one morning, for he broke his left arm when he fell off his horse in Park Street, but with his arm in splints and sling he continued his lectures on glanders. Many who knew McFadyean commented on the twinkle in his eyes. There is a general report that he laughed little (once only at *Charley's Aunt*) and seldom smiled, but he is said to have chuckled occasionally in his lectures.

It has been said that McFadyean's greatest service to the veterinary profession was as a teacher. He taught undergraduate and postgraduate courses, used his journal to educate the profession, and his influence was felt far beyond the confines of this country. He was generally held to be outstanding as a lecturer to undergraduates. He seemed to have an instinct for the right word. McFadyean lectured on four days each week. He spoke in concise, lucid phrases at dictation speed, and students prized their notes as informal textbooks long after they had qualified. Many lectures were appropriately illustrated by fresh or preserved specimens brought into his class on trays. Clifford Formston found him a brilliant teacher — articulate, deliberate and painstaking. It has been claimed that he would resume a lecture exactly where he left off last time, even in the middle of a sentence. There was no fooling about in his classes, although the dissecting room was inevitably the site of unruly behaviour at times. It is hard to imagine how he contrived to cope with the work involved in his courses, and he did not get an assistant to help with demonstrations and practical classes until 1903.

McFadyean realised that, if the College was aiming to improve the standard of training, there would have to be much tighter entrance requirements. He fought a suggestion by the Royal College that the College should accept applicants who had not passed all parts of the College Preceptors (or equivalent) entrance examination at one sitting. He strongly promoted the idea that students should spend some months seeing practice before they took their final examination (it had of course been the custom for some prospective students to spend time with practitioners before they came to College). The first written Royal College examinations were held in 1892, and the four-year course was introduced in 1895. The winter session ran from October to Christmas, and the spring session from January to the end of March. The summer session, from 1 May, was thought by some members of the profession to be a mistake, as it deprived the students of some of the time they might have spent in agricultural practice.

McFadyean also realised that, if veterinary research was to progress, and specialist posts at home and abroad were to be adequately filled, there was a need for a postgraduate course in veterinary pathology and bacteriology. He initiated this course in 1904, and ran it even during the First World War — it was advertised, for example, in the 1917 Royal College register. The

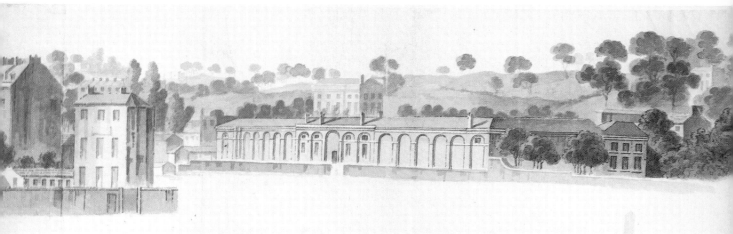

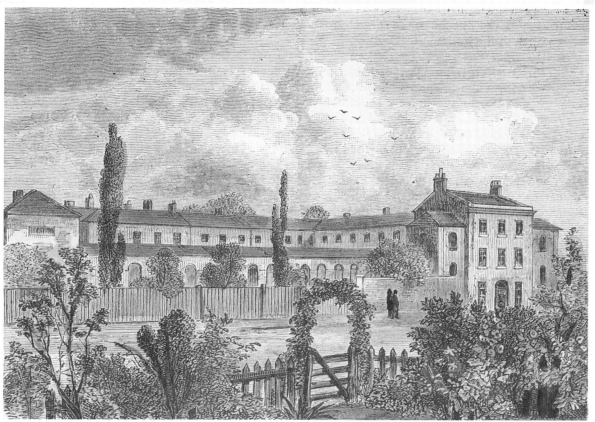

ABOVE: Water colour of the College, 1805. (GLRO) BELOW:
Hand-coloured drawing of the College, 1825.

classes were of two months' duration and were conducted at first once, then twice, yearly. The course was under the supervision of the Principal, and was specially directed to the requirements of officers of the army veterinary service, colonial veterinary surgeons, veterinary inspectors under the Contagious Diseases of Animals Acts, and candidates for the fellowship diploma of the Royal College. Some idea of the extraordinarily wide scope of the course, considering the limited time available, is given in lecture notes recorded by P. Offord in 1910.

The introduction of a special degree — BSc (VetSci) — offered by the University of London, was also supervised by McFadyean, who became chairman of the relevant board of studies in veterinary science in 1906. The course covered preclinical and paraclinical subjects, classes being given by members of College staff who became recognised teachers, supplemented by teachers in other schools of the university. This degree died with the institution of the BVetMed degree, and undergraduate teaching is now supplemented by students who choose to take an intercalated BSc degree in such subjects as anatomy and physiology before embarking on the clinical part of the BVetMed course. A degree of specialisation in the College course was much later to be provided by the system of electives introduced into the clinical years.

In addition to more or less formal courses, McFadyean also trained research workers who were employed in, or attached to, his laboratory. Being essentially a lone worker, he did not establish any extensively flourishing school of disciples.

The pathology laboratory was established in 1890 with the aid of a grant of £500 from the Royal Agricultural Society of England. It was placed under the charge of P. D. Coghill, who referred to it as 'the research institute' as early as 1891. When Coghill died in 1894, McFadyean said he could carry on with the help of a boy to do the rough work. Pathological specimens were accepted from veterinary surgeons and members of the Royal Agricultural Society, but most of the reports were perfunctory. Professor John Penberthy, who had been teaching pathology until McFadyean's arrival, helped with laboratory and field investigations. McFadyean carefully fostered the College/Royal Agricultural Society relationship. He was for several years a member of the society's influential veterinary committee, and he was appointed its consulting veterinary surgeon in 1905. After McFadyean's retirement in 1927 the society elected him a life governor.

It was in the pathology laboratory that most of McFadyean's work was done — the Research Institute in Animal Pathology was only opened in 1925, two years before McFadyean's retirement. The old laboratory has been described by A. E. Mundy, McFadyean's later laboratory technician.

McFadyean interviewed Mundy in December 1920 for the post of laboratory assistant. The Principal called him Jack, which became his name thereafter. McFadyean asked him to show that he could light a fire, and told him his working hours would be 6.30am to 6.00pm, six days a week (and if required for photographic work, on Sunday mornings) for 6s 6d weekly. The research institute was then a building with two large rooms on the ground floor and three smaller ones above. One of the ground floor rooms was for the reception of pathological specimens and for washing glassware; the second contained McFadyean's office, a photographic bench, a microscope bench, a dark-room, and the dispatch area for tuberculin, mallein and vaccines. There were some 2,000 bottled pathological specimens on shelves. Two ancient microscopes served the whole department, along with a freezing microtome and about a dozen Petri dishes. The animal room was in a loft over stables, up a steep staircase. The duties of the animal unit were carried out by one man, George Radbon, who was also post-mortem room attendant, and washer-up of laboratory glassware.

The general conditions were far removed from the hygienic laboratories of the present day, yet a strict routine enabled McFadyean to work with dangerous pathogens, and to produce a large number of papers of an extraordinary range, many of which appeared in his own *Journal of Comparative Pathology and Therapeutics*.

The complete list of his works is staggering, covering half a century of endeavour. McFadyean admittedly worked in an age when discoveries in the field of pathology and bacteriology were there for the asking, but the range of his interests — bacteria, viruses, parasites, neoplasia, morbid anatomy — was immense, and his contributions to knowledge are striking. Particular mention can be made of his work on tuberculosis — surely his greatest contribution — Johne's disease, anthrax, glanders and contagious abortion.

The famous occasion on which McFadyean publicly rebuked the great Koch for his view that human and bovine tuberculosis were distinct diseases, and that no special precautions need be taken against the ingestion of tuberculous milk, has been dealt with in detail by Pattison.

This historically important tuberculosis episode occurred at the International Tuberculosis Congress in 1901. McFadyean's special knowledge of tuberculosis was recognised by an invitation to present one of the only three papers to be given in plenary session — by Koch, on combating tuberculosis, by Brouardel, Dean of the Faculty of Medicine, Paris, on public health aspects of the disease, and by McFadyean on the danger to man of tuberculous milk from cows. At that time 30% of cattle in Britain were tuberculous, and 2% of these were excreting tubercle bacilli in their milk. Koch asked rhetorically if the most rational methods were being used to combat tuberculosis? He thought not. Too much importance was attached to the hazard for man of contact with tuberculous animals. 'Human tuberculosis differs from bovine and cannot be transmitted to cattle.' He would 'estimate the extent of human infection by the milk and flesh of tubercular cattle, and butter made from their milk, as hardly greater than hereditary transmission, and I therefore do not deem it advisable to take any measures against it.' Two days later, McFadyean said 'The greatest living authority on tuberculosis — the world renowned discoverer of the tubercle bacillus, and the man to whom we are mainly indebted for our knowledge of the cause of tuberculosis — has declared his conviction that human and bovine tuberculosis are practically distinct diseases . . . I am overwhelmed to find myself in a position which compels me to offer some criticism on the pronouncement of one the latchet of whose shoes I am not worthy to unloose . . . The almost entire absence of any law dealing with tuberculous udder disease is a scandal and a reproach to civilisation'.

Pattison comments 'Experiments to test Koch's statement were initiated in many countries. In Britain, a Royal Commission, with McFadyean a member, was set up to determine whether tuberculosis in animals was the same disease as in man, and whether it was communicable from man to animals and from animals to man . . . over the next 10 years, with McFadyean always deeply involved, classic experiments were carried out which amply vindicated McFadyean's views'.

This work, and his services on related commissions and committees, fully warranted the award of a knighthood to McFadyean in 1905. It is difficult to understand his failure to be elected a fellow of the Royal Society, although it is possible that he had offended some of the fellows by his outspokenness. It is ironic that McFadyean is now chiefly remembered by present-day students as the discoverer of the 'McFadyean reaction' of anthrax blood films — a property of which he was not in any case the first observer — and by the McFadyean prize.

While he was Principal, the number of students coming into the College varied, but was often above 70. Numbers fell off considerably during the First World War, being as low as 11 in 1916, but there was a sharp recovery after the war — 111 entered in 1919. The system of funding meant that small student numbers brought lean times. An important supplement to College funds was the sale of mallein and tuberculin — the sale of the former tending to increase in wartime. McFadyean decided to make mallein in 1892, in which year he and

Hunting first tested it (it was made by the method developed at the veterinary institute at Dorpat, Estonia, where tuberculin was first tested in cattle) and from 1893 mallein was provided free to veterinary practitioners in Britain. In 1901 a scheme was devised whereby half the profit from the sale of mallein and tuberculin was to go to McFadyean, and half to the College. In the first year the profit was £2,424 and in the second year £5,894. Reliance on these sales meant financially restricted times. In 1906, for example, a fall in mallein profits coincided with a reduced grant from the Royal Agricultural Society.

In 1921 the registration committee of the Royal College found that McFadyean had no case to answer against J. C. Coleman, who had accused him of unprofessional conduct regarding the provision of tuberculin and joint-ill vaccine direct to farmers. Coleman renewed the charge at a meeting of the Royal Counties division of the National Veterinary Medical Association (NVMA) on 22 July 1921. McFadyean sued him for slander, but the jury said the occasion was privileged. The general secretary of the NVMA, J. B. Buxton (later to succeed Hobday as College Principal) wrote expressing the association's strong disapproval of the method of distributing the vaccine, in reply to which McFadyean sent in his resignation from the association.

In his inaugural address at the opening of the winter session in 1896, Professor James (Jimmy) Macqueen set out the College curriculum — the four-year course was introduced in 1895, with written and oral examinations. 'The first year is given to junior anatomy, chemistry — theoretical and practical, botany and zoology. The second to senior anatomy and dissections, physiology and practical histology, stable management, and the principles of shoeing. The third to morbid anatomy, pathology and bacteriology, with demonstrations and practical work, therapeutics, *materia medica*, and practical pharmacy, toxicology, hygiene and dietetics. The fourth year is devoted to the principles and practice of veterinary medicine and surgery, meat inspection, obstetrics, shoeing, operations, clinical work, and examination of horses for soundness. To qualify for the Diploma a student . . . must give his attention to nearly 700 lectures, 200 demonstrations, and more than that number of clinical and tutorial classes . . . He must attend the treatment of 1,800 or more animals . . . at the Free Clinique, where 5,000 horses and dogs are treated each year . . . he must take an active interest in the examination as to soundness of from ten to eleven hundred horses of all classes . . .'

There can be no doubt that the actual fabric of the College steadily deteriorated during McFadyean's régime. He was adamant that any funds provided for research (which meant effectively in his own research department) must not be used for the general purposes of the College — this was his stated policy in 1910. He concentrated on developing the pathology department, and surplus funds which became available from time to time tended to find their way to that department. The Development Commissioners allocated to the College for educational purposes £800 (1909-10) £1,300 (1910-11) and £1,300 (1911-12).

The last major rebuilding had occurred in 1890-1891, but it was only towards the end of McFadyean's long reign as Principal, after the fabric of the College had suffered years of neglect, that a rebuilding fund was set up to finance a programme of improvements.

An idea of what the College looked like at that time is given in an anonymous typescript, presumably written by Professor James McCunn, which was found in his office after his death. In meticulous detail, the writer describes the old facade of the College, and continues: 'The main doors were opened at 8.00 am and closed at 5.30 pm. They gave access to a vaulted archway which led to the main quadrangle. In the archway a doorway on the right opened on to a passage leading to the grooms' kitchen. In the passageway was a bench on which bandages from strips torn from unbleached calico were rolled by students during the day, and by the nightwatchman at night ready for the next morning . . .

. . . 'On the northern side of the quadrangle, almost in the centre of the facade, was a large stable door, leading into six stalls furnished with beautiful "St Pancras ironwork" and paved with small narrow Staffordshire blue bricks, except for the passageway, which was paved with small greyish-yellow bricks. This was the main reception stable, generally occupied by horses awaiting examination for soundness. This stable was ventilated by the original system devised by Coleman.

. . . 'There were many open fires about the College — in the bone room, botanical class room, dissecting-room, students' cloakroom, grooms' kitchen, office and governors' room, pathological laboratory, in all the professors' offices, in the house surgeon's quarters, and in the two flats. Coal was always in plentiful supply.

'George Radbon kept the dissecting-room clean. He also had to look after the cattle and sheep, and the slaughterhouse, assist at post mortem examinations, clean the chemistry laboratory and McFadyean's pathological laboratory, attend to the boiler which heated the library, pathological classroom, central lecture theatre, museum and biology classroom. He looked after the small experimental animals and was on call to assist in the casting of large animals. There was no hot water to wash one's hands, even in the dissecting room.

'The middle quadrangle was surrounded by loose-boxes. All these had affixed to their walls brass shield-shaped plates, on which were the names of those veterinary surgeons who had contributed to the costs of repair and reconstruction of the boxes. These plates were polished daily.' [Most of them were retrieved by G. Pennington (clerk of the works) and Professor Formston when the boxes were demolished, and are now in the College library at Camden Town.]

. . . 'On the left-hand side of the archway leading to the middle quadrangle was a small-animal operating theatre constructed and furnished by Frederick Hobday in memory of his brother John, a veterinary student who died before qualifying. Beyond the entrance to the middle quadrangle a door opened into a loose-box used for examining horses' eyes.

'On the left, beyond this box, was the "bed" where large animals were cast and operations performed. It was in the centre of a yard surrounded by buildings and a relatively wide causeway . . .

. . . 'Overlooking the "bed" was the anatomy lecture room, called the "long classroom", which could seat about 100 students. Beyond the long classroom, in the north-west corner of the quadrangle, was another room, its long axis east/west, which was for many years the students' common room. When, for some unknown reason, they set fire to its furniture and contents, McFadyean reacted vigorously — the students lost their common room, and kennels for the experimental laboratory animals were erected in it' [this happened long before McCunn's time].

'The quadrangle which enclosed the "bed" had a massive glass roof supported on iron columns. At the northern end was a table at which small-animal patients were attended to between 9.00 am and 12.00 noon. Whilst waiting for attention the owners sat on a long three-tier stand which stood on a causeway on the east side of the quadrangle. Behind this was the Dollar equine operating table.

'The roadway from the tradesman's gate to the arch under the professor of anatomy's room had a gentle slope downwards until it reached the "bed". This slope was used for trotting horses being examined for lameness. The granite sets at the side of the "bed" were irregular — Professor Penberthy, with tender feet, had over the years learned where the smooth spots were. Except for Saturday morning, when third-year students were permitted to attend, the "bed" was the domain of final-year students. In their clinical work, the final-year students worked in pairs. Each pair had a number of loose-boxes and kennels allotted to them, and they were responsible to a professor for the application of the treatment prescribed and for keeping case records in a book inspected from time to time by the professor.

'Students had to interview owners, examine patients, make a diagnosis and propose a line of treatment. If treatment included an operation [actually only castrations and spayings] students went off and did the job, taking it in turns to act as surgeon and as anaesthetist, using their own instruments. The professor was always at hand in case of need. In the forge, students were taught how to remove shoes, prepare the foot, and nail on shoes. There were always cattle, sheep and pigs needing attention in the yard behind the central lecture theatre and museum. The accommodation for small animals was rather limited.'

The subscribers' clinic survived until the Second World War. In 1939 there were over 1,000 subscribers. They were received at the 'front gate' between 10.00 am and 4.00 pm. Two professors were in charge, taking duty on alternate days. Each professor was assisted by a house surgeon. Students were allocated to each professor for duty at the clinic and changed twice a term. They played a full part in the examination of patients, and made up prescribed medicines. They assisted in operations and acted as clinical clerks for animals admitted into the infirmary. A further group of six students did duty in the pharmacy. McCunn commented that the great feature of the educational system of those days was that students were not so burdened with the classroom and with the spoken word.

Many amenities did not exist — there was no hot water tap, no refectory, no common room, no central heating except in the new buildings, and as often as not that did not work. There were two wash-basins in a small alcove under the library. The hot water came from the heating system, but at some time or other a student had left the hot tap running, so McFadyean had the supply cut off. In winter, staff and students had to wear overcoats in order to keep warm.

The main quadrangle was laid out with flowers and ornamental bushes, and there were two grass lawns, with a large circular flower-bed in the centre, surrounded by a grass verge. The quadrangle resounded to the clatter of shoes and the cracking of whips as horses were trotted along the granite sets and examined for lameness.

Professor Formston recalls an incident which took place in one of the old buildings shortly after he joined the staff in 1928 as lecturer and demonstrator in 'animal management and the shoeing of horses'. Lectures were given in the chemistry lecture theatre which backed onto Great College Street. It had tiers of steeply rising seats, with middle and lateral gangways. 'Very early in my career as a teacher I was giving a lecture in this theatre when the strains of God Save the King were heard, ostensibly coming from a band of musicians in Great College Street. All the students stood to attention. When the band ceased the students resumed their seats amidst silent chuckles and knowing winks, all waiting for my reaction. I resumed my lecture, when once more the band played an encore God Save the King. This diversion was repeated on three occasions. I knew where the band was situated, namely in the basement of the theatre and I also knew of the trap door through which they had gained access. During one of their renditions I sent a student to the forge for a hammer and nails and nailed down the door. There was no further disturbance. Eventually the "musicians" were released and a very dishevelled and grubby bunch of students emerged. Honours were even. It was all good fun. An original prank, but never repeated.'

McFadyean did not take part in the clinical work of the College, but he knew what was going on. He selected Hobday, Motton and Male as outstanding clinical assistants. Hobday was later to follow McFadyean as Principal of the College, and Motton and Male became successful general practitioners.

In April 1896 a pensions committee was set up — staff were to pay 10% of their salary into the pensions fund, and the College 5%.

The staff in McFadyean's time included George Druce Lander (1874-1939), who succeeded Bayne as professor of chemistry and toxicology in 1903. Lander's *Veterinary Toxicology* appeared in 1912. The following year he was appointed consulting chemist to the Jockey

Club; he also became consulting chemist to the Royal Calcutta Turf Club and the Royal West Indies Turf Club. During the First World War he was a technical adviser on a government committee on the production of explosives. He resigned his College post in 1921 and retired to Kent, and in 1923 he was examiner in chemistry for the Royal College.

James Thomas Edwards (1889-1952) entered the College in 1907. he qualified in 1911, obtaining his BSc in 1912, and his DSc in 1926. After a brief spell of practice in Llanelly, he became junior research assistant to McFadyean. He held a three-year research scholarship (spent partly at the Pasteur Institute in Paris, and partly at Alfort). He joined the Royal Army Veterinary Corps in 1914 and was called back to the College in 1916 as research assistant, demonstrator in pathology, and lecturer in veterinary protozoology. In 1920, when the hitherto basic subject of stable management burgeoned into veterinary hygiene and was accorded a chair, he was made first professor of veterinary hygiene. In 1921 Edwards went to the Imperial Veterinary Bacteriological Laboratory in Muktesar, India. His main and outstanding contribution to veterinary science was the attenuation of the rinderpest virus by passage in rabbits and goats.

E. Brayley Reynolds was born in 1879, one of 11 children in a long-established veterinary family in Daventry. He served as a trooper in the South African War and qualified from the College in July 1912, aged 33. He was commissioned in the Royal Army Veterinary Corps and served in France and Mesopotamia, commanded the military veterinary hospital in Baghdad, and was awarded the OBE. After the First World War he was professor of *materia medica* and head of the outpatients' clinic at the College until 30 September 1922. He was held to be an inspiring teacher and an experienced logical scientist. He left the College for Newmarket practice and became a renowned equine consultant. He served as examiner in surgery for the Royal College and was awarded the Dalrymple-Champneys Prize. He died in 1967, in his 89th year.

Edward Simpson (Teddy) Shave (1857-1949) was born at Springfield, near Chelmsford, where his father was in veterinary practice. Shave was at the College under Simonds, qualifying in April 1879, having won the Coleman Bronze Medal and the Fitzwygram prize. (He became FRCVS in October 1890.) In 1879 he was appointed assistant demonstrator of anatomy and, after being promoted to lecturer and demonstrator, he was given the title of professor in 1886. This was a part-time appointment, as some professors were permitted to leave the College at 2.00 pm unless emergency duty required their presence. Shave went into veterinary practice as a young partner, specialising in Fleming's operation for the relief of 'roaring', and in neurectomy. In 1888, in addition to anatomy, he lectured on histology and morbid anatomy, at the same time giving private coaching classes.

In July 1894 professors were told they must relinquish outside activities, so Shave gave up his coaching classes and his practice. He enrolled as a medical student at the Middlesex Hospital and in 1899, aged 42, he qualified MRCS, LRCP. Principal Robertson had encouraged Shave in this venture, whereas McFadyean did not know of his medical training until Shave's plate was up in Camden Town. In practice as a doctor, Shave apparently excelled in midwifery. He continued to teach anatomy at the College until 1920, when he was told his post would be full-time at £600 per annum, so he resigned from 30 September. In the same year, he was appointed a Royal College examiner in anatomy, serving until 1942. It was he who examined the author in anatomy in 1937, informing him, in passing, that the volume of the contents of a cow's rumen could be usefully described as 'a wheelbarrowfull'.

Shave was noted for his wit and repartee. He was always in charge when lecturing, never lost his temper, and never reported anyone to the Principal. He had to sit in on a zoologist's lectures to preserve order. That unfortunate man (presumably Lowne) had once taken his class to Golders Green, and mounted a small straw stack as a rostrum, to which the students then set fire.

Shave left for his medical practice after his morning veterinary lecture, but was back in the dissecting-room by two o'clock. In class, he often used the nearest student's finger as a pointer, but curiously, for an anatomist, never used the blackboard.

Professor Share-Jones recalled spending many hours of happy association with Shave and Macqueen in the little common room behind the long classroom, the converted hayloft. In Shave's department there were about 60 students spread over the first and second years, yet he had only one demonstrator and two porter assistants (one in the bone room, one in the dissecting room.) Henry Power took classes in physiology, and his son D'Arcy ('Sunny Jim'), in histology. In Share-Jones's view, Shave's period of tenure at the College was probably its peak period for horse practice.

John Share-Jones (1877-1950) qualified at the College in 1900, becoming tutor in surgery and later demonstrator in anatomy. In 1904 he was appointed lecturer in anatomy at the newly-founded veterinary school in Liverpool University. He served on the Martin committee on the reconstruction of the College. The Royal College received £1,000 from his estate to establish a Share-Jones Lectureship, and since 1959 a biennial lecture has been given, usually at the College, on a subject associated with veterinary anatomy.

James Macqueen (1853-1936) professor of surgery, was allegedly inspired to become a veterinarian by seeing Clement Stephenson in Newcastle, in uniform as a veterinary officer in the Yeomanry. He took the Royal College diploma at Glasgow in 1877 and stayed on at Glasgow with Professor McCall for nearly 12 years as house surgeon and later as lecturer on anatomy, *materia medica* and surgery, obtaining his fellowship of the Royal College in 1886. In 1888 he was invited by Brown to teach junior anatomy at the College. He lectured on many subjects (botany, histology, hygiene, surgery, pathology of farm animals) before occupying the chair of surgery in 1895. He was a pioneer of equine abdominal surgery. He held that neurectomy was the last resort of a baffled veterinary surgeon and was not an operation to be proud of, merely ensuring a quick sale of a lame horse. It is interesting, in view of Macqueen's long service to the College, that in 1891 he said no teacher was fit to teach for more than 10 years, as enthusiasm for teaching was apt to die out within that time.

Macqueen was much in demand as an expert witness. He had many years' association with the Jockey Club, the Shire Horse Society, the Royal Agricultural Society and the Hackney Horse Society. He was examiner for the Royal College fellowship diploma for 36 years. He held many offices in the NVMA but had to retire from the presidency owing to ill-health. He assisted in the foundation of the Victoria Veterinary Benevolent Fund (now the Veterinary Benevolent Fund) in 1892. In 1915 the Royal College awarded him the John Henry Steel Medal, and in 1927 he received the Victory Medal of the Central Veterinary Society.

McCunn (a member of a sept of the Macqueens) wrote that for many years Macqueen reigned as the Socrates of the English-speaking veterinary world. Slow and deliberate in speech (except, it seems, in class) his language was virile and his sarcasm could cut to the bone. He was a teacher unsurpassed. In his inaugural address in October 1886, Macqueen said that few men who had not been teachers ever made satisfactory examiners. Encyclopaedic knowledge had no market. A bankrupt veterinary surgeon was a rare sight. 'You will meet with men whose word is as good as their bond. Prefer the bond, it is safer.'

A. W. Stableforth graduated in March 1923 and became demonstrator of pathology under McFadyean. From 1926-1933 he worked with F. C. Minett and S. J. Edwards on mastitis in the research institute in animal pathology. He then took charge of the division of preventive medicine, before going in 1939 to the Central Veterinary Laboratory, Weybridge, becoming director there in 1950.

In 1908 kindly and avuncular Professor John Penberthy resigned from the chair of medicine. Penberthy is recorded as brimming over with good humour. It is said, teasingly, that all his treatments of cattle ailments were the same — one pound of magnesium sulphate. He was a humane man — 'If we are not humane, we are nothing'. He died in May 1927 aged 69, and was succeeded by H. A. Woodruff. G. H. Wooldridge, coming from his post in the Royal Veterinary College of Ireland, succeeded Woodruff in the chair of *materia medica* and hygiene.

McFadyean is reported as saying at a meeting in October 1907, that 'probably at no time in its history had the College stood so much in need of benefaction'. The College 'could do very well with about £10,000 to satisfy its most pressing needs and requirements.' No such windfall was forthcoming but, on a more modest scale, 13 loose-boxes were entirely renovated, at a cost of £540, through the generosity of individuals and groups of veterinary surgeons, some of whom dedicated boxes to the memory of dead colleagues. A former benefactor, Stephen S. Ralli, agreed to contribute £270 towards the cost (£320) of a new range of dog kennels, and to help equip 'an up to date dog infirmary'.

Harold Addison Woodruff BSc Melb MRCS MRCVS died on 1 May 1966 in Edinburgh, at the age of 88. He qualified at the College in 1898, becoming a tutor in surgery. The following year he was appointed professor of veterinary science at the Royal Agricultural College, Cirencester. In 1900 he returned to the College in London in the chair of hygiene and *materia medica*. From 1908 to 1912 he was professor of medicine, during which period he studied human medicine at University College Hospital, qualifying in 1912. He went to Australia the following year, to become professor of pathology and director of the veterinary institute at the University of Melbourne. He took his BSc in 1933, and from 1935 to 1945 held the chair of bacteriology.

McFadyean was elected to the council of the Royal College in 1893. He was third in the list with 686 votes, behind his father-in-law, Walley (who died of tuberculosis in 1894, possibly from infection picked up at a post-mortem examination) and W. J. Mulvey. McFadyean was president of the Royal College in 1906, 1907, 1908 and 1930. An interesting sidelight on his work for that body is given by Dr Fred Bullock, who was appointed registrar of the Royal College in 1907 and called on McFadyean soon afterwards.

He found him 'at 9 o'clock after breakfast in the cosy study at the south-eastern corner of the old quadrangle. The study led down by three steps to a small conservatory with the garden beyond, which included a tennis lawn, and the tall trees of which only two now (1937) remain. His study struck me as being the workshop of a very busy man, and I could not see how the desk could be used or even closed, every inch of it being covered with letters, papers and journals. They covered also two small tables and overflowed to the floor. He was sitting before the fire correcting a galley proof. He disembarrassed a chair for me, piling the papers on to another, and bade me be seated. I do not remember our conversation, but I knew that I had met a gentleman, who would understand the difficulties of a secretary coming new to a strange job. During the remaining period of his Presidency, which to my great satisfaction lasted until July 1909, I was a frequent visitor at 9 o'clock in the morning before going on to my office. Sometimes I found him in his laboratory, and I learned that he was frequently there at 7 o'clock in the morning. He would not keep me long waiting, and I found that I could take every problem to him and be sure of receiving wise and unbiased advice. In later years, the study overflowed into the conservatory and many a difficult report or memorandum has been argued out and polished up there.

'When the Council decided in 1907 to promote a Bill in Parliament to authorise payment by members of an annual fee, Sir John McFadyean was appointed Chairman of the Committee. That Bill aroused unexpected controversy with the Royal Agricultural Society and especially the Highland and Agricultural Society of Scotland, who interpreted one clause as giving new powers to the College [RCVS] to prosecute unregistered practitioners and as menacing the liberty of stock-owners to employ unqualified persons to attend to minor ailments in animals. It was a complete misunderstanding, but to answer their objections it was necessary to obtain opinions from eminent legal authorities, and in this very difficult and delicate business the Chairman's clear understanding of the position, his ability to express his point of view in the clearest possible manner, and his readiness to interrupt his own work to help me in the drafting of the voluminous correspondence which the controversy entailed, saved me much anxiety and placed me under a debt to him which can never be repaid . . . It was a most precious advantage to be able to consult one who knew the mind of the Council; for in those days Sir John McFadyean was already an acknowledged leader of the Council's policy.

'Later when he was President of the Organising Committee for the 1914 International Veterinary Congress and the preliminary work had been done by the Honorary Secretary, Sir Stewart Stockman, Sir John asked me to organise the necessary administrative work in preparation for the meetings . . . No one in this country knew better than he the veterinary organisations in different parts of the world . . . We succeeded in enrolling, in spite of the troubled conditions in Europe, a record number of members. But we were doomed to the bitterest disappointment. The Congress, planned with so much anxiety, had to be abandoned on the day after its opening owing to the outbreak of the Great War. Our Reception at the Natural History Museum was spoilt by the absence of many foreign delegates, some of our own members were already in uniform and one of Sir John's own sons was called up. Sir John had to meet this unprecedented situation and undertake the responsibility of closing the Congress. This difficult duty he performed with calm dignity but with a clear appreciation of the seriousness of the occurrence. He told me that it would be 16 years before a new congress could be organised. His forecast was uncannily exact, but the whole profession is proud and glad to remember that he was able in his 78th year to undertake the double duties of President of the College and President of the Congress in 1930.

'He retains in his semi-retirement the esteem of the whole profession and this symposium (*Festschrift*, 1937) is the spontaneous expression of the affection in which he is universally held.'

The word 'affection' in Dr Bullock's last paragraph comes as a surprise, but we English do seem to have a soft spot for the old. It is strange, too, that in 1949 his son-in-law, Dr J. T. Edwards, was to record that McFadyean in 1935, at the age of 82, had said to a grandson who had voiced a wish to enter on a veterinary career — 'You had better put that out of your mind at once: the veterinary profession has now sunk as low as it can ever sink'.

One further major development during McFadyean's regime was the building of the research institute in pathology in the Principal's garden, which effectively involved abandoning any idea of relocating the College.

The Advisory Committee on Research into Diseases of Animals was appointed by the Development Commission in November 1920, and it reported in 1922. Its terms of reference were 'To report on the facilities now available for the scientific study of the diseases of animals, to indicate what extension of those facilities is desirable in the immediate future in order to advance the study of disease whether in animals or man, and to advise as to the steps which should be taken to secure the aid of competent scientific workers in investigating diseases in animals'. The chairman of the committee was Lt Col Sir David Prain, and its members were Professor O. Charnock Bradley of the Royal (Dick) Veterinary school, Captain Walter Elliot MP, Sir Willam Leishman,McFadyean, Charles J. Martin (subsequently to chair the 1929 committee on the rebuilding of the College) and Frederick Braybrook Smith of Downing College, Cambridge (an agriculturalist with 18 years' service in South Africa.) The committee, which held 15 meetings, noted that the research institute in animal pathology at the College was the only independent institution in the United Kingdom wholly devoted to the investigation of animal disease to which the name research institute could be applied. The Principal gave his services voluntarily, and was helped by an assistant director and two junior research assistants. The professor of hygiene (J. T. Edwards) also devoted part of his time to research. Accommodation both for laboratory work and for experimental animals was provided at the expense of educational facilities and without any State assistance. The United Kingdom veterinary colleges received in 1920-21, in the aggregate, a State subsidy of £3,696 for research purposes; such a condition of affairs constituted a national disgrace. In the period 1911-1920, the four holders of development fund studentships had justified the expenditure on their training. There was a need to ensure recruitment of a cadre of research workers with reasonable prospects of tenure, pay, promotion and superannuation. One important immediate step would be to bring salaries and superannuation in the institute into line with scales at agricultural research institutes.

For financial reasons, it was not the time to set up a reasearch institute in comparative pathology, and it was probably premature to establish chairs of comparative pathology and comparative medicine. The research institute in animal pathology at the College should get new laboratories at the earliest practicable date, and its annual maintenance grant should be increased. Having set out the current four-year course, the committee noted that Williiam Bulloch, professor of bacteriology in the University of London, had said that veterinary students were better grounded in pathology than medical students.

Veterinary colleges should get increased government assistance, and it might be an advantage for them to be affiliated to universities. A proposal was made that a diseases of animals research committee (or board) be set up by the Development Commission, which would consist of seven to 10 members and be advisory and not executive.

The report was dated 15 February 1922. There were three statements of reservation: Sir Walter Fletcher thought two matters (new laboratories for the research institute, and research studentships) should be submitted to the proposed research committee before implementation; McFadyean opposed the proposed research committee. F. B. Smith thought no additional grants should be made to the research institute until the inquiry as to the adequacy of accommodation and situation of the existing veterinary colleges, recommended in the report, and with its scope extended to included suitability for research as well as education, had been made. He regretted the establishment of a chair of comparative pathology at Cambridge or some similar institution was not recommended . . . 'it seems to me that it would be very wrong to fail to utilize as far as possible the exceptional facilties already existing at Cambridge, or which with slight extensions could be provided there for veterinary research and comparative pathology. Owing to its situation in the midst of an agricultural district thickly populated with livestock, and its nearness to Newmarket, the greatest centre of light horse breeding and training in the world, and to the relations the School of Agriculture has established with farmers, Cambridge is well adapted for bringing investigators into touch with the livestock industry . . . During the past ten years a considerable area of land close to the town has been acquired by the University through the efforts of certain departments interested in experiments with animals, and well equipped with field laboratories, animal houses, paddocks and other conveniences for experimenting with horses, cattle, sheep and pigs, and any further land that might be required could be got nearby.'

He drew attention to the university's great schools of pure science, the medical school 'which has devoted much attention to the study of tuberculosis in animals as well as in man', the agricultural school 'which has specialised in the physiology of farm animals in the direction of both nutrition and reproduction', the institute of parasitology whose researches had already proved of great value in dealing with certain diseases of livestock in South Africa, the biochemical school, 'which has successfully attacked the group of ailments known as deficiency diseases', and institutes for the study of the principles of plant and animal breeding. The collaboration of the many distinguished workers already engaged in branches of science directly or indirectly relating to diseases of man or of animals would be of the greatest assistance to the profession. In addition the science schools turned out every year between 200-400 honours graduates. If opportunities were forthcoming many of these could undoubtedly be attracted to veterinary research, 'and probably at no other centre do better facilities exist for training investigators or creating the cadre of research workers advocated in the Report than at Cambridge. Nor would any place be more favourable for the fundamental research . . . upon which progress so much depends, or for bringing about the closer co-operation of pure scientists and members of the medical and veterinary professions, the desirability for which was referred to by several witnesses'.

Following up F. B. Smith's proposals, the College received a letter dated 3 April 1922 from F. C. Floud, secretary of the Ministry of Agriculture, which suggested that, before any other steps were taken on this report, the governors of the College should seriously consider the question of transferring the College and all its work (both teaching and research) to Cambridge, and relinquishing the buildings in Camden Town. The latter were ill-adapted for teaching and research, and had the disadvantages of a highly urban position. Smith's arguments were largely made with reference to research, but they applied almost equally to the teaching of veterinary science. The Ministry thought the training of veterinary students should be in close association with agriculture and the breeding of livestock. The Camden Town leasehold interest was presumably not inconsiderable. A site free of charge might be available near the school of agriculture in Cambridge, and the Ministry would be prepared to recommend the Treasury and the Development Commission to make a large grant in aid of the cost of new buildings and the transfer of the College thereto.

It seems the Ministry had not done enough to persuade McFadyean of the advantages of this offer. McFadyean was now an old man, and he did not take kindly to F. B. Smith's scheme. He wanted, and got, his new institute building, but in so doing he missed probably the greatest opportunity the College has had of escaping from the trammels of Camden Town.

To complete the sorry tale, on 21 June 1922 the College governors replied to the Minister of Agriculture: the governors were of the opinion that the difficulties in the way of removing the College to Cambridge were so great as to render such action almost impossible. Furthermore, they had come to the conclusion that the removal of the College would be seriously detrimental to its efficiency, and they were therefore unable to agree to the proposal. Students would not benefit by association with the school of agriculture, which could not give its own students necessary acquaintance with farm stock. Transfer to Cambridge would entail the loss of subscribers' income — subscribers did not pay their subscriptions with a view to the advancement of veterinary education, but to obtain advantages with regard to the treatment of diseased animals in London — and there was no prospect of a similar source of income in Cambridge. The Ministry might provide extra money, but nothing would compensate for the loss of practice, which could not be transferred to, or created in, Cambridge, where there would be conflict with local practitioners; Cambridge could not provide as many diseased animals in a month as London did in a day. It would of course be possible to close London and open Cambridge, but success was not assured.

The governors claimed (on unstated evidence) that the urban location of all the large veterinary schools of the world was the result of deliberate choice, to ensure adequate clinical material. The cost of living in London for veterinary students (of whom two-thirds were sons of veterinary surgeons or farmers) did not exceed £100 (including College fees) for each of the four years of study, but would amount to nearly twice that amount for the average undergraduate in Cambridge. The average income of veterinary practitioners was modest, and any enhanced prestige from a Cambridge qualification would not allow higher fees to be demanded. Again, the advantages the College derived from its situation in a city which was the chief centre of medical education and research, and from its connection with the University of London, far outweighed any that could be reasonably expected if it were transferred to Cambridge.

The end of the matter came in July 1923, when the *Veterinary Record* noted that the College had been granted £25,000 for the erection of a new research institute in animal pathology. The foundation stone was laid on 30 May 1924 by the president of the College, the Duke of Connaught, who presided at the opening of the institute on 14 July the following year. McFadyean was present as director, with A. L. Sheather as assistant director. Among the illustrious academic and scientific guests was the veterinarian-sculptor, Adrian Jones. The architect was H. G. P. Maule, later to design the new College in Camden Town. Lord Glanelly and Mr Roberts each gave £1,000 towards the cost of equipment, and Professor Crookshank, a vice-president of the College, presented his magnificent library of over 1,000 volumes and 400 reprints, pamphlets and journals. The institute as such closed in 1950, with the incorporation of the College into London University, and became the department of pathology. Its directors were McFadyean (1924-1927), Minett (1927-1939) and Bosworth (1939-1950).

McFadyean received many honours. He shared the first award of the Steel memorial gold medal with Sir Frederick Smith. (As the medal was meant to encourage young workers, this award to such well-established figures was subjected to some criticism.) He became Hon LlD of Aberdeen University in 1906, was made DVetMed (*hon. causa*) by the Budapest Veterinary Academy in 1925, and was elected (top of the poll) a foreign corresponding member of the French Academy of Medicine. In 1933 he was awarded the Weber-Parkes Prize by the Royal College of Physicians for his work on tuberculosis. After his resignation from the College, he became an honorary associate of the Royal College, and a life member of the Royal Agricultural Society. In 1933 he was elected a fellow of the Royal College, the first to be so honoured.

In 1926 students became involved in the General Strike, serving as drivers, looking after the 'railway horses', and even enrolling in the special constabulary. Their exploits are described in *A Veterinary Student's Experience of the General Strike* (*Veterinary History* New Series No 3, Summer 1983).

On 22 July 1927 the general purposes committee received McFadyean's resignation. He was sadly upset by the subsequent appointments of Tom Hare as professor of pathology and Minett as director of the research institute, as he thought his assistant Sheather had a rightful expectation of one or even both these posts. McFadyean was elected to the board of studies in veterinary science as 'another person', and he continued to serve on the general purposes committee of the College.

At a meeting of the general purposes committee in October 1927, McFadyean expressed doubts as to Hare's competence to teach pathology. A few months later McFadyean stopped the research institute from being used for teaching purposes. He was particularly upset because a number of his pathological specimens were destroyed by Hare; a question was even asked about this in the House of Commons by the Liberal MP, R. J. Russell. Hare said he had retained some specimens for teaching, but others had been discarded because they were dried up, or there was no space to store them. In a letter to Principal Hobday, Hare said McFadyean had neither handed over the pathology department to him, nor had he said that any of its contents might be of value to him in future. McFadyean clearly found it difficult to give up the trappings of power.

McFadyean died in February 1951 at the age of 87. A McFadyean memorial lecture was established in the College in 1963, the first lecturer being Sir Peter Medawar in May 1966. A McFadyean prize for students for excellence in pathology was instituted in 1971 as a result of a gift by his daughter, Mrs Constance Edwards.

In 1902 a letter was received from the conjoint examining board of the Royal Colleges of Physicians and Surgeons asking the College governors to nominate a representative to serve on the general as well as the executive committee of the scheme for cancer research. This was the genesis of the Imperial Cancer Research Fund. McFadyean was nominated. Since then, the College has had a nominee on the council of the fund and it also nominates a representative governor.

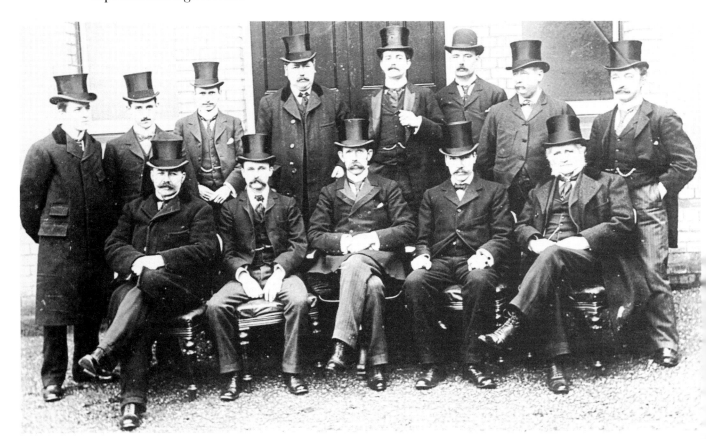

Teaching staff, 1895; back row (from left): H. Woodruff, J. B. Walker,
E. Percey, Professor Hobday, Wild, Powys, Professor Bottomley; seated:
Professors Penberthy, Shave, McFadyean, McQueen and Power.

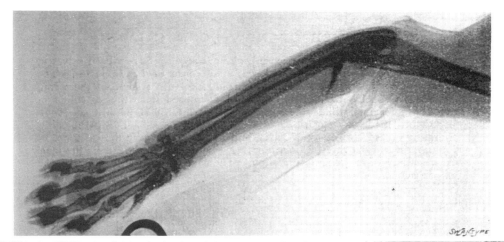

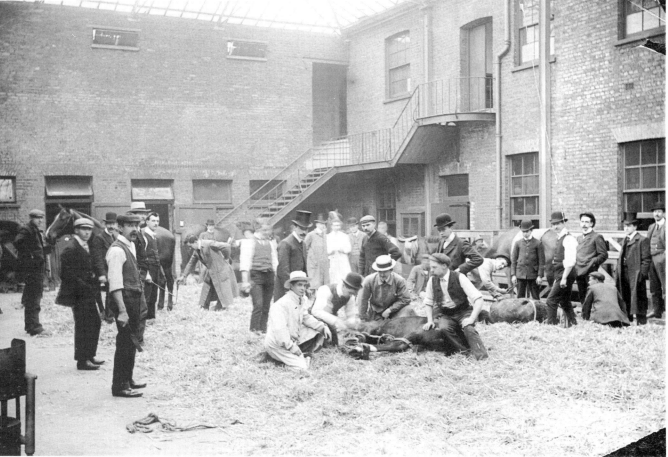

ABOVE: Believed to be the earliest diagnostic X-ray picture in veterinary literature, illustrating one of three cases described by Hobday in the 1896 *Journal of Comparative Pathology and Therapeutics*. To obtain this picture of a cat's leg, which reveals a foreign body (a piece of metal) in the soft tissue below the elbow joint, an exposure of 2½ minutes was necessary, the animal being immobilised with chloroform and hobbles. BELOW: The operating bed, about 1901. Note the use of 'X' hobbles, front to hind legs.

135

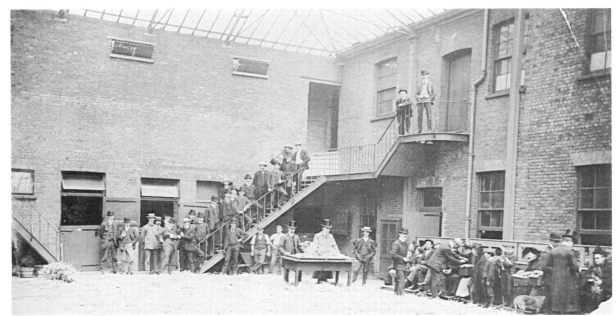

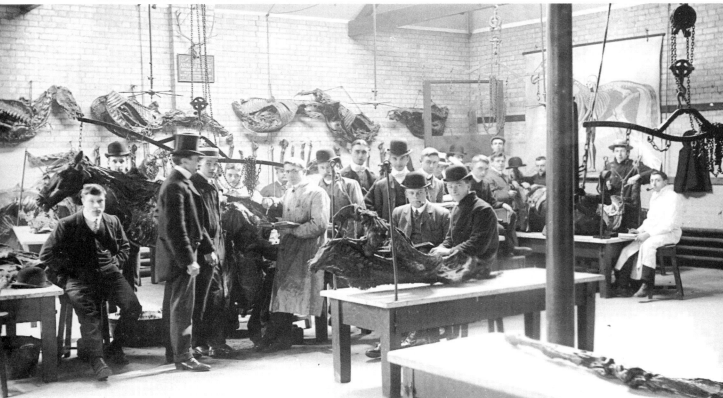

ABOVE: Outpatients queue up (on right) for treatment, about 1901.
BELOW: The bone room, 1901, with a member of staff identified by his
top hat.

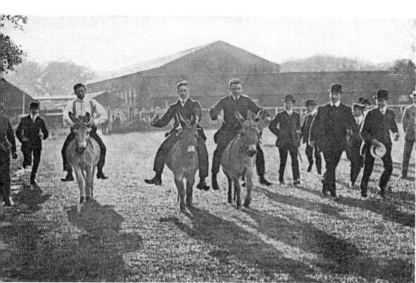

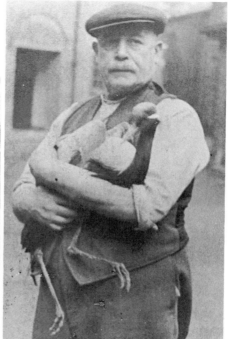

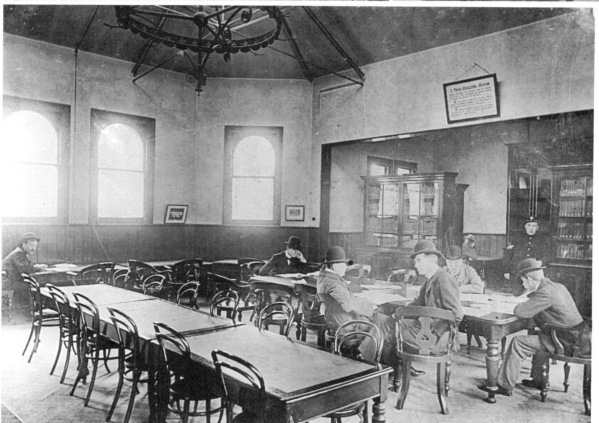

LEFT: Donkey race at the students' annual sports day, June 1906, held at Wembley Park. RIGHT: George Radbon. BELOW: The College library reading room, 1910.

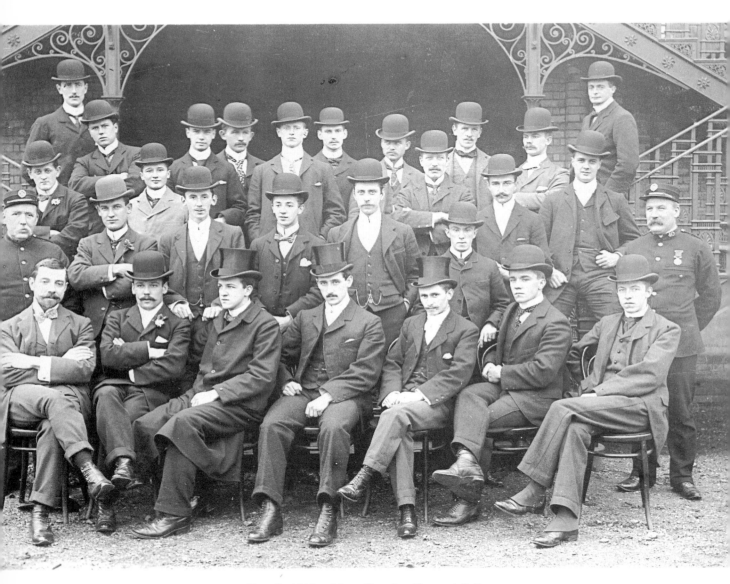

Class D, 1910, with staff and uniformed College servants.

FREDERICK GEORGE THOMAS HOBDAY

Principal 1927-1937

Only a few months after Hobday took over the reins from McFadyean, he was faced with a dire situation. Following years of deterioration, several of the buildings had become so seriously dilapidated that the College was served with a dangerous structure notice by the London County Council, and faced closure in 1928. The rebuilding fund set up by McFadyean had reached only £21,000. The future looked bleak, and the prospect of raising the huge sum needed to rebuild the College seemed almost hopeless. Fortunately, the new Principal was more than equal to the challenge.

Frederick George Thomas Hobday was born in 1870 at Burton-on-Trent, where his father was employed by Bass the brewers. He is known to have had a good career at his local grammar school, but little is recorded about his early days. It is said he was an enthusiastic cyclist, and that a fall from a penny-farthing cycle prevented him from attending what could have been for him a triumphant prize-giving day when he left school.

Although he was a great admirer of the local veterinary surgeon, Mr Wartnerby, who attended Bass's horses, Hobday confessed that it was a mere chance which directed his interest towards the veterinary profession, as he had long wanted to be a farmer. After he left school, his father took him to visit two veterinary practices, and it was arranged that Hobday should go for a probationary month with S. Hodgkins and Son of Hanley. He made a good impression and was soon indentured for three years' apprenticeship. He spent two years with his preceptor before going up to the College, working out the third year of his apprenticeship during College vacations. In later years, based on this experience, Hobday advocated a pupillage of at least six months in a veterinary practice before a student came to the College and, when this proved to be impracticable, he became a vigorous proponent of the six months compulsory 'seeing practice' before the final examination of the Royal College was taken.

For a time Hobday, who qualified on 18 May 1892, was house surgeon at the College. He left to act as a *locum tenens* or assistant in various practices, and spent a period with Arthur Blake in Redhill before returning to the College in 1893 as lecturer (junior professor) in *materia medica* and therapeutics. He also worked in the poor people's out-patient clinic, and lectured in animal hygiene and dietetics. During that period he became interested in developing the use of local anaesthetics and in chloroform as a general anaesthetic, and greatly extended his surgical skills. He soon developed his modification of Williams's plastic operation for 'roarer' horses — the 'Hobdaying operation' which, he claimed, he eventually performed over 4,000 times. Within 12 months he had two qualified veterinary assistants, and a senior student helped in the dispensary. He gained his fellowship of the Royal College by examination in 1897.

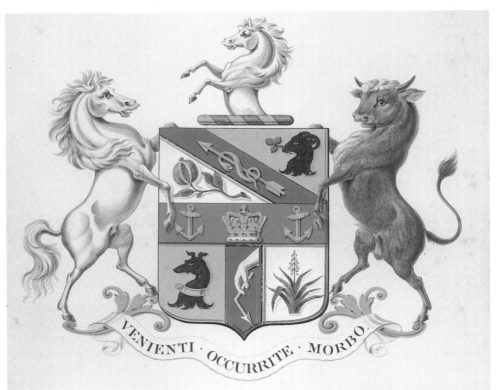

VENIENTI · OCCURRITE · MORBO

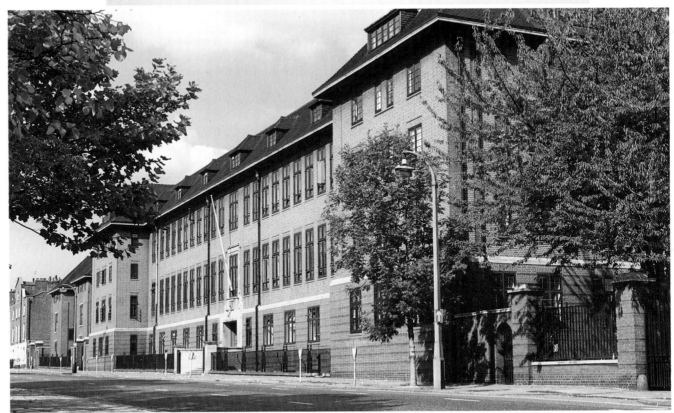

ABOVE: The College Coat of Arms. BELOW: The main College
building, Camden Town, 1988.

Hobday held his College posts for five years, but at the end of 1899 he found the financial rewards too meagre and, to the regret of McFadyean, he decided to go into practice in Church Street, Kensington, as a junior partner of Frank Ridler. On leaving the College he was presented with a handsome bronze timepiece and two tazzas (ornamental cups). H. A. Woodruff succeeded him at the College. Hobday now began to further his experience of horse practice. At that time there were horses everywhere — well-filled carriage stables of millionaires, commercial stables, horses for cabs, omnibuses, coal carts, dust carts, hearses, and so on. The practice had contracts with large stables, and undertook shoeing as well as advising on the purchase of horses and their general management.

At the outbreak of the First World War, Hobday, who was in the army reserve, was called up immediately by telegram and ordered to collaborate with the remount officer in the West End of London. The scale of use of horses in that war is impressive. In the first 12 days, 165,000 horses were imprest, and between 1914 and 1918, 450,000 horses were bought in the United Kingdom. Hobday was posted as veterinary officer to King Edward's Horse, a regiment of irregular cavalry billeted in the grounds of Alexandra Park, before being moved to Grove Park in Watford.

He went to France as surgical consultant to veterinary hospitals but, on receiving his majority, he was appointed to command No 22 veterinary hospital at Abbeville, the largest reception hospital for horses and mules on the Western Front, and given oversight of the farriery school. At this hospital, in the years 1915 and 1916, more than 120,000 sick and wounded animals were dealt with. Hobday noted that glanders was stamped out within two years of the start of the war. After the disaster of Caporetto, he was ordered to remove his hospital to Italy, entraining in December 1916 and settling down at a forward reception hospital in Cremona. For meritorious war service, Hobday was awarded the CMG; he was twice mentioned in despatches, and was appointed Officier du Merité Agricole in France, and Cavaliere dei SS Maurizzio e Lazarro in Italy.

After the war Hobday returned to Kensington, where he developed a small-animal consultative side to the practice. He continued as editor of the *Veterinary Journal*, a post he held from 1905 to his death in 1939. He also served as an examiner for the Royal College. He was elected to the council of the Royal College in 1910-14, and again from 1925 until his death. He served as vice-president in 1911.

Hobday was greatly attached to the idea of comparative medicine. With like-minded colleagues he was largely responsible for founding the comparative medicine section of the Royal Society of Medicine. Sir Clifford Allbutt was the first president of the section, and Hobday succeeded him in 1924 as the first veterinary president. He became an honorary fellow of the society.

Another initiative in which Hobday took pride concerned research on canine distemper. Supported by the Masters of Foxhounds Association, Sir Theodore Cook (editor of the *Field*) and Hobday made a public appeal in 1925 for funds for research into the disease. McFadyean was approached, but it was thought impossible to carry out the work in the conditions prevailing at the College. An approach was then made to Sir Walter Fletcher of the Medical Research Council. The breeding of the necessary disease-free dogs was carried out there by Buxton (later to succeed Hobday as Principal) and when he left for Cambridge the distemper vaccine was perfected by Laidlaw and Dunkin.

In the closing years of McFadyean's principalship, a building and development committee had been set up by the College, of which Hobday, still in practice, was a member, as he was of the College's general purposes committee. The rebuilding scheme that the building and development committee had in mind was at first modest. In 1927 the fund amounted to only £13,000. In that year Hobday was appointed (out of 10 applicants) Principal and dean in succession to McFadyean, and was given the specific task of raising sufficient funds to qualify for a government grant. The situation soon became desperate. In 1928, with the College threatened with imminent closure because of severe dilapidatoin, the building fund had only reached £21,000. Sir Archibald Weigall, treasurer of the College, said the time had come for a departmental committee to be set up to report on the whole future of the College.

On 30 July 1928 the Martin committee was appointed by the Minister of Agriculture and Fisheries, Walter Guiness, to 'consider and report generally on the reconstruction of the Royal Veterinary College and the probable cost; and in particular on the question what accommodation should be provided, having regard to the training to be given; whether that accommodation should be provided on the present site; if not, where the College should be transferred; and what arrangements should be made in respect of the Animal Pathology Research Institute now situated at the College, if it appears necessary to change the existing arrangements'. The members of the committee were Sir Charles Martin (chairman) Charnock Bradley (of the 'Dick' school), Merrik Burrell, Henry E. Dale, A. Weigall and H. Y. Sawyer. Of these Bradley, Fletcher and Martin were members of the Prain committee of 1920, whose report led to the building of the research institute in animal pathology and was followed by the College rejecting the Ministry's suggestion that the College move to Cambridge.

The Prain committee had held 15 meetings and heard evidence from 23 witnesses, while the Martin committee held 12 meetings, but took evidence from only seven witnesses; six from the College — including Clough, Hobday, McFadyean, Sir John Moore (a governor) and T. C. Wight (secretary of the College). No other members of the teaching staff appear to have been asked to give evidence, still less any students.

The Martin report quoted the Lovat report of November 1928 by the colonial veterinary services organization committee, which was appointed in 1927 and had visited the College at the invitation of the Principal (presumably McFadyean): 'We do not hesitate to say that we were dismayed with what we saw'. The Martin report goes on: 'Suffice it to say, therefore, that with the exception of one building which is of fairly recent date [the 1891 building] the College is in a state of dilapidation and the work is being carried on under conditions which are a national disgrace' (an echo of the Prain report) '. . . The end of the current year will find the College void of all resources . . . the pass to which affairs have been brought has not been due to any lack of enthusiasm on the part of those few members of the Governing Body who for many years have been sufficiently public-spirited to devote attention to the affairs of the College, or to the small staff . . . small salaries . . . wholly inadequate facilities . . . who continued loyally at their work . . . extraordinary that the College has been able . . . to turn out year by year a regular flow of qualified students. This apparent adequacy . . . obscured from public attention the gradual decay which was creeping over the College . . . the process of degeneration had set in years ago.'

In 1922 'the Ministry made a definite suggestion to the Governors for the transference of the College to Cambridge. For reasons which on consideration we are bound to say appear to us to have been adequate, the Governors could not see their way to accept the suggestion'. It was noted that the College had a considerable professional connection at Camden Town which provided material for teaching, and a substantial income from subscribers.

The Martin report next turned to a suggestion that the first year's study (of preclinical subjects) should be taken elsewhere before students entered the College. This was not thought a good idea and would produce little financial gain. It was felt that students should come directly into a veterinary environment, and that even if studying elsewhere, they would have little contact with other students because of the time-engrossing nature of the veterinary course. The committee proposed nine departments (at that time there were, in addition to the Principal, only three full-time and three part-time professors). The committee noted that the number of students in 1924-25 was 128, but in the 1929 session was 157 (including 17 women). The committee suggested an annual intake of 75, with total accommodation for 250 on a four-year course (assuming that only 80% would proceed beyond the first year).

Next came the vexed question of the location of the College. 'Unfortunately the feeling had arisen that the decision of the governing body not to transfer to Cambridge . . . was influenced to some extent by personal considerations and the desire to preserve the individuality and independence of the College . . . the conclusion to which we have come, has been arrived at solely from consideration of the interests of veterinary education . . . It is significant that the most successful veterinary colleges have been situated in the vicinity of cities . . . ample facilities should be available for the demonstration of actual sickness and disease . . . in veterinary science, through the clinic which must always be associated with the veterinary college . . . ready flow of sick animals . . . only be secured in a thickly-populated district . . . the city has advantages from the stand-point of accessibility to students, and more important still . . . makes possible the intermingling of teachers and students of various faculties and so obviates the dangers of intellectual isolation. A city veterinary clinic is largely composed of horses, dogs and cats . . . more than doubtful if (in country) large animals in any numbers would be forthcoming . . . practitioners would not look kindly on intrusion of such a serious competitor as a veterinary college clinic . . . treatment and principles of surgery are successfully taught with the smaller animals . . . relatively slight acquaintance with farm animals can be supplemented by residence with practising veterinary surgeons and farmers . . . we hardly think it necessary that the College should own a farm . . . the weight of evidence is in favour of an urban site . . . we have taken the opportunity of exploring the conditions under which the College might become a school of the University of London . . . a transfer to another city would be inimical to its best interests.'

The report then turned to the location of the College in London. The Camden Town site was admitted not to be an ideal one for an educational institution — in a congested district, with noisy traffic (those trams!) and an uninspiring outlook.

However, the site was readily accessible from most parts of London. It was close to the metropolitan cattle market in Islington (now long since closed). The clinic was able to secure an abundance of small animals and there was still an appreciable number of horses. The site was reasonably near the central university, University College and the London School of Hygiene. Finally, there was no other area of sufficient size available in the neighbourhood.

The matter of retaining the Camden Town site was settled when Major Maule, the architect of the research institute and the Beaumont animals hospital, decided that, with the purchase of additional land to the north of the College, he could accommodate 300 students on an admittedly limited site. According to Burrell, the only thing the College would lack would be 'the greater amenity, which nearly all the continental colleges possess, of gardens, trees and more spacious layouts'.

The die being cast, the old College was totally demolished by 1935. The new main building was declared open on 9 November 1937.

The Beaumont animals hospital, completed as the first part of the rebuilding programme, was the result of a favourable legal interpretation of the will of a wealthy Yorkshire lady, Mrs Sarah Martin Grove-Grady, daughter of J. Beaumont of Huddersfield. She had helped establish the first horse ambulance service in London. Her will was proved and made public in 1926. Substantial bequests to various animal charities included one of £10,000 to the RSPCA, which was refused by that society because the will stipulated that all members of council and headquarters staff must be, and must always have been, antivivisectionists: these bequests totalled £110,000. The residual estate of £200,000 was to be devoted to founding the antivivisectionist Beaumont Animals' Benevolent Society, which should purchase land to provide a refuge or refuges for all animals on such land at the time of purchase, or otherwise placed on the land, safe from maltreatment or destruction by man. A further clause in the will provided for 'founding, establishing, supporting, maintaining or providing of hospitals or homes for animals in Great Britain, having no declared vivisectionist upon the governing body or bodies thereof, or in any way connected with the management thereof'.

The will was disputed in July 1928. Mr Justice Romer, in the Chancery Division of the High Court of Justice, upheld the will, as in his opinion the trusts were valid and charitable. The matter went to appeal on 13 February 1929, before the Master of the Rolls and Lords Justices Laurence and Russell, who reversed the previous decision. Notice of appeal to the House of Lords was given, but was withdrawn because the Attorney-General, the next of kin, and the trustees of the will had agreed to a compromise whereby the next of kin offered to provide £25,000 under a scheme to be settled in the Chancery Division. The scheme was approved by Lord Justice Maugham on 24 November 1931; the money was to be handed over, under certain conditions, to the College governors for the purpose of erecting, as part of their building scheme, a hospital for the treatment of animals, to be known as the Beaumont animals hospital. It appears that the Grove-Grady legacy was allocated to the College largely due to the efforts of Lord Knutsford and the Research Defence Society. In the event, £18,,500 was spent in building and £1,500 on equipment, and £5,000 was invested to assist necessary maintenance. An illustrated account of the hospital is given by Hobday in the *Veterinary Journal* for 1934. The Beaumont animals hospital building was completed in 1933, the pathology museum block, designed to link the research institute with the new main building, also in 1933, and the 'canine hospital block' in 1934.

Hobday's task as fund-raiser for the rebuilding of the College was a truly daunting one. Whether it should ever have been imposed on him is a matter for consideration. The amount of government money involved in the rebuilding programme, even if the Ministry had agreed to pay the whole sum required was, in the context of national expenditure, small indeed. It is obvious now that, however minimal the outcome of the College's fund-raising effort, the government would have had no option but to pick up the final bill for reconstruction. Still, the task was set — raise £100,000 and the government will provide £150,000 — and Hobday got to work with a whole-heartedness and energy that soon brought the plight of the College to the attention of the traditionally animal-loving British people. Every rank of society, from the King (who, as Patron of the College, gave £100) to the humblest costermonger, contributed.

The greatest variety of means was used to tap public goodwill. Lord Harewood raised the problem in the House of Lords. Hobday made two successful radio broadcasts. An appeal for 250,000,000 farthings in the Giant Nosebag Fund caught the public's imagination. The Nosebag Fund was the idea of a journalist, Mr Devise, and the nosebag was presented by G. Villiers Parker of St Martin's Lane. It toured shows, circuses, hunts, and other events. Its padlock astounded those who saw it. Made by F. Byrne of the Worshipful Company of Farriers in his forge at Burton-on-Trent, it weighed 15 lbs and had two keys. Benefactors included Spratts and the Tailwaggers' Club, the Kennel Club, Spillers, *Horse and Hound* and Bumpus the booksellers. Private veterinary enterprise raised funds too — Herbert Buckingham, a small animal practitioner in Norwich, collected £500. Sir Edward Stern's £10,000 was the last major contribution. It is perhaps ironic that Richard Daubney, whose £5 donation was the final one received, had been in favour of moving the College to Cambridge.

The target of £100,000 was raised by 1932, and donations eventually reached £135,000. By 1931, when the fund stood at £39,000, the College had purchased the freehold of its site for £16,875.

Two major efforts by the students helped swell the fund and bring the College to public notice — the carnival, eloquently described by McCunn, and the College float in the 1931 Lord Mayor's Show.

McCunn noted that the carnival on Thursday 5 March 1931 was a great day in the history of the College. It was organised by two students, Raymond Holmes and his assistant Sam Pole, to raise money for the re-building of the out-patients' hospital and clinic. They were given a room next to the Principal's office to serve as their own office. Holmes excelled as an organiser and administrator and Sam was the ideal adjutant. For over three weeks they were never in a proper bed, snatching a few hours' repose on the floor. In the end they organised a procession which was 1½ miles long.

The first event of the day was judging the fancy dress costumes worn by students and others, in the College quadrangle at 9.30 am. The Metropolitan Police band led the procession, which assembled at 10.00 am in Prince of Wales Road — decorated private and trade carts, vans, motor vehicles, Messrs Hugon's oxcart, coaches, including Mill's midget coach, men on stilts, men on decorated cycles, mounted men dressed as cowboys, Red Indians, cavaliers, and a galaxy of students dressed as monkeys, cats, clowns, policemen, soldiers, sailors, and so on. The procession moved off at about 11.45 am down Adelaide Road to Finchley Road and Golders Green, to a halting place on the Great North Road. McCunn reports that 'the animals were superb; they ran along the pavement, they climbed the lamp-posts and sat on pillar-boxes delousing each other to the delight of admiring children who attached themselves to the procession'. 'Oscar' Ottaway, dressed as a monkey, chased girls, clambered up lamp-pots and trees and generally behaved in monkey-like fashion. A film was made for the College archives. Robert Barley provided mounts for marshals, of whom one was house surgeon Clifford Formston.

At lunch at 1.15 pm British Movietone News, Gaumont News and Paramount News took photographs and made recordings. The procession returned through East Finchley, Tufnell Park and Kentish Town, peacefully disintegrating as tired individuals made their way home.

McCunn noted that, as the day ended and the procession wended its way back to the College, the bands still played, but not with the precision of the morning; the refreshments at the marquee that had been set up in the Finchley Road had a soporific effect on the players.

The report ends with a flourish. Robert Barley's coach and four had a world-renowned whip and guard. They tarried at the marquee, and drove back to College at a smashing trot. They came down College Street like a fire engine, and the spectators' cheers stimulated the coachman and the horn blower to further efforts — even the horses seemed to be under the carnival influence. At full trot the coachman turned his horses at right angles into and through the College entrance, and then with post horn blowing and to the cheers of the students, they went round the College quadrangle. This was, says McCunn, a feat of driving he had never seen surpassed.

One of the bands started to play in the ring which had been set up on the 'bed'. The students sang and danced until they were exhausted. Holmes then took everybody off to a Camden Road hall where there was dancing until 4 o'clock in the morning. The College float in the Lord Mayor's Show was also a great success.

As to student/staff relations, Hobday made the claim that he relied on the discipline of honour and not of fear. It seems true that some of McFadyean's students did fear him — Professor Formston recalls seeing displayed on the board a notice signed by the secretary, T. C. Wight, warning that any student committing a misdemeanour would be sent down 'without compassion, hesitation or remorse' — whereas the students felt a great affection towards Hobday. He increased the number of students in the College (120 in 1928, 345 in 1936) and in particular encouraged the entry of women students who, although not overtly ineligible, were tacitly barred until near the end of McFadyean's rule. According to the College minute book, on 9 September 1927 — McFadyean's last month as Principal — it was decided that, as there was nothing in the regulations to deter women from entry, they would henceforth be freely admitted. This move was much debated in the profession, and was not universally approved. T. J. Bosworth, on 13 May 1929, wrote that he agreed women should be allowed into the profession, but he insisted they should not, as he put it, be inveigled in with specious promises of fame and fortune. Miss Aleen Cust, who on 20 December 1922 became the first woman to be admitted to membership of the Royal College, had spent a short revision period at Camden Town. She died on 29 January 1937 in Jamaica and left £29,915, donating £5,000 to the Royal College for a scholarship in research — women were to be preferred of candidates of equal merit.

The first major intake of women students was in 1928 (three in January and 12 in October) with one previous entry (Miss Greener) in October 1927 — the month in which Hobday became Principal of the College. The student entrance record shows that Averil Wynnifred Greener, aged 21, came from Class B, Liverpool Veterinary College (sic). In 1928, the three women entrants in January were Linda Gerda Gillies, aged 19, a Class C student from Glasgow; Gwendolen Muriel Heap (20), holding the Cambridge school certificate; and Jean Mary Forbes Kinnear (18), with the certificate of the Educational Institute of Scotland. Most of the 12 women entrants in October that year were 17 or 18-year-olds straight from school, although 25-year-old Beatrice Locke came with an external BSc(Agric) of London University.

A London graduate, Joan Joshua, first woman fellow of the Royal College, and first woman member of Royal College council, qualified at the College in 1938. She gained a high reputation in private practice and in the Liverpool school's veterinary clinic.

Olga Uvarov, first woman president of the Royal College, qualified at the College in 1934. Born in Russia, she came to England as a child when both her parents had been killed; she was adopted by her uncle, the noted entomologist Sir Boris Uvarov. After a period in mixed practice, she started a small animal practice in Surrey. Joining Glaxo laboratories in 1953, she became head of their veterinary advisory department, and in 1971 she was appointed technical information officer to the British Veterinary Association. She was a member of the veterinary products committee from 1971 to 1978, and of the medicines commission from 1978 to 1982.

She was elected a member of Royal College council in 1968, serving for 20 years. Made a fellow of the Royal College in 1973, she was elected president in 1976. In the same year she was awarded the degree of DSc(hc) by the University of Guelph in Canada. She was active in professional affairs in many capacities and received numerous well-deserved honours. Olga Urarov has been a fellow of the College since 1979. Appointed CBE in 1978, she became DBE in 1983.

Hobday increased the number of staff in the changes which followed McFadyean's retirement. C. Formston, G. B. Brook and J. W. H. Holmes were appointed house surgeons.

Geoffrey Bernard Brook qualified in Edinburgh in 1926, and transferred to the College in 1928. He made great contributions to the use of epidural anaesthesia in practice. His publication *Experimental and Clinical Studies of the Spine of the Dog* (1936) was a classic. Brook left the College in 1929 and went into practice with Robin Catmur in Abingdon, Berkshire. Eventually he had his own practice in Leamington Spa. He died in January 1988.

On 24 October 1927 Macqueen accepted the office of dean, and his appointment was continued beyond the age of 65, until Hobday became dean on 31 October 1928. Macqueen at that time asked unsuccessfully for financial assistance as he had no pension, and to help out he was allowed to give a course of lectures in the 1929 summer session for 25 guineas.

Great interest centred on the disposal of McFadyean's chair of pathology and his directorship of the research institute. McFadyean was strongly of the opinion that the post should be a combined one and that it should go to A. L. Sheather, but the College decided to make two separate appointments. On 2 September 1927 a selection committee recommended that Dr Tom Hare be appointed professor of pathology. Dr F. C. Minett was appointed director of the research institute. He also became professor of pathology after Hare's dismissal in August 1933.

Tom Hare (1895-1959) was the son of a Nottingham chemist. He was enrolled as a student at the Liverpool University veterinary school in 1912. His determination to be always well-groomed, almost dapper, was already in evidence. Later, as professor, he was invariably dressed in morning coat, striped trousers and spats, and modelled himself on Anthony Eden as regards hat and moustache. He served in the Cheshire Regiment throughout the First World War, reaching the rank of captain, and returned to Liverpool, qualifying MRCVS in July 1921 and MB, ChB in 1924. It is recorded that he was good at many sports and was chairman of the inter-university athletic board of Great Britain and Ireland. He was also active in student affairs. Academically, he held fellowships in pathology and surgery, and received his MD degree in 1926.

In March 1927 Hare was appointed research officer on foot-and-mouth disease by the Ministry of Agriculture at the Lister Institute in Chelsea. There had been nothing in his career to suggest he was in any way fitted to become professor of pathology in the College, but he was so appointed in September 1927. He was anathema to McFadyean, who told the College that Hare was not up to the job. One of the main complaints about Hare was that the pass list in pathology was unacceptably low. There is some indication that Hare was thought by the RCVS examiners Bosworth and Maitland not to be acceptable as a teacher. Fear of the pathology examination prevailed in the College while Bosworth and Maitland were examiners. Hare was given notice in 1933 and, on leaving the College, he set up veterinary research laboratories in the Finchley Road. He was joined by A. B. Orr (whose resignation as demonstrator in pathology was reported in 1937.

Another staff change was of future significance. A. R. Smythe, professor of *materia medica* from 1926-1929, left on 13 December because of his father's severe illness. J. G. Wright (one of two interviewed from among 12 candidates) was appointed to succeed him.

In the early 1930s, Mr and Mrs Courtauld each generously gave the College £10,000 to found the Courtauld chair of animal husbandry and, when the relevant government stock fell from 5% to 3½%, they each donated a further £2,500. William C. Miller, lecturer in genetics at Edinburgh University, was appointed to the Courtauld chair on 3 November 1934. He qualified as a veterinary surgeon from the 'Dick' school in 1919, became lecturer in zootechnics and animal management at the 'Dick', and in 1921 lecturer in hygiene and animal management at the East of Scotland Agricultural College. He occupied the chair until 1946, when he left the College and became director of the equine station of the Animal Health Trust in Newmarket. He died in December 1976.

Hobday's interest in animal welfare was shown by his service as treasurer of the Metropolitan Water Troughs Association, on the council of Our Dumb Friends' League, and on the council of 'Justice to Animals'. He was largely responsible for the birth of the Universities Federation for Animal Welfare, and was its president from 1927. He took a leading role in the endorsement of the Weinberg casting pen for the slaughter of cattle.

Hobday introduced radiography into the College. H. J. Ede FSR (1869-1948), who was appointed radiographer to the College when Hobday became Principal, suffered eye trouble due to X-ray damage in his later years, and developed a progressive paralysis agitans. His fingers were also affected, as with other early radiographers. He X-rayed racehorses for Mr Burton, an Epsom veterinary surgeon, and serviced Hobday's practice.

The Martin committee reported in 1929 and set out the conditions of affiliation as a school of the University of London: the College must be reasonably solvent; the professors and lecturers must be appointed by special boards of advisers; salaries must be not less than £1,000 (professors), £500 (readers) and £300 (recognised teachers); departments must be properly equipped for teaching and research; an academic board must be established, and consulted on all educational matters; and College accounts must be submitted to the court of the university.

Hobday had established an academic board in 1927; minutes of the board date from 3 October 1927 to 27 September 1938, after which there is a lapse of some years. At the first meeting it was agreed that students could attend the railway (LMS) stables to the east of the College, when lame horses were being examined.

In January 1928 the secretary and registrar of the Royal College, Dr Fred Bullock, agreed to lecture on jurisprudence. It was agreed on 1 May 1928 that Derby Day (on which day the King's official birthday was celebrated) should be observed as a College holiday (a tradition later reintroduced by Sir John Ritchie, and approved by the Queen Mother when she met students at the opening of Northumberland Hall). In the same year, the perennial problem of who should pay for laundering white coats was raised — the governors could not provide any money.

On 25 June 1931 the resignation of the witty biology teacher, 'Tryp' Evans MA of Guy's hospital (who succeeded Marett Tims MA MB in October 1915) was marked by the presentation of a silver cigarette lighter. On 2 October 1933 it was decreed that smoking should be allowed only in the quadrangle, dissecting room, post mortem room, common rooms and staff dining room.

The minutes of the meeting of the academic board of 10 June 1936 bear mute witness to an event which shook the College and the profession to their foundations. At that time Hobday was in the chair. Only 14 days later, J. B. Buxton was chairman, the governors having decided that Hobday was to be Principal and dean in name only, until the opening of the new buildings in 1937. Buxton would be acting Principal and dean, taking over the full title on Hobday's retirement. The *Veterinary Record* of 16 May 1936 wrote: 'We have received the following announcement officially approved for publication by the Board of Governors of the Royal Veterinary College: "The impending retirement of Sir Frederick Hobday through reaching the age limit is causing the Governors to be confronted with the all-important task of selecting a successor to Sir Frederick at a very critical time in the history of the veterinary profession. The new Principal will have to take over the new College buildings, which will be completed next year, and be responsible for their equipment and staffing. On his powers of organisation and of administration will turn to a very large extent the efficiency of the profession in future years. The Governors are seeking a new Charter from the Privy Council, under which will be formed a new Court of Governors and a new Council. This new governing body will have no easy initial task in making the appointment of a Principal. In order that the change over may be gradual, Sir Frederick will remain, it is understood, in office until the opening of the new buildings, but will go on leave as from October 1st next in order that his successor may be responsible for the organisation of the buildings which will be under his control in future. The Governors have felt that Sir Frederick Hobday's official connection with the College should not be terminated until the new buildings, for the erection of which he has worked so hard and successfully, were completed and formally opened. Large sums are still needed for their completion, equipment and endowment.'

This announcement had clearly caused its draftsman considerable difficulty. Members of the profession voiced their alarm and concern, but some of them misunderstood the position so much that they pleaded with Sir Frederick to reconsider his 'decision to resign'. Letters flowed in to the *Veterinary Record*, but something appears to have caused the journal to take a cautious line, for on 11 July the editorial committee said the correspondence would be closed, although the contents of letters would be referred to in leading articles from time to time.

The full story of the so-called retirement of Hobday remains untold. Professor Clifford Formston offers one explanation later in this chapter. It is, however, clear that Hobday was asked to relinquish the functions of his office, ostensibly on having reached the age limit. Hobday specifically claimed that the age limit did not apply to Principals of the College. A College minute of 2.9.1927 reads: '. . . with the exception of the Principal of the College, the retiring age of Officers of the College in the future, and this shall be retrospective, should be 65 with power to the Governors in exceptional circumstances to extend the period'. (Hobday might have called in aid the names of Coleman, Sewell, Simonds and McFadyean). Hobday clearly felt he had been treated in an extremely shabby fashion, and two governors resigned, while a third wrote a letter of protest.

Hobday felt his honour and honesty had been brought into question, which elicited a letter dated 28 September 1936 from Burrell, chairman of the board of governors, who wrote — 'The Governors have never made the slightest imputation against either your honesty or honour'. Hobday was to go on leave on full pay until he finally relinquished office at the opening of the new buildings.

A question about Hobday's retirement was asked in the House of Commons by Mr Richard Short, MP for Doncaster, but the Minister of Agriculture, W. S. Morrison, replied that age was the sole reason.

At a general purposes committee meeting on 2 November 1936 the chairman, Merrik Burrell, said he wished to bring to the notice of the committee certain recent correspondence which had passed between him and Sir Frederick Hobday on the subject of the latter's retirement. The correspondence having been read, the chairman stated that although Sir Frederick in his letter of 5 April had expressed himself as satisfied with the offer made to him by the governors in their minute of 30 March 1936, it was clear that he had changed his attitude. (It has been suggested that Hobday, who seemed at one point to have thought of letting the matter lie, was persuaded by certain well-wishers, in particular James McCunn, to resist). According to the committee minutes: 'He [the chairman] had, therefore, particularly in view of Sir Frederick's last letter, dated 26th October, 1936, thought it better to ask Sir Frederick to meet the Commitee today [Burrell, Danesbury, Gilbey, Brassey, Stanyforth, Watson, Gilmour plus Buxton] and make any statement he desired for the Governors' consideration. Sir Frederick Hobday was then introduced, and after making a statement to the Committee regarding the grounds on which he had been requested to resign, which he considered inadequate, said he was suffering both privately from his total severance from the College, to whose interests he was devoted, and publicly from the impression which had got abroad that there was some undisclosed reason for his retirement. He suggested that if the Governors would confer on him the title of Emeritus Professor it would go a long way to restore the past confidence of the General Public, as well as the members of the Profession, and to reduce the present feeling of grievance against the Governing Body. Sir Frederick was asked to draft a letter to the Chairman expressing his views of the status and implications of such a title. Sir Frederick then withdrew. His letter, dated 2nd November, 1936, having been shortly received and considered, the Chairman proposed, and Professor Watson seconded, and it was unanimously resolved, that the title of Emeritus Professor of Surgery be conferred on Sir Frederick Hobday on his retirement from the Chair of Surgery at the College. The

Secretary was instructed to send an announcement to that effect to the *Veterinary Record*, noting that, as far as the Governors were aware, this was the first occasion on which such a title had been conferred by a British Veterinary College.'

Some consolation was given to Hobday by the presentation to him of his portrait in oils by John Hassall RI, at the Connaught Rooms on 18 February 1937. The presentation was made by the Duke and Duchess of Portland — the Duke had been a senior governor of the College during Hobday's term of office. The portrait, now hanging in the College library in Camden Town, shows Hobday in court dress, as honorary veterinary surgeon to the King.

After his full retirement, Hobday became lecturer in comparative medicine in St George's Hospital. When he went to India in 1938 the scene at the railway station, when virtually the whole student body went to see him off, was an unprecedented demonstration of affection to a greatly-loved man. Before leaving, Hobday was presented with a silver model of the racehorse Solario by J. E. M. Ridge, president of the students' union. An appeal to endow scholarships in comparative medicine, open to medical and veterinary workers alike, was launched, and no doubt Hobday's dream of a chair of comparative medicine would have been realised had the Second World War not intervened.

In May 1939 Hobday went to Droitwich to stay with his old friend Arthur Blake MRCVS and to take the cure. He suffered a heart attack a few weeks later, and died on Saturday 24 June. At his funeral service at St Mary Abbott's church, Kensington, the King was represented by John Willett MVO, his honorary veterinary surgeon. Hobday had asked that instead of flowers, friends might send donations to the poor students' fund of the College. His wish was that his ashes should be scattered in Putney Vale Cemetery, near the graves of his brother, John and his old friends, Henry Gray and William Hunting.

Hobday's lecture notes (of which the College has examples) were kept in small black books, or even on the backs of old envelopes. At meetings, he often sat near the door — last in, early out. He was a friendly man and very clubbable, being a member of the City Livery Club and the Savage Club (of which Hassall was a fellow member).

In his will, Hobday left £11,676. Had he remained in practice, he would no doubt have become a rich man. In the matter of fund-raising, the College got the benefit, while Hobday's health paid the price.

Hobday earned many honours. He was an honorary fellow of the Hunterian Society, delivering the Hunterian Oration in 1938. He was honorary veterinary surgeon to Queen Alexandra, King George V, Edward VIII and George VI. He was honoured by veterinary and scientific organisations in India, Switzerland, America, Belgium, Italy, Norway and Sweden. His greatest honour came in 1933, when he was knighted for his work on behalf of the College.

Commenting on the events which led up to Hobday's 'retirement', Professor Formston writes: 'When I retired from the College in 1974 I had witnessed many changes under the guidance of six Principals. As a student in 1924 I entered an institution unbelievable in its state of dilapidation yet basking in the aura of its Principal, Sir John McFadyean. As I write, I have in front of me the College calendar of 1928. It bears the names of the governors of the day, along with other members of the British aristocracy who were vice-presidents or committee members, all presumably with the interests of the College at heart. How was it possible for the College to fall into such a deplorable state? In 1924 the teaching staff, some part-time, could be numbered on the digits of both hands and the student body, all male, was approximately 100. There was no student common-room, no cloakroom, no refectory — for a cup of tea or coffee one had to traipse to a café in Camden High Street — no hot water even in the dissecting room and little warmth outside the library. There was a single toilet and the only telephone was in the gateman's office. The gateman — janitor in today's language — eked out a living by selling College headed notepaper to the students.

'Great (now Royal) College Street reverberated with the clanking of tramcars and the clicking of horseshoes on tramlines and granite sets. A few hundred yards up the street the local refuse destructor belched forth black smoke and a dirty grey fine ash, which on a foggy day produced a yellow haze, later to be termed "smog". However, once through the portals of the College there was peace and tranquility enhanced by a relatively large quadrangle divided into two lawns bordered by lilac trees and flower beds. In the background was the "ride" and the centrepiece was a double iron stairway leading to a platform and the main lecture theatre, with the College clock set in its pediment. Despite the lack of amenities, following the pedantry of school the College spelled emancipation. We were masters of our own destiny. For me these were the happiest days of my life. We had a deal of affection for our teachers who were all affable, friendly and helpful; we regarded McFadyean with awe, almost reverence. We saw him daily crossing the quadrangle from his laboratory to his residence yet never did we see him stop to speak to anyone and no one approached him. He was a brilliant lecturer but outside the classroom he appeared aloof and remote.

'In contrast, Hobday was a wiry little man, effervescent, bounding with energy and always in a hurry. He brought change. The College became alive. Student numbers, including women, were increased; clinical facilities were improved by converting loose boxes into operating theatres; hot water became available and students were given common rooms and a refectory. Hobday's skill as an equine surgical specialist, in particular his ventriculectomy operation, brought an influx of horse patients. His reputation in small animal surgery further increased the numbers on the subscribers clinic. He introduced radiography which he had pioneered before the turn of the century, and demonstrated the use of film in teaching.

'Affectionately dubbed "Freddie" by the students, Hobday was undoubtedly the most popular Principal we ever had. He had the full support of the academic and lay staffs. "Communication", by letter or word of mouth, was an important word in his vocabulary. Like his predecessor he lectured — somewhat erractically maybe — to the students and one of his first acts was to give the staff a voice by creating an academic board. He helped to established a lay staff social club and in the new buidings provided a spacious clubroom. He also gave the club a full size billiard table. This he had bought in Italy and, having a problem in exporting it as such, had packed and consigned it to his home as an "operating" table. This was an era when the whole College was on one campus with complete harmony between academic, administrative and lay staffs. The dichotomy which has ensued from the outbreak of war in 1939, with the College on two sites, has marred this close relationship.

'The profession first learned of Hobday's "retirement" from an announcement in the *Veterinary Record* of 16 May 1936. He was to retire under the age limit as from 1 October 1936 and from this date until the opening of the new buildings in 1937 he would "go on leave". He was to be, for his last year, Principal in name only.

'The general public heard the news when it made headlines in the *Sunday Express* of 13 September 1936: "SIR FREDERICK HOBDAY MYSTIFIED. I HAVE BEEN TREATED LIKE A CRIMINAL".

'In an interview with the paper's representative, Hobday is reported as saying "the whole subject is a mystery to me. Until I received a letter from Sir Merrik Burrell asking me to resign, I was unaware of any trouble, neither had I any reason to anticipate anything of the kind. I have been shown no mercy at all. If I had been a criminal I could not have been treated worse. I have never had any complaints and I cannot understand why, as Principal of the College, I was not informed about any inquiry."

'The news broke the day before the official opening of the NVMA congress in Scarborough. I was there to assist my professor, J. G. Wright, in a series of demonstrations on small animal euthanasia and I well remember the consternation the news caused amongst the congress delegates. It became the main topic of conversation throughout the congress and was embarrassing to Hobday (who was due to demonstrate the cryptorchid operation) and all those with whom he came in contact. The news item clearly indicated that Hobday had been "sacked".

'There were those who thought Hobday — never one to shun publicity — had instigated the report, but in a subsequent letter to the *Veterinary Record* of 26 September he issued a disclaimer. In the same letter he expressed his bitterness at the action of the College governors. Two of them, Sir John Moore and Professor Lovatt Evans, resigned in protest. Hobday reiterated his feelings in his book *Fifty Years a Veterinary Surgeon* published a year before his death.

'It is more than likely that the newspaper report was prompted by a question in the House of Commons when the matter of Hobday's retirement was raised. There was further embarrassment for Hobday and his well-wishers when things did not go right with his cryptorchid demonstrations. The first patient was a two-year-old Shire colt, not previously operated upon. The right testicle was speedily retrieved but a prolonged search of "fully an hour" by Hobday and two other "cryptorchid surgeons" failed to find the other testicle. By this time surgical asepsis had gone by default and it came as no surprise when the colt died three days later from peritonitis. A post mortem examination proved the patient to be a "monorchid". The second case, a six-year-old Shire, was operated on with the usual Hobday acumen and skill.

'I must make it perfectly clear that I consider the governing body had no authority to dismiss Hobday — for dismissal it was — under the age limit, because Principals were exempt (McFadyean was 74 when he retired).

'A minute of the general purposes committee of 4 February 1935 reads: "The Chairman reported that the Finance Committee had met that forenoon, owing to the absence of Mr G. L. Martin, the Assistant Secretary, from duty, it had not been possible to prepare the usual financial statements for the information of the Committee. In the circumstances it had been left to the Secretary to get what assistance he thought necessary to bring this work up to date and for the Principal to pass the accounts for payment. The circumstances of Mr Martin's case having been explained, it was decided that he be given due notice to terminate his engagement at 31st March 1935 and that his salary be paid monthly in arrears until that date."

'A further minute from the quarterly meeting of the general purposes committee dated 30 July 1935 states: "A letter was read from the Secretary resigning his post. He was asked to withdraw from the meeting and on his return the Chairman informed him that his resignation had been accepted with regret, but owing to the difficulty of obtaining a successor during the holiday season, the Chairman expressed the hope that the Secretary would remain in office until the end of the year. The Secretary stated that he would try and arrange to carry on until then." T. C. Wight had been secretary for 22 years. He was a well-known breeder of Chows, and was perhaps more interested in them than in routine office work.

'George Martin, the assistant secretary, was a dapper, smartly dressed, suave individual. He was a master of copperplate writing and spoke French fluently. he had the assistance of a typist, Miss Plant, a lady prim and proper and undoubtedly efficient. Early in 1935 Martin went sick. In his absence his office was found in some disarray. The accounts were in a state of chaos, bills had not been passed for payment, the cash book had not been written up and no posting had been done in the ledgers for six months. There was evidence of "discreet" drinking. For one reason or another Martin had sought solace in alcohol. This was the state of affairs discovered by Miss M. Benton when appointed accountant in February 1935.

It became evident that the secretary, T. C. Wight, had not exercised the supervision normally expected of him. It was his duty to endorse all cheques. This had not been done. His resignation was inevitable, but the ultimate responsibility rested with Hobday, who paid the penalty. A little more time given to overseeing the administration of the old College and less effort towards building a new one might have saved the day.

'Hobday's last official appearance, at the opening of the new College buildings by King George VI, was a sad day for all of us. In the first Hobday memorial lecture I said of the occasion:

"At the opening ceremony the students were in good voice. They greeted Their Majesties with enthusiastic loyalty and decorum. That they should reserve their most vociferous demonstration of affection for their retiring Principal was surely understandable. The reception accorded the Chairman of the College's Board of Governors was one of unmistaken hostility — a little unseemly but perhaps in the circumstances, pardonable." The clarion call of the students still rings in my ears: "We want FREDDIE".'

The opening of the new College buildings by the King and Queen was described in the *Veterinary Record* of 13 November 1937. To quote from the account:

'A new era in the history of the Royal Veterinary College, London, and one so pregnant with possibilities of achievement as to be virtually unrelated to the past and its conditions, was triumphantly inaugurated on Tuesday last, November 9th, 1937, by His Majesty King George VI when, accompanied by Her Majesty Queen Elizabeth, he visited the College to open the magnificent new buildings, described below, erected on the site of the former College to the plans of Major H. P. G. Maule FRIBA.

'The great occasion was favoured with "royal" weather, and the citizens of North London seized avidly upon this latest most eagerly awaited opportunity to welcome Their Majesties. The route of approach in the neighbourhood of the College, in the reconstruction of which the people of St. Pancras have manifested much interest, satisfaction and pride, was lined with a cheering throng, the extra-mural recognition culminating in Great College Street, loyally beflagged, where the students acclaimed the arrival, first of the Duke of Gloucester, President, and other members of the Court of Governors, the Mayor and attendant civic dignitaries of the Metropolitan Borough of St. Pancras, and finally of the King and Queen, to whom they formed a guard of honour.' (This guard of honour, in which the author was included, was reasonably cheerful, but there was more than a rumbling of discontent when it became known that there was no room inside for any significant number of students. Principal Buxton had explained that the Main Hall was only big enough for representatives of official bodies, but members of the profession, alumni or not, had the opportunity of visiting the College on the afternoon before the official opening.)

Shortly after 11.00 am, the Mayor, Mayoress and Town Clerk of the borough arrived at the main entrance, where they were met by Sir Merrik Burrell (chairman of governors), Weigall (treasurer), Hobday (Principal — what was he thinking?), Buxton (acting Principal), and McLaren (bursar and secretary.) The same reception group, plus the Marquess of Crewe (HM Lieutenant of the County of London and senior vice-president of the College) and the Mayor, welcomed the Duke of Gloucester, who arrived at 11.20 am. Ten minutes later Their Majesties arrived, accompanied by the Minister of Agriculture and Fisheries (W. S. Morrison). Inside the building they were greeted by the Earl of Harewood, a vice-president of the College, and in the hall a bouquet of flowers was presented to the Queen by Burrell's granddaughter, the Hon Barbara North.

Their Majesties being seated on the dais, they were addressed by the chairman of council, Sir Merrik Burrell, as follows: 'These buildings replace old buildings erected in 1791 during the reign of King George III.' (This is a somewhat misleading statement, as over the years there had been quite a lot of new building, notably in 1891.)

Burrell continued: 'The College is fortunate in the possession of portraits of King George III and Queen Charlotte' (these had been donated by Burrell himself) 'and will be even more fortunate when it possesses the portrait for which your Majesty has so kindly undertaken to sit, and which is to be painted by Mr Philip de Laszlo, and most generously presented by him to the College in memory of Your Majesty's presence here today'. The two large portraits, of a remarkably insipid character, hang in the main hall. 'The College has had the honour of continuous Royal Patronage since 1830, and received its first Royal Charter in 1875; this was regranted in a revised form in 1936. HRH the Duke of Connaught was its President from 1904 to 1932, when HRH the Duke of Gloucester honoured us by succeeding him. Some 14 years ago, the old buildings had become so out of date, so inadequate, and so dilapidated, that it was resolved to demolish them completely and to rebuild on the same site, with additional adjoining land — the whole purchased from the Ecclesiastical Commissioners. The wisdom of the Governors' decision was confirmed by a Departmental Committee.' This is somewhat ambiguous, as it telescopes events in relation to the Martin Committee.

'The Governors have had a very hard task in trying to collect necessary funds, but with the assistance of a grant of £150,000 from the Government and with the help of many generous subscribers a sum of £285,000 has become available. A further sum of £40,000 is still needed to build the large animal hospital and operating theatre, so completing the building scheme, and to provide the full scientific equipment of the College.' This was the time for the College to acknowledge the supreme fund-raising effort that Hobday had made, yet his name was not mentioned.

The King then declared the new buildings open. Various people were presented to Their Majesties, including McFadyean, Hobday (named Principal), Buxton, J. Ridge (president, Students' Union Society) and Major Maule. The platform party then toured the College, with students as guides. To occupy the audience in the main hall, J. G. Wright delivered without notes a short address on the history of the College. He had tried this out on his colleague, Clifford Formston, on a number of occasions — Wright had a great facility for preparing 'impromptu' speeches. In the evening, the students held the first of the long series of commemoration balls.

The architect's comments on the new buildings include the following: 'The buildings may be classified under two heads. Firstly, the central teaching and administrative block, with which is incorporated the Research Institute in Animal Pathology built in 1924 at the extreme south-east corner of the site. This latter is now connected with the main building at the ground floor level by a wing containing the large pathological teaching museum, with animal quarters beneath at the lower ground floor level. Secondly, the buildings which comprise the various hospital quarters and operating theatres, etc., for the animal patients. These buildings, at present five in number, include the Beaumont Animals' Hospital, on the left-hand side of the main block facing Great College Street, which is a free clinic, corresponding to the out-patients' department of a general hospital.

'Immediately behind the Beaumont, and connected thereto by a subway, is the canine hospital and animal husbandry department. This building is a combination of a hospital and teaching department, which includes not only laboratories and a small museum, etc., but also, on the ground floor, quarters for agricultural stock used for teaching and demonstration purposes. Exercising yards for dogs, both covered and open, are a feature of this building, which is also so planned as to admit of the maximum amount of light and air both to itself and the adjoining buldings.'

Maule described some further buildings and, after referring to the plan to construct a large animals' hospital to the north of the site (never built): 'It may be of interest to note that the principle here adopted of grouping all the main teaching departments in one building differs widely from the continental practice, where, in many of the great veterinary colleges, the various departments are detached and self-contained units, necessitating a far larger area of land for their accommodation'.

The architect took particular pride in the mezzanine floors at the back of the building. These are in fact the greatest defect of the plan. It is nowhere possible for a trolley to be pushed round any one floor of the building without encountering stairs. The two courts at each side of the main hall are dead ground, and the location of the library, and the flats above, mean that the south side of the building effectively blocks easy circulation above the ground floor. The main entrance door is at the top of the steps, and the separation of the hospital from the teaching and administrative parts of the building virtually ensured that preclinical and clinical work would appear unrelated.

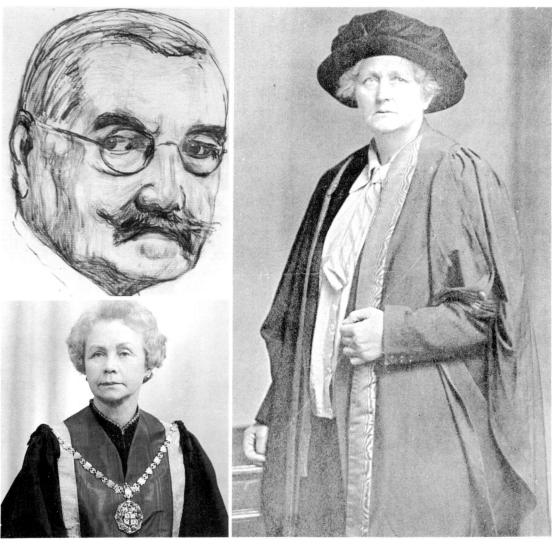

LEFT: Sir Frederick Hobday. RIGHT: Aleen Cust, who took a revision course at the College before qualifying as the first woman to hold the MRCVS diploma in 1922. BELOW: Dame Olga Uvarov, the first woman president of the Royal College of Veterinary Surgeons, qualified at the College in 1934.

155

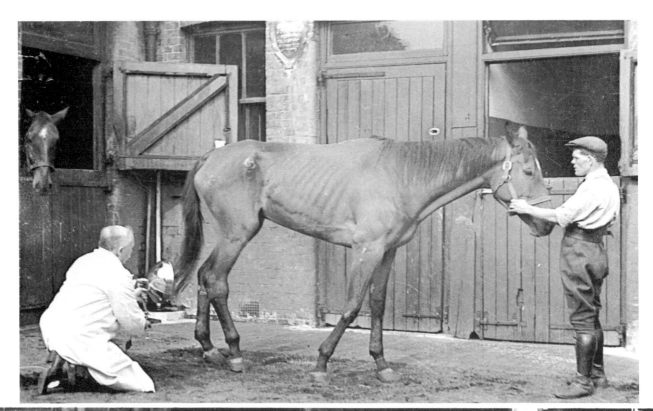

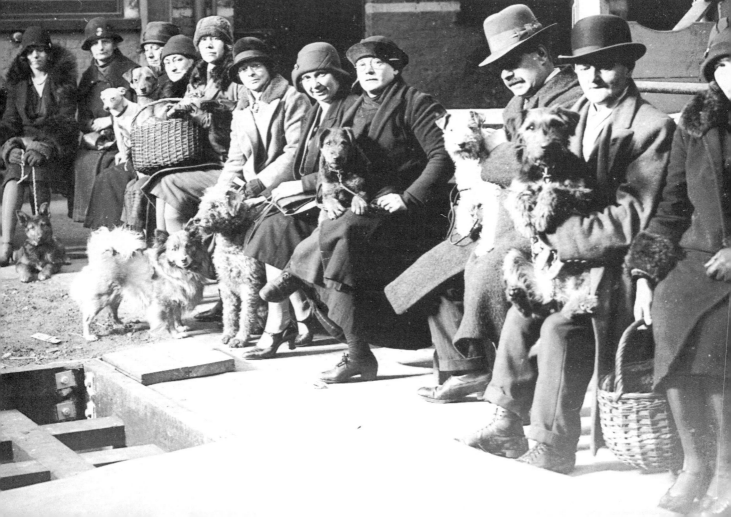

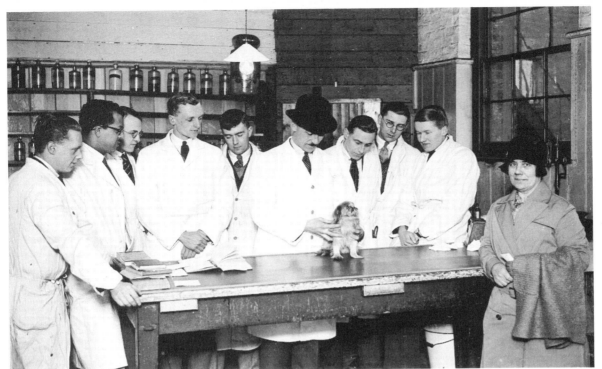

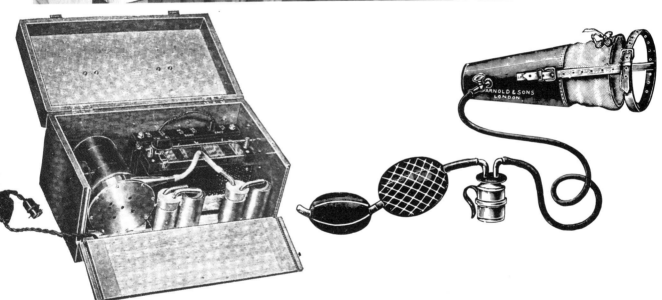

OPPOSITE ABOVE: Fred the groom and Mr Hitchings, applying ultra-violet ray treatment to a swollen hock on an emaciated patient. Note the polished shield on the wall. BELOW: Owners wait patiently for the Poor Patients' clinic in 1930. The hole in the ground was for installation of the new operating bed, which could be raised hydraulically at its four corners. ABOVE: Hobday examines a patient in the clinic, 1930. BELOW: Two of the many items of equipment designed by Hobday.

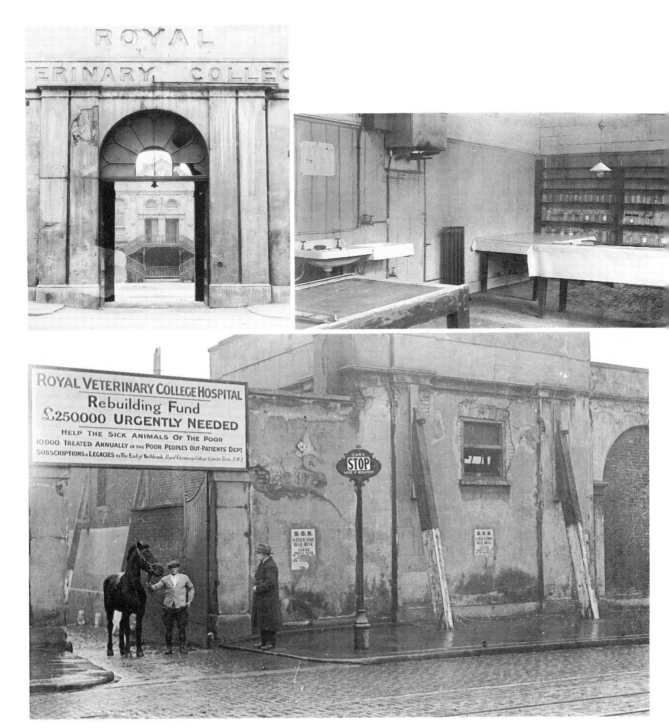

LEFT: The dilapidated front entrance to the College, about 1928.
RIGHT: Converted loose box in use as an operating theatre, 1929.
BELOW: The service gate at the north-west corner of the main block,
shored up, with peeling stucco and torn appeal posters.

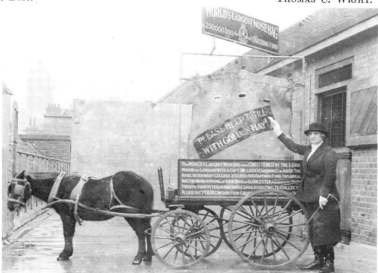

ABOVE: The College calendar, 1928 — a glittering roll-call of the aristocracy. BELOW: Appeal to fill the 'World's largest nosebag' with 250,000,000 farthings.

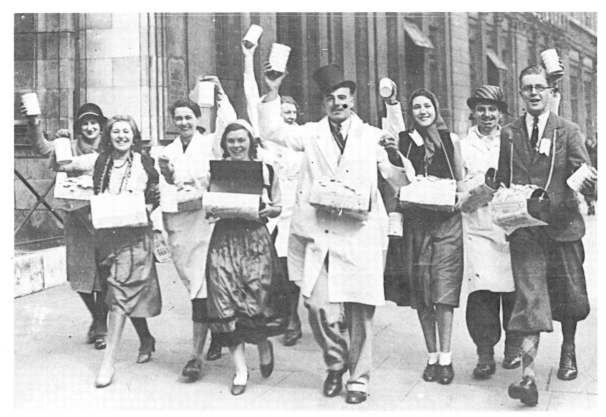

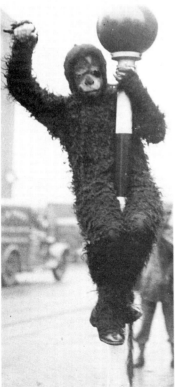

ABOVE: Students setting out on a street collection. LEFT: 'Oscar' Ottaway's gorilla impersonation was one of the star turns in the students 1931 carnival procession. After qualifying, he taught at the College for a time, eventually becoming professor of veterinary anatomy at the Bristol school. RIGHT: A contrast in size and style, showing the original College entrance block dwarfed by the newly built Beaumont animals hospital, 1933. (CL)

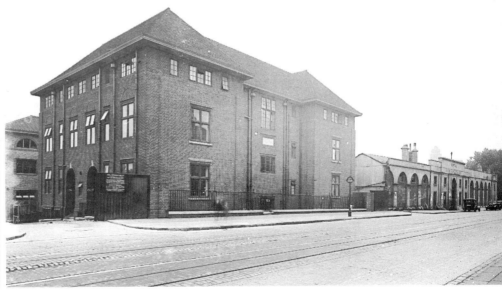

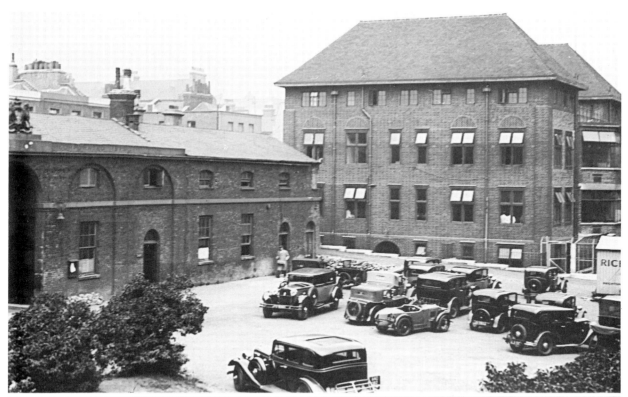

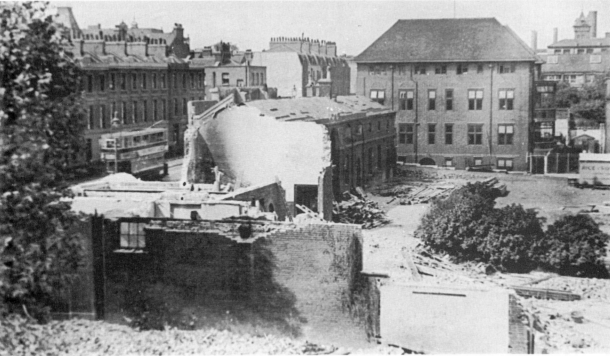

ABOVE: The Beaumont animals hospital replacing the north side of the quadrangle, with the entrance block still intact. The bell hanging beside the main entrance used to sound at the end of lectures. Car parking was obviously a problem even in the 1930s. BELOW: Partial demolition of the original entrance block. On the left, note the roof of Maple's Repository and the passing tram in Great College Street.

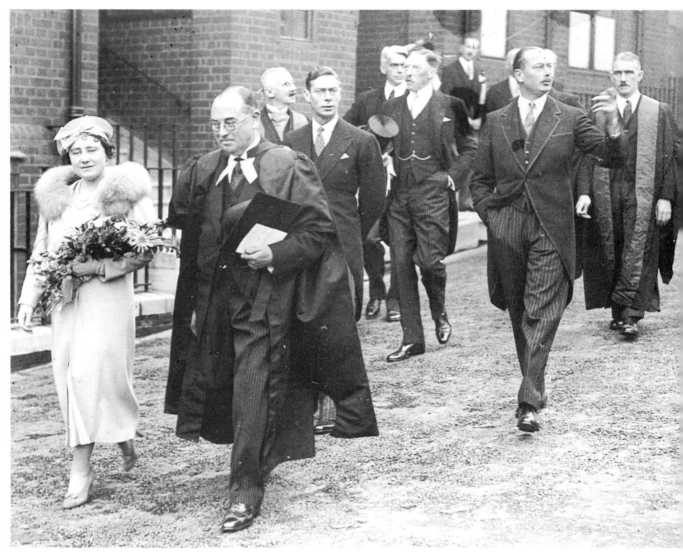

King George VI opens the new College buildings in Camden Town, 1937. From the left: Queen Elizabeth, Professor Buxton, Professor Wooldridge, King George VI, W. S. Morrison, Viscount Lascelles, Duff-Cooper (on step), the Duke of Gloucester, Professor Wright. Where was Sir Frederick Hobday?

PART IV

A University School — with a Campus at Last
JAMES BASIL BUXTON

Principal 1937-1954

The controversy surrounding Hobday's enforced retirement sent shock waves through every level of College activity. In this environment, it was not surprising that Buxton's appointment as Principal was at first not universally popular. There was even some surprise that such a distinguished scientist should wish to leave the prestigious chair of animal pathology at Cambridge and come to London. Buxton was, however, an ideal choice.

He was known to be a superb organiser who could speedily get to grips with a difficult situation. He had been active in professional affairs for many years, and he possessed great tenacity of purpose. These qualities helped him steer the College through one of the critical periods in its history. During Buxton's eventful reign, the College coped with wartime evacuation to Berkshire, agreed (at long last) to establish a permanent field station at the Hawkshead site in Hertfordshire, and became fully incorporated into the University of London.

James Basil Buxton was born in 1888, the son of a veterinary surgeon in Highgate; his brother was also a veterinary surgeon. He was educated at Highgate School, and qualified from the College on coming of age on 3 March 1909. He received the diploma in veterinary hygiene from Liverpool University in 1910, and also passed the examination for membership of the Royal Sanitary Institute. He went to the 'Dick' school in Edinburgh in 1911 to be lecturer in hygiene and stable management. This appears to have been his only period of employment as a teacher in a veterinary school; an obituarist said it was a matter for regret that his administrative duties as Principal of the College precluded his active participation in teaching (as, indeed, subsequent Principals have found).

In 1912 Buxton became veterinary superintendent at the Wellcome Physiological Research Laboratories, then at Brockwell Hall, Herne Hill, under Henry Dale. He was responsible for building and equipping the new laboratories at Beckenham in Kent, where he remained for nine years. Here he showed to the full his great ability to organise facilities for the execution of research. During the First World War he was one of the key group of men organising the production of anti-gangrene and other sera.

In 1922 he became director of the farm laboratories at the National Institute for Medical Research, founded at the old Mount Vernon Hospital in Hampstead, to further the *Field* canine distemper project. He planned the investigation, subsequently brought to a successful conclusion by Laidlaw and Dunkin, into developing a method of vaccination. Buxton devised the double intradermal tuberculin test here, and worked (with R. E. Glover — his successor as Principal of the College) on BCG vaccination against tuberculosis in calves.

Following on the Prain report, Buxton was appointed in June 1923 to the chair of animal pathology at Cambridge University, also becoming director of the Institute of Animal Pathology in Milton Road. Here his team included Bosworth and Allen, who later followed him to the College after Hobday's retirement. The reports of the institute contained important research papers, but Innes, the pioneer veterinary pathologist on the staff, claimed that, while the reports added to the prestige of the institute and its director, they were not the ideal location for research papers by younger men hoping for scientific recognition.

Buxton was offered the post of acting Principal of the College on 27 July 1936, assuming the full office of Principal and dean on the day King George VI and Queen Elizabeth opened the new buildings — 9 November 1937. Surprisingly enough, the selection committee that recommended Buxton did not actually meet but, after consultation by letter, Burrell, Weigall, Gilmour and Watson recommended Buxton's appointment. The post carried a salary of £1,200 plus superannuation, and a flat in the new building. He was to commence duty on 25 September 1936.

While still a young man, Buxton began taking a prominent part in professional affairs. At the Royal College, of which he became a fellow on 3 March 1914 (at the stipulated minimum time of five years after graduation) he was elected to council in 1920, serving as a member for 34 years. He was chairman of the examinations committee in 1925, and in 1932 as president, he was involved in launching the new five-year course, having been a most active participant in its planning. In his year as president he had the privilege of presenting the honorary fellowship of the Royal College to McFadyean. He was awarded the John Henry Steel Memorial medal in 1934, and served as treasurer of the Royal College from 1948 until his death.

Buxton was one of those concerned in keeping alive veterinary societies threatened with extinction in the First World War. In 1919 he became honorary secretary of the National Veterinary Medical Association (now the British Veterinary Association) serving for three years. In 1925 he was elected the association's president. The Central Veterinary Society, of which he was president in 1920, awarded him its Victory medal in 1923. He was president of the Royal Counties division of the NVMA in 1923, and of the Eastern Counties division in 1929. In 1934, at its meeting in Llandudno, the NVMA awarded him the certificate of honorary associateship. He held office in many other societies including the Royal Society of Medicine, the Victoria Veterinary Benevolent Fund and the Veterinary Research Club (he took a prominent part in its foundation, and was its president in 1926). In the last year of his life he was master of the Worshipful Company of Farriers. He served on many official committees, including the foot-and-mouth disease research committee appointed by the Ministry of Agriculture, the Lovat committee on veterinary services in non-self-governing dependencies, the Medical Research Council committees on distemper and on tuberculin, and the development commission's Advisory Committee on Agricultural Science.

An obituarist (one of his closest friends and colleagues) succinctly described Buxton as dignified yet genial, with a keen sense of humour. He was generally liked and respected by students and by most of his colleagues, once he had weathered the difficult period after Hobday's enforced retirement. He had a first-class brain, capable of a rapid grasp of a complicated situation, possessed formidable powers of concentration, and pursued orderly methods. Like all good administrators, he delegated tasks with shrewd judgement, asking for, and usually being cheerfully granted, full co-operation by colleagues. Buxton made a phenomenally rapid rise to eminence in his profession, and showed his skills at their best as honorary secretary of the XIth International Veterinary Congress in London in 1930. He appeared to be somewhat shy of students, but he and his wife threw themselves wholeheartedly into their sporting, dramatic and other social activities. There was never any doubt that Buxton was in charge of College affairs.

The three great matters with which Buxton had to deal were the evacuation of the College to Berkshire in the Second World War, the search for a site for a field station, and the full incorporation of the College into the University of London.

By the summer of 1939 it had become obvious that war with Germany was imminent. Arrangements for carrying on in the event of war were first considered by the College on 3 May and by the 16th of that month it had been decided that evacuation was preferable to attempting to carry on as usual in Camden Town, even with considerable strengthening of the already strong building. Although not universally accepted — one critic wrote of the College suffering an attack of the jitters — this decision proved sound. On 22 May the chairman of council, the Principal and the bursar visited Reading University for preliminary discussions on a possible transfer there in the event of war. The bursar was C. G. Freke, who had just retired as financial secretary to the Bombay government. The chairman was Sir Merrik Burrell (1877-1957) who had been elected in 1929 and was to continue in office until 1946.

On 11 October a war emergency committee was formed, consisting of the chairman, Principal, bursar and treasurer. On 26 October Professor Miller asked for staff representation on this committee, but this was refused. The University of Reading, due to a last-minute change of plan, was able to offer facilities only for the preclinical first and second years. The third year was rapidly accommodated at Holme Park, Sonning-on-Thames, and the fourth and final years were installed at Streatley House, Streatley-on-Thames. The only part of the College left to function at Camden Town was the Beaumont animals hospital with Gordon C. Knight in charge, assisted by two house surgeons.

The College's teaching programme started in January 1940. Initially there were difficulties with some members of staff. At a council meeting on 23 January 1940, Buxton emphasised that most of his colleagues had co-operated wonderfully, but he regretted that certain senior colleagues had not done so, and it would be necessary for him to deal firmly with them in order to ensure the efficient teaching of the students.

Although the start had been delayed until January, the 1939-40 session was completed in time for the Royal College examinations in June 1940; the course took 24 weeks instead of the usual 30, and there were no vacations for staff or students. The examinations were held in G.P. Male's yard in Reading (surgery), and at Reading abattoir (medicine). A short course in small animal surgery was held in the Beaumont animals' hospital by C. Formston just before the summer examination. It was reported that there were 31 new students in January 1940, and 72 in October 1940. Bomb damage was caused at Holme Park on the morning of 28 August, and at Camden Town on 25 September and 16 October.

The move to the country was a difficult operation and it necessarily meant that fewer staff were needed. The summary dismissal of most of the outside lay staff did not redound to the credit of the College. R. C. G. Hancock and four others appealed for assistance for four old servants of the College (among some 40 staff who had been dismissed) namely Messrs Radbon, Hitchings, Sibley and Nash. Donations were to be sent to H. E. Bywater, the appeal raising £51 11s. Several letters of protest at the dismissals were published in the *Veterinary Record*.

Some of these men had given years of loyal service to the College. For example, Henry Hitchings (1876-1962) became foreman at the College in 1921 after 27 years' service as a farrier-sergeant and senior veterinary NCO in the army. Professor McCunn noted: 'He not only supervised the general care of the animals and attended to the requirements of the professional staff, but was called to do all those tasks which fall to the lot of a maintenance engineer — heating, water, gas and electrical supplies. He could turn his hand to carpentry, slating and tiling and brick-laying. When we were short of loose boxes, due to the demolition and rebuilding work, he constructed with the aid of two of his men, Stanley Bryant and Fred Nash, a row of six boxes which would have been a credit to a professional builder. He perfected the well-known "Hitchings Hoof Saw" which is probably one of the most useful instruments in a horse veterinary surgeon's armamentarium. After the war, he was asked to teach and demonstrate the mysteries of the handling and restraint of animals.'

George Radbon joined the staff as assistant to 'Harry the slaughterman' and worked for the College for well over 50 years. He cared for any farm animals housed in the College, and also looked after the post-mortem room and the dissecting room. Radbon was essentially McFadyean's man and was responsible for opening carcasses under his direction. As one attending these classes it was not unusual to hear from McFadyean: 'Now, George, you've done it again!' as George's knife was wont to slip at the wrong moment. Radbon helped Lander, and later Clough, in the chemistry department, did rough work in the pathology department, cared for the experimental animals, and stoked the boiler. He helped cast animals on the 'bed', did turns of night duty at the front gate, boiled out skeletons and helped prepare specimens for dissection. He died in 1950.

Percy Septimus Sibley (1882-1950) was for many years gateman at the College. He joined the staff in 1927 when he retired from the Metropolitan Police, serving until the College was evacuated in 1939. One of his self-imposed duties was to persuade obviously well-to-do clients seeking the out-patient department to become subscribers. He was a splendid figure in his porter's uniform, and seemed to know everything that was going on in the College; at one time the only telephone in the College was in his office. He once tried unsuccessfully to stop an elephant escaping through the College gates.

Fred Nash was odd-job man at the front gate of the College.

Another servant of the College was Samuel David Fitt, who succeeded J. G. Fotheringham as librarian in December 1923, serving until 1941. He had run his own stationer's and bookseller's business and a circulating library before being called up into the army. He saw action at Ypres and the Somme, and was wounded and gassed. After the war, he worked for a time with the Ministry of Information and then had a bookshop in Hampstead. Fitt was a friendly and helpful man who served as unofficial banker to many students, always handing over a beautifully written IOU for their cheques. He also did brisk business selling new and secondhand books to students.

On 28 February 1941 the war emergency committee became the war executive committee. A meeting of the committee (actually, of the chairman, Sir Archibald Weigall and the Principal) refused a request from Clough for travelling expenses between London and Reading, which led to his resignation. (Sir Archibald Weigall Bt KCMG was gold medallist at the Royal Agricultural College, Cirencester in 1894. A great horseman, he served the College as governor, treasurer and chairman. He died in 1952, aged 77).

George W. Clough (1881-1944) worked for 11 years in the chemistry department at Birkbeck College and, after a variety of appointments, succeeded G. D. Lander in 1920 as professor of chemistry and toxicology at the College. He was a great lecturer. His most biting comment was 'I don't know what you came here for, Mr So-and-So'.

In 1941 Professor J. G. Wright (always known as 'John George') left the College to take up the chair of veterinary surgery in the Liverpool veterinary school. Born in September 1897 he served in the ranks in the Royal Artillery in France and Flanders in the First World War, later being commissioned at Sandhurst where he was awarded the Sword of Honour. He came to the College in 1919 and qualified MRCVS in 1923, having won many distinctions, including the Fitzwygram first prize. From 1923 to 1928 he was in general practice, mainly in Cardiff. He obtained the fellowship diploma of the Royal College in 1929. In 1928 he had been appointed to the chair of *materia medica* in the College, and with the retirement of Hobday he transferred to the chair of surgery.

There followed the era of 'We, in the Beaumont', when he developed intravenous barbiturate anaesthesia in the clinic, and impressed his vivid personality on his students. His lectures were like theatre turns and often extended long after the hourly bell. His reading was wide, and his energy unlimited. Few resisted his charm. The *Veterinary Record* noted: 'He entered academic life in 1928 when he accepted the chair of *materia medica*. His outstanding qualities as a teacher became at once apparent when he succeeded in infusing this traditionally dreary subject with interest and held the attention of his students by the sheer magnetism of his own personality and dedication. The decade during which he taught on the clinical material of the Beaumont will live for ever in the minds of those lucky enough to be students at that time. His keenness of observation, meticulous attention to history-taking and clinical observation, the desire to record and analyse, became the model of the ideal clinician which many of his students sought to emulate'.

At Streatley, J. G. Wright became interested in reproduction in horses and cattle, and at one time the *corpus luteum* was his favourite subject of enquiry. He saw the opportunity for a further great contribution to the veterinary profession when he transferred to the chair of veterinary surgery at Liverpool. There, he formulated and put into operation the first veterinary field station in a rural area to provide practical tuition in the husbandry and diseases of farm animals, offering a totally new concept and dimension in veterinary education in this country. Not satisfied with this achievement, he then obtained faculty status for veterinary science at Liverpool in 1952, so recording yet another first. He died in 1971, honoured by his profession, but surely deserving some recognition by the State.

Another colourful character was J. W. H. Holmes, who qualified from the 'Dick' school in 1927. He obtained his DVSM in 1928 and in the same year joined the College staff as house physician, soon becoming known to the students as 'Enema Joe'. Holmes was a pioneer dermatologist at a time when skin diseases, in particular sarcoptic and demodectic mange, were much in evidence. He was one of the first to demonstrate the value of a Wood's lamp in the diagnosis of ringworm in cats. In 1937 he succeeded J. G. Wright as lecturer in veterinary pharmacology. He moved to Streatley-on-Thames when the College was evacuated in 1939, and in 1945 took charge of the College practice in Wallingford, becoming the principal supplier of clinical material to the departments of medicine and surgery. When in 1958 the final year students were transferred to the new field station at Hawkshead, Holmes resigned from the College after 30 years' service and bought the Wallingford practice. At the time of his death in August 1985, it was one of the most flourishing practices in Berkshire.

In 1942 the senior teaching staff was served with notices of dismissal and offered re-engagement on new terms of service, already applicable to the junior staff. One effect of this was to provide clearly for a definite retiring age.

By this time most of the main block and the research institute in Camden Town had been requisitioned by the government. Parts of the premises were eventually de-requisitioned in the last quarter of 1945, allowing the teaching of first and second year students to resume in Camden Town in 1945, the third year classes following in 1946.

Professor Formston, who was at Streatley with the College from 1939 until 1958, vividly recalls that period.

'Streatley House, a large square brick-built house of three storeys became the administration headquarters of the College. It provided office accommodation, dining and common-rooms and, with an annexe, a hostel for some 50 students. Other students lived in houses rented by the College or with local residents. The College also leased the Home Farm, the Beeches, which became the department of pathology, the Cottage, Vine Cottage and Fern Cottages. In 1940 the College bought all these premises with the exception of the Cottage — the Principal's residence. Childe Court was purchased for the Principal along with three semi-detached cottages at the farm. The farm buildings consisted of a huge oak-timbered barn with adjacent cow byre and outbuildings, all now demolished to make way for extensions to the Swan Hotel. The College also had two paddocks opposite Streatley House.

'Professor J. G. Wright was appointed warden of the hostel and lived in Vine Cottage. Miss Yona Marshall, daughter of an East Anglian veterinary surgeon, became the resident bursar. Miss Marshall, who died in 1978, served the College for 28 years as domestic bursar at Streatley and later at Hawkshead.

'Local residents appreciated the new life engendered by veterinary students and the student "revues" and dances held in Goring parish hall. Sports days and cricket matches were added attractions. Privately-owned squash courts were put at the disposal of students and the local golf club welcomed students and staff.

'During the war most of the Streatley students became members of either the Streatley or Goring platoons of the Home Guard while a number joined the Wallingford branch of the Upper Thames Patrol. Most, if not all, had initial training with Reading University Student Training Corps and latterly with the Holme Park platoon of the Home Guard. This was led by Lieutenant C. Ottaway (lecturer in anatomy and warden of Holme Park) and was colloquially designated 'Oscar's Army'. Some of the College staff, of which I was one, signed on as special constables.

'Initially being faced with two classes of students to teach at Streatley, with no access to clinical patients was, to say the least, dispiriting. At Camden Town we had at least dogs and cats and some horses but here we had nothing apart from a small dairy herd of 10 cows and a dozen pigs. Most of the teaching was a course of lectures given in a hut, erected for that purpose in the grounds of Streatley House. We approached G. P. Male of Reading, a governor of the College. Male at that time had the biggest practice in the country, and he appeared to view the close proximity of the College with some concern. However, he did allow his premises to be used for the forthcoming final examination. His son, Normal Male, was appointed local secretary for the RCVS.

'The first breakthrough came in 1940 when E. B. Savory, a stockbroker who had taken up farming in the Streatley area, asked if the College would take on his veterinary work. He had three farms in Rectory Road which led on to the Berkshire Downs and the start of the ancient track to the Ridgeway. Here, at Warren Farm, he had his residence and a stud of Suffolk mares and a stallion. At the other end of his estate, adjacent to the present golf course, was the dairy farm with a herd of approximately 30 Guernsey cows and followers. He kept his own bull. Between these two was a smaller unit, the pig farm of 20-30 Large White sows and offspring. It was agreed that students would be allowed to attend and that any fee would be in the form of an honorarium.

'The most valuable teaching asset was undoubtedly the dairy farm. When we came on the scene, abortion was rife. At that time dead vaccines had given little satisfaction but a live vaccine S19, produced in America, had shown greater promise. T. J. Bosworth, who had succeeded F. C. Minet as professor of pathology in 1939, was consulted and as a result he obtained an S19 culture from the United States and prepared a vaccine for us. It proved eminently successful and I think we were the first to use this vaccine on a farm. Later, workers at the Agricultural Research Council (ARC) farms at Compton proved the efficacy of the S19 vaccine. This campaign alone with its serial blood examinations warranted frequent visits to the farm which fortunately was just beyond the Streatley golf club. At a time of petrol rationing this was a bonus. Savory also kept a flock of 100-200 Cheviot-Border Leicester ewes. Running with them were four Hampshire Down rams. In 1940, 22% of lambs, at birth, rapidly developed entropion. In the majority of cases only the lower lids were involved. By 1943, by careful selection of rams the incidence [232 lambs] had dropped to 3.4%.

'Savory's farms provided a welcome source of clinical cases when the outlook was grim. At the end of the war Savory offered the College the whole of his estate (with the exception of Warren Farm) with nine cottages, for roughly £22,000. The Ministry turned down the offer.

The only viable unit, the dairy farm, was taken over by G. McCulloch and the College practice did his veterinary work.

'The departure of J. G. Wright for Liverpool towards the end of 1941 was a severe blow to the College and to me personally. He was probably the most dynamic teacher since McFadyean. Given control of the Streatley section of the surgery department I needed help and Albert Messervy was appointed as lecturer. We had been students together. He had fled from Jersey where, with his brother, he had a flourishing practice, escaping with his wife and family literally as the island was being invaded by the Germans.

'When Professor G. H. Wooldridge reluctantly retired in 1942, J. W. H. Holmes took charge of the medicine department until the arrival of H. Burrow two years later. It was in 1942 that the College purchased (for £1,375) eight acres of hillside land and buildings at the Coombe, a little way up Streatley Hill and about seven minutes' walk from Streatley House. The buildings were constructed on two sides of an enclosed yard and comprised a coach house which became an operating theatre, two open forage bays, a small loose box (office and pharmacy) on the one side, and two loose boxes and four stalls and a groom's kitchen (tack room) on the other. A loft over one side provided kennel space for dog and cat patients. Large animals, mainly horses, were operated upon on the grassy slopes — on occasion under the protection of an umbrella. Later we had an operating barn erected. We could now say that we had a surgery department, albeit makeshift. What we needed next were patients, and in this we were singularly fortunate.

'I had heard that John Hunt, a veterinary surgeon with a practice at Crowmarsh near Wallingford and six miles from Streatley, was thinking of retirement. I went to see him in May 1942 and, subject to approval by the College, agreed a price of £1,000 for the goodwill, drugs and equipment and use of the surgery until other premises could be found. The College agreed the purchase. We now had to find someone to run the practice — and this had to be Messervy. He was an instant success, particularly with farmers with Channel Island herds of which there were quite a number. (Before the war, Reading had been the principal market for these breeds.) The practice did not reach its full potential until the clinical departments were more adequately staffed and student transport was provided. Nevertheless, from the beginning students were taken on to farms and the slaughterhouse at nearby Cholsey for pregnancy diagnosis and other classes. Messervy returned to Jersey in 1945 and J. W. H. Holmes took charge of the practice.

'As a result of the war, farming produce, in particular meat and milk, assumed a new importance. Cattle increased in value to the extent that surgery was now more economical than slaughter. Surgery for the relief of traumatic reticulitis, for example, was now worthwhile. With the careless use of baling wire, this condition was a serious and far too common event. In 1949 I presented a paper on this subject to the International Veterinary Congress by which time I had operated upon 181 cattle of both sexes. More than 500 patients had been operated on by members of the department before baling twine was eventually substituted for wire. Towards the end of the war, with the advent of the German 'doodle-bug' or flying bomb, there was a temporary increase in their flying pathway in the number of acute cases of reticulitis, due to exploded fragments of steel wire contaminating pastures and hayricks. As an aid to diagnosis the Rank Organisation in 1946 presented us with a 'Cintel' metal detector.

'We were able, then, to convince dairy farmers that in severe cases of dystocia, a caesarian operation was preferable to dismemberment of the foetus. We thus pioneered the operation on the standing animal under paravertebral nerve block.

'Farmers also began to realise the disadvantages of cows' horns and we became involved in dishorning herds of cows and heifers. Ultimately the somewhat gory process resolved itself in the less noxious surgical or chemical disbudding of the young calf.

'As time went on we became increasingly in demand for all forms of large animal surgery, most of which was done at the Coombe hospital. On the other hand, it could entail a journey to the Midlands or the south coast. On one occasion, we went to a farm on the outskirts of Swansea to "Hobday" two shire geldings, each weighing almost one ton.

'We were indebted to many veterinary surgeons for employing us but two were particularly helpful — Keith Everett of Farnham in Surrey, and Clement Fennell of Odiham in Hampshire. A visit to the George Inn at Odiham for lunch never failed to remind me that this was the place "where it all began".

'During the war, milk became a valuable commodity and it occurred to Dr Folley of the National Institute for Research in Dairying (NIRD) at Shinfield, near Reading, that to increase the milk supply, virgin heifers could be brought prematurely into milk by the administration of a synthetic oestrogen, stilboestrol. The project, which later included ovariectomised cows, was promoted in collaboration with the Agricultural Research Council (ARC) at Compton and my department. The oestrogen was initially given to the heifers in their food, the mixing of which was done by land girls who, after a while, began to notice bodily changes within themselves and, it was said, became more "vivacious". It was then decided to implant the stilboestrol in pellet form subcutaneously. The extra supply of milk fell short of expectations and frequently left the recipient with cystic ovaries.

'Our first contact with the ARC farms at Compton came through the director, George Dunkin, a College governor and brother-in-law of Principal Buxton. The Compton manor estate of 1,600 acres and several farms on the Berkshire Downs, seven miles from Streatley, had been purchased in 1937 for development as a farm animals research unit. The outbreak of war in 1939 brought things to a halt. Dunkin died in 1942 and was succeeded by W. S. Gordon. It is impossible to exaggerate the help and co-operation we had from Gordon and his colleagues throughout our stay at Streatley. Compton, with its several dairy farms, pig and poultry units, a flock of Hampshire Down sheep, and its research projects, never failed to produce something of clinical interest almost on a day-to-day basis. The clinical liaison which the surgery department had with colleagues at Compton — S. J. Edwards, I. H. Pattison, A. McDiarmid, A. Brownlee, A. W. Taylor, J. L. Taylor and E. A. Macmillan (farm manager) are names which readily come to mind — was so successful that, when the College left Streatley, the ARC appointed a veterinary clinician to carry on where we left off.

'In 1944 Harold Burrow was appointed professor of medicine. He was a Lancastrian, latterly in practice at Derby and an examiner for the RCVS; a farmer by nature and a good judge of horses and cattle. When he arrived he was disappointed to find that his departmental buildings consisted of an office in the Cottage (retained until the lease ran out) and a coach house converted into a clinical laboratory. It was some time before he had erected, to his own design, a unit woefully inadequate by today's standards in the grounds of Streatley House. For teaching material he had to rely on cases from the College practice, supplemented by visits with students to agricultural institutions and estates. Burrow, who founded the Student Agricultural Society, was a bluff character, popular, sincere and an amiable colleague. He was assisted by J. C. Greatorex who had joined the College staff as lecturer in medicine in 1943. In Greatorex he had a loyal servant who undertook an onerous teaching load which included clinical pathology, meat inspection, parasitology and applied pharmacology. Greatorex was appointed senior lecturer in 1954 and reader in equine medicine and veterinary public health in 1962 — a post he held until his retirement in 1977.

'Preventive medicine was in the hands of H. R. Allen who came to the College as a reader with Buxton in 1937. He headed the diagnostic laboratory at Streatley which concerned itself mainly with bovine mastitis control and brucellosis. He died in April 1961 within five months of retirement, aged 67.

'From 1941 to 1947 the principal source of assistance came from house surgeons appointed on a yearly basis. It was only in 1947 that a senior appointment was made when John Hickman came in as reader in surgery. Unfortunately, within a year he had left to join what is now the Animal Health Trust. He was replaced in 1949 by G. H. Arthur who, for the previous seven years, had worked with J. G. Wright at the Liverpool school. Arthur was well versed in all aspects of farm animal medicine and surgery and undertook the teaching of veterinary obstetrics and diseases of reproduction. He was made professor in that subject in 1965, and left the College in 1973 to become professor and head of the department of surgery at Bristol veterinary school.

'Geoffrey Arthur's arrival at the College coincided with the appointment of L. C. Vaughan as house surgeon, later to become lecturer, reader and ultimately professor and head of the department on my retirement in 1974. Leslie Vaughan was one of the pioneers in the field of veterinary orthopaedics. These two formed the hard core of the surgery department of the morrow, which was further strengthened by the inclusion of W. D. Tavernor as lecturer in 1957. Tavernor, who became senior lecturer in 1968, left the following year to join the Home Office as a senior inspector.

'Following the return of most of the students to Camden Town, social contact between Streatley and London was maintained by interchanges of student concerts, pantomimes and revues. A Streatley highlight was the resuscitation of the student athletic club by J. C. Greatorex and his coleague E. F. Lewis. The first sports meeting was held on the Goring recreation ground in May 1947, the principal trophy being the Greatorex cup.

'The last decade at Streatley was the most productive. Most of the academic staff had become members of the Royal Counties Veterinary Association and we had a close working relationship with practitioners over a wide area, with our colleagues at Compton and to a lesser extent with the NIRD at Shinfield. We also had contact with the thoroughbred racing world through veterinary surgeons and training establishments at Compton, Newbury, Lambourn and Wantage. It was to the College practice, however, that we had to turn for the bulk of our routine clinical work. One fruitful source was Gatehampton Farm, immediately on the opposite side of the river, which provided us with every type of surgical exercise likely to be encountered on a mixed dairy farm.

'In our last year, 967 surgical patients were admitted to the Coombe hospital, most of which came from the practice, and 130 visits were made to Compton and neighbouring farms. We undertook items of clinical research on a broad basis in gynaecology, orthopaedics, anaesthesia, ophthalmology and general surgery, details of which are enshrined in the College's annual reports and in published work. Here one must acknowledge the assistance given to the clinical departments and the College practice by P. L. Ingram of the department of pathology. Ingram was a meticulous, painstaking worker and in terms of clinical pathology he was a walking encyclopaedia.

'To leave Streatley, a dairying centre, for suburban Potters Bar and the Hawkshead site, was not unanimously welcomed. Some of us would have preferred a return to Camden Town, where provision had already been made to accommodate the departments of medicine and surgery before the war. However, Hawkshead had been purchased in 1955, and from the university's point of view it was a sound investment. When McCunn was appointed acting Principal, he occasionally visited Streatley, which he disliked. He always scathingly referred to it as Shangri-la.'

The first attempt to establish a permanent field station was made in November 1944 when, following a memorandun from Burrell, the College decided to negotiate for a 99 years lease on West Grinstead Park Estate in Sussex, at not more than £1,000 per annum. Senior staff were not happy about this: G. H. Wooldridge said the estate was too far away. McCunn agreed, and was also concerned that staff should not become divided into 'town' and 'country'.

Nevertheless, on 29 September 1945 the estate was taken on a 99 years lease: it was recognised that this would involve considerable expenditure later. In 1946 a practice was bought at Steyning, to form part of the estate plan. At that time, too, heads of College departments had expressed interest in the Hawkshead site at North Mymms, although two thought it was too close to London. In December the Steyning practice was sold. The College was now investigating Hawkshead and Boltons Park in detail. It was decided on 30 March 1949 to dispose of the lease of the West Grinstead Park Estate, and it was assigned to the Ministry of Agriculture on 29 September 1949.

On 15 February 1950 the heads of departments recommended that negotiations to purchase Hawkshead and Boltons Park should not be pursued as the Ministry was only allowing 150 acres of land. Then the Principal of Wye College enquired if the College field station could be set up near them, but on 26 July the academic board said Wye was too far out of London, and the College accepted this on 21 September 1950. There followed a look at various sites. In November 1950 the Principal inspected a property at Wheathampstead. The question of the Wye location was again considered in March 1951, at the request of the Principal of the university, Sir Douglas Logan, but without effect. In February the College just missed a property at Virginia Water, and South Hill Park, Bracknell was visited too late in June 1951. In March 1952 in was learnt that two properties were available near Maidenhead — the Islet Park Hotel and the Weir Bank Stud Farm. The hotel was unsuitable but the Stud Farm had some attraction to the University Grants Committee visitors. McCunn, Amoroso and W. R. Wooldridge urged that Hawkshead should be reconsidered, but Buxton said they should first try for Weir Bank. No suitable accommodation for staff or students being found, this plan was abandoned. On 24 March 1954 the purchase of the Hawkshead and Boltons Park properties was recommended to the University Court, and their purchase with a grant of £100,000 was recorded on 8 February 1955, the price being set by the district valuer.

The incorporation of the College as a school of the University of London was an outcome of two reports on veterinary education, known as the first and second Loveday reports.

The committee on veterinary education in Great Britain was appointed on 3 November 1936 to 'review the facilities available for veterinary education in Great Britain in relation to the probable future demand for qualified veterinary surgeons, and in particular to make recommendations as to the provision which should be made from public funds in the five years 1937-1942 in aid of the maintenance expenses of institutions providing veterinary education'.

The committee, which would report to the Minister of Agriculture and Fisheries and to the Department for Agriculture for Scotland, was originally chaired by Sir Thomas Moloney. On the death of two members (Sir John Robertson and Sir James Currie) and the resignation of Moloney, the committee came under the chairmanship of Thomas Loveday, vice-chancellor of Bristol University who, along with John Smith, continued as original members of the committee, joined by Sir Joseph Barcroft of Cambridge school of agriculture, W. L. Burgess, Sir Louis Kershaw, and W. R. Wooldridge. The committee now became known as the Loveday committee, which produced two reports, and which increased the number of veterinary schools in this country, moving them fully into the university system.

While the committee rightly bears Loveday's name, many gained the impression from the reports that they were largely the outcome of deep convictions held by W. R. Wooldridge, who thus has a strong claim to be the architect of the modern British veterinary educational system. His work in establishing the Veterinary Educational Trust at Newmarket (later re-named the Animal Health Trust) did not receive due public recognition, and the College shamefully failed to honour him by the award of its fellowship.

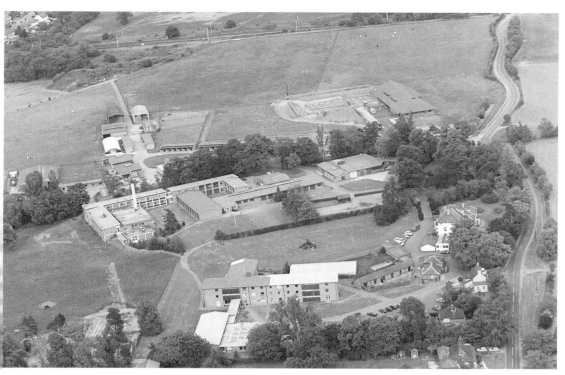

ABOVE: Aerial view of Hawkshead campus, June 1990. Hawkshead House, the white building extreme right, faces the lawn and Duncan's Horses, with Northumberland Hall in centre foreground. The Queen Mother hospital, with extensions in progress, is top right of picture, with the Sefton equine hospital, clinical and administrative blocks below.
BELOW: Aerial view of Boltons Park farm.

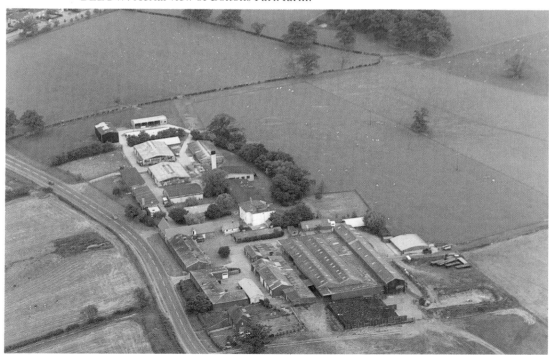

Walter Reginald Wooldridge (1900-1966) graduated MRCVS in 1924, being in 1922 an honours graduate in chemistry in the University of London. He received his PhD in 1929 for work on bacterial enzymes and then became lecturer in biochemistry at the London School of Hygiene and Tropical Medicine. He founded the Veterinary Education Trust in 1942, becoming its scientific director one year later. He was awarded the CBE in 1954, and received the degree of DSc (hc) from Bristol University.

In the first Loveday report, dated 8 July 1938, the committee set out its view of the then state of veterinary education: 'The system of education and conditions in the Schools are unsatisfactory. The basic sciences are in general not adequately taught. The prescribed courses of study concentrate on animal sickness and treat the maintenance of health altogether too lightly. Attention is focussed too completely on the curative aspect to the neglect of the preventive: animal husbandry in its wider sense — that vital section of veterinary education — is not stressed. The farm animal receives too little consideration relatively to that given to the horse, dog and the cat. The particular system of external examination in force must tend to deflect teaching into channels prejudicial to sound education. At the Schools, the teaching staffs are inadequate and in many instances the stipends are low and out of all proportion to the responsibilities which the posts carry; proper facilities for clinical training and for the practical side of animal husbandry are everywhere lacking; under the pressure of financial stringency students have been admitted in excessive numbers, with the result that the classrooms and laboratories are overcrowded; and teachers have neither time nor facilities for research'.

The committee was concerned to get the balance right between the schools, the universities, and the licensing body (the Royal College). The Royal College conducted the qualifying MRCVS examinations, although it did not teach. The schools had no right of representation on Royal College council (although in practice many teachers were elected to council) or its examination committee. The Royal College examiners could not be members of its council nor teachers from the schools (although at each school the principal teacher in each subject was added as an internal examiner, who had no official part in setting the written questions).

It was noted that the College had recently (1937) received a new charter under which its governing body included one member appointed by the senate of the University of London, with which it was loosely connected as an institution, having recognised teachers for the degree of BSc(VetSci). The university gave no financial support to the College and it had no say in the appointment of its teachers.

The committee recommended: (i) that the charter of the Royal College should be amended in order to provide for the inclusion on its council and examination committee of representatives of the schools and universities teaching veterinary students; (ii) that the council of the Royal College, thus reconstituted, should be entitled to send observers to those university examinations which exempted candidates from preclinical Royal College examinations; (iii) that the universities should consider the institution of three-year veterinary science degree courses.

The committee considered that the 'one portal' system of entry to the profession — that is, by registration by the Royal College — should be maintained. Other recommendations covered farm pupillage, the provision of field stations and large animal hospitals, and the period of 'seeing practice'. The committee put forward a revised curriculum for the five-year course of study which, it rightly claimed, provided a logically progressive system leading from the study of the normal animal to clinical patients.

Commenting on the size and location of the College, the report stated: 'None of the Schools in Great Britain is ideally situated. The College, lately built in Camden Town, lacks effective contact with the related sciences, and is remote from farms. The decision to rebuild the

College on its old site was, in our opinion, mistaken and portends increasing embarrassment over a long future. But the College has been re-built at a cost exceeding £300,000; the buildings are well-designed and constructed, and the Treasury has made a contribution of £150,000 towards the capital cost. We feel bound, therefore, to accept the continued existence of the College in Camden Town as a datum of our survey of the general situation, noting that this school is particularly well situated to provide a training in the treatment of small animals and horses of an urban population'. The committee noted that the College, apart from a grant of £1,500 per annum in the period 1795-1815, received no Government aid until 1907, when a maintenance grant of £800 per annum was made; the last grant made, in 1936-37, was £9,000.

There were two references to what the committee took to be a problem of training 'town boys' as compared with the sons of farmers and veterinary surgeons. 'In every branch of the profession the first essentials are a liking for animals, a thorough knowledge of their ways, and ability to handle them and gain their confidence. The boy who comes from a farm learns almost unconsciously the signs of health in animals and the methods adopted to maintain them in health; and he obtains an insight into the very intimate relationship between the care of animals and agriculture. All this knowledge, which comes to him as a normal part of his experience in his early years, admirably suits him for training as a veterinarian. The son of a practising veterinary surgeon enjoys similar advantages. Lack of such early contacts in veterinary students coming from towns is a serious handicap during their years of study and one which it is difficult to remove later in life.' (This opinion was not shared by those students whom McCunn disparagingly called 'suburbanites'.)

The committee did not see a great role for women practitioners, and it 'could not justify the expenditure of public money on the training of women for work among dogs and cats; the number of women students admitted by the schools should be small'. It is not clear whether the committee considered the same stricture might apply to the training of men students who planned to work exclusively in companion animal practice.

The unsettled conditions of 1938 and the outbreak of war in 1939 meant that no more than preliminary consideration could be given to the committee's recommendations, and it seemed reasonable to expect that further action would have to be deferred until peace was restored. However, on 13 January 1943 the Minister of Agriculture wrote to Loveday pointing out that the government had announced its intention of maintaining a healthy and well-balanced agriculture after the war. The committee was therefore asked to review its former recommendations in the light of this policy.

The committee then came to the conclusion that it had underestimated the number of veterinary students that would be needed in the implementation of this policy. It thought the number of students in London and Edinburgh should be increased, a new school should replace the old Glasgow school, and new schools should be established in the universities of Bristol and Cambridge.

To all these university schools, the following conditions should apply: the necessary financial assistance would be provided by the State; the degree in veterinary science or medicine awarded by the university would be a registrable qualification for membership of the Royal College; and the university would have control over the courses and the examinations, generally similar to that exercised over medical degrees.

The two Loveday reports laid the foundations of modern veterinary education in this country. The schools have adapted themselves well to the new situation. Research has taken its rightful place alongside teaching as a required function of a teacher, and the placing of the senior appointments of reader and professor in the hands of university boards has led to a general up-grading of the academic standing of veterinary teachers. The tenure and salaries of staff were brought into general alignment with those of universities in 1927.

In December 1948 it was decided to apply for admission as a school of the University of London. This was achieved in 1949, when on 1 October the College became a school of the university in the faculty of medicine, for five years in the first instance. The report of the university inspectors was received in 1949. The Ministry of Agriculture grant continued until 30 September 1950 and from then on the grant became the responsibility of the University Grants Committee. Six members of staff were given the title of professor (Bosworth, Formston, Burrow, Amoroso, McCunn, Scorgie) and one of reader (Lovell — subsequently to become titular professor). Teaching for the degree of Bachelor of Veterinary Medicine (BVetMed) began in the session 1952-53.

During Buxton's reign, the staff included several noteworthy individuals.

Professor Legge-Symes retired from his part-time unpensioned post of professor of physiology in 1938 at the age of 72. Symes qualified at St Mary's Hospital in 1892. He was one-time director of physiology at London University and was examiner for the Royal College before becoming professor of physiology in the College. He was well known as a research worker, for his papers on digitalis and luminal, and as the inventor of the Symes cannula.

An even more distinguished professor of physiology was E. C. Amoroso, appointed in 1947. Emmanuel Cyprian Amoroso, always and everywhere known as 'Amo', was born in Port of Spain, Trinidad, on 16 September 1901. He was educated at St Mary's college there, leaving school at 18. He enrolled at the age of 21 in University College of the National University of Ireland, and led the field in science and medicine. His outstanding career has been the subject of a memoir written by his colleague and disciple, R. V. Short: *Biographical Memoirs of Fellows of the Royal Society*, Vol 31, November (both were Fellows of the Royal Society). In 1933 Amoroso was appointed demonstrator in histology at University College London and in 1934 he obtained his PhD. While unemployed, he went to Folkestone for the day and gained inspiration by looking at the statue of William Harvey, born there on 1 April 1578. Coming back by train, he got into conversation (as was his wont) with a fellow passenger, who turned out to be the notorious 'Red' Dean of Canterbury, Dr Hewlett Johnson. The Dean told Amoroso he had seen an advertisement for a senior assistant in charge of histology and embryology at the Royal Veterinary College, and encouraged him to apply for the post. This Amoroso did, and he was appointed from 1 October 1934. He was a brilliant lecturer, although his classroom attendances tended to be erratic according to the exigencies of his research work. His students listened with awe to his descriptions, as it might be, of the 'terminal arborizations' of a nerve (why, they wondered, not 'end branches'?) He seemed to be Maximow reincarnate. He was an inspiration to colleagues and students alike, and he brought news of the broad outer world of science to the College. His desk overflowed with papers, as did his hut at Reading University; he once asked for some help in his labours, but the College gently countered by suggesting that he limit his activities somewhat.

Amoroso was appointed professor of physiology in 1947, succeeding O. G. Edholm, and he retained this post until his retirement in 1968. His work on placentation earned him his FRS, and he received numerous other honours — to name just a few, he was FRCS, FRCOG, FRCP, FRCPath, and FInstBiol. He exemplified in this respect the biblical saying 'to him that hath shall be given'. At one time Amoroso entered on the veterinary course, but could not keep this going. He must surely stand as a unique phenomenon in the history of the staff of the College. After his retirement he was appointed visiting scientist at the institute of animal physiology at Babraham. He died on 30 October 1982.

Following Professor Wright's transfer to Liverpool in 1941, C. Formston was placed in charge of the department of surgery. In 1942 Buxton announced his intention of forming a clinical department embracing surgery and medicine, with himself as its head, but nothing came of this. The College thought it might delay filling the surgery chair until after the war, to allow full scope for getting the best man for the job, but a year later it was decided to advertise three chairs — surgery, medicine and physiology, and these were filled by Formston, Burrow and Edholm.

Clifford Formston taught at the College for 46 years. He became Vice-Principal in 1963 and in 1971 was the first chairman of the division of veterinary clinical studies. His specialised subject was ophthalmology, for which he received numerous awards and international recognition. Under his influence, several College graduates went on to become outstandingly successful ophthalmologists, among them Geoffrey Startup (qualified 1946), Keith Barnett (1956) and Peter Bedford (1966). Professor Formston was given the title of emeritus professor when he retired in 1974, and was made a fellow of the College in 1975. Among other awards he received the John Henry Steel memorial medal from the Royal College, and the BSAVA Blain and Simon awards. A plaque originally identifying one of the operating theatres at Camden Town, but now in the Queen Mother hospital at Hawkshead, reads: The Formston Theatre, in recognition of 46 years service, 1928-1974, as a member of academic staff by Clifford Formston FRCVS, professor of veterinary surgery.

Harold Burrow, who died in October 1987, was professor of medicine in the College from 1944 to 1963, when he retired at the age of 60. A brilliant student, he graduated from the 'Dick' school in 1926, winning the first Fitzwygram and the Walley memorial prizes. He was a fluent and graphic lecturer, full of appropriate anecdotes, his main interests being meat inspection, veterinary public health and the humane slaughter of animals. He was a council member of the Royal Society of Health and in 1956 become its first veterinary chairman.

All through the war, the Beaumont animals' hospital continued to function under the unruffled and determined leadership of G. C. Knight, supported by his loyal and able lieutenant, S. W. Douglas.

Gordon Charles Knight was born in Wimbledon in 1900. He became a lay worker in Middleton Perry's practice there, entering the College in October 1926 and qualifying in 1930. He returned to Perry's practice until 1938 when he replaced Chamberlain as senior assistant in the department of surgery at the College, for duty in the subscribers' department. On the evacuation of the College in 1939, Knight assumed control of the Beaumont animals' hospital. He was appointed university reader in veterinary surgery in 1952, and retired in 1968. He served on Royal College council from 1958 to 1972. Formston wrote that Knight had the finest pair of surgical hands he had seen. Knight, who died in 1987, made many contributions to the development of surgical techniques, especially in orthopaedics, thoracic surgery and ophthalmology (he was an early advocate of cataract surgery in the dog). Among his many awards were the Dalrymple-Champneys cup and medal in 1954.

In the department of medicine, Professor G. H. Wooldridge was deemed in 1942 to have reached the age limit for his appointment. He, however, held that he was under no obligation to resign at 65. He had declined to disclose his age to the war executive committee, but had then told it privately to Buxton who, not feeling bound to secrecy, had passed on the information to that committee. Counsel's opinion having been sought in December 1942, Wooldridge's appointment was terminated on 30 September 1943. At the end of the summer term, the students gave him a silver statuette of a hunter as a token of their affectionate regard. They chaired him across the lawn of Streatley House, then took him to the 'Swan' for refreshments. Then back to Streatley House with Mrs Wooldridge to dine with Miss Marshall, the president of the students' union and fellow students, and on to a dance at the Goring village hall. George Henry Wooldridge, 'Uncle George' to generations of College students, was born in Stoke-on-Trent in 1877, the son of a farmer. He entered the College in October 1895 and qualified with first class honours in 1899, his many prizes including the Coleman medal and the centenary scholarship. He was for a year a tutor in the clinical departments of the College, and continued to see dairy practice with J. Wilson of Nantwich, where he had been a pupil before entering the College. In 1900 he was appointed professor of veterinary science at the Royal Agricultural College, Cirencester and three years later was appointed to the chair of medicine at the young Royal Veterinary College of Ireland in Dublin. At this time, he was elected to membership of the Royal Irish Academy. He became FRCVS in 1905.

In 1908 Wooldridge was appointed to succeed Harold Woodruff as professor of *materia medica*, hygiene and dietetics at the College, later moving to the chair of medicine when Woodruff left. He was an active consultant and, among his many publications, perhaps the best known is his *Veterinary Encyclopaedia*, produced with the help of many colleagues. He was treasurer of the National Veterinary Medical Association for 16 years, and was its president in 1926. He was a member of council of the Royal College from 1924 until 1956, and served as president in 1939; in 1928 he received the John Henry Steel medal of the Royal College. He served as president of the Central Veterinary Society, and of the section of comparative medicine of the Royal Society of Medicine.

Wooldridge was considered to be an extremely competent veterinary surgeon. His operations were conducted in a deft, accurate and above all gentle manner. Students often wondered whether the ash falling from his perpetual cigarette did not have a stimulating effect on wound healing. In 1931 he contracted psittacosis while conducting a post mortem examination on a diseased parrot. The 'vector' was a cigarette he was smoking at the time. Little was then known of the disease or of any specific treatment; he was treated for broncho-pneumonia and recovered after a protracted illness. Wooldridge constantly urged students to handle tissues with great gentleness. He was tall and thin, with pince-nez at an angle above the waxed spikes of his moustache and deep starched collar. His pet phrase was 'Quite so!' Trim, precise, and tidy as was his work, his study was chaotic. He held high rank in Freemasonry, having Grand Lodge Honours, London Grand Rank, being a founder member of London Staffordshire Lodge No 4474 and its Chapter; he was also a member of Supreme Grand Chapter. He died in 1957.

F. C. Minett left the College for the veterinary research institute at Muktesar in India in 1939, and was succeeded as professor of pathology and director of the research institute by T. J. Bosworth. Minett, born in 1891, qualified at the College in 1911 and obtained his BSc degree in 1912. From 1911-1912 he was junior assistant in the department of pathology. He served with the Royal Army Veterinary Corps from 1914 to 1924, gaining the OBE. He joined the staff foot-and-mouth disease research group of the Ministry of Agriculture and Fisheries at Weybridge, and then in 1927 was appointed director of the research institute of animal pathology at the College, adding the chair of pathology and succeeding Tom Hare in 1933. The main work of the institute under him was on bovine mastitis and Johne's disease. Lecturing was not Minett's strong point. His lectures were largely based on Muir's *Pathology*, and his manner, perhaps because he was a shy man, suggested that he was not interested in teaching.

Eustace George Coverley Clarke succeeded G. W. Clough as lecturer in chemistry in 1942. Clarke was particularly involved in toxicological and forensic matters, and was especially interested in ricin and in testing for alkaloids. He received the title of professor of chemical toxicology on 1 January 1968 and retired in 30 September 1972 after 30 years at the College. He died in 1978.

Buxton died suddenly at his desk in Streatley House on 25 May 1954. His memorial service in the Church of St Mary Woolnoth on 23 June was conducted by the rector and two assistants, one of whom, Rev George Willis, had served briefly on the College staff in the department of hygiene, leaving in 1952 to take Holy Orders.

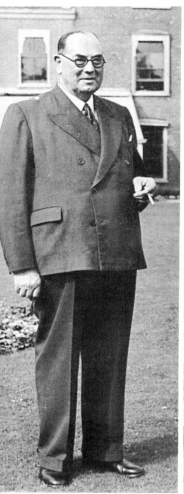

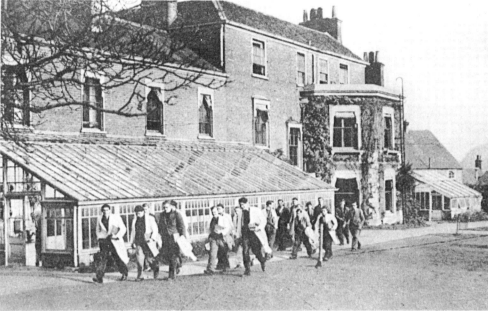

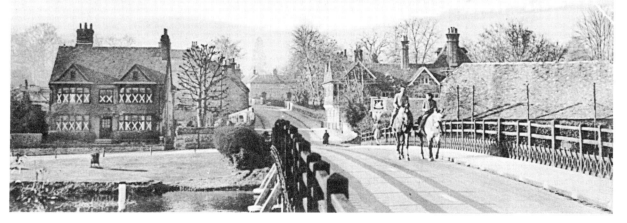

LEFT: J. B. Buxton on the lawn at Streatley House. BELOW: Bridge linking Goring with Streatley (far side). The inn sign of the Swan hotel is visible on right. Streatley House was on the left, a little way up the hill. RIGHT: Conservatories, outbuildings and nearby houses in Streatley were adapted as lecture rooms and laboratories, often involving a brisk walk between sessions.

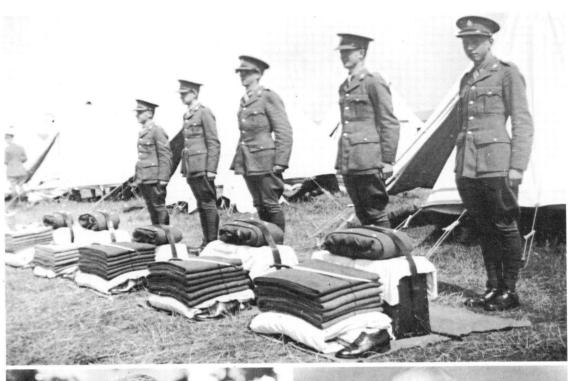

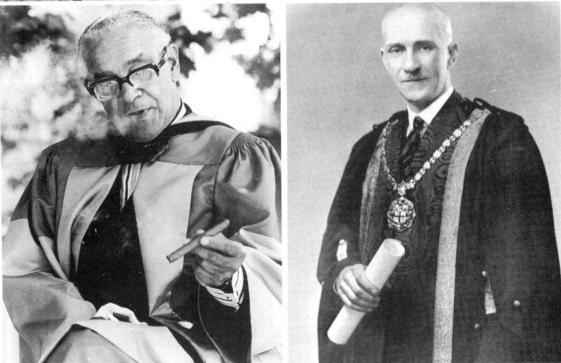

ABOVE: Volunteers from the College at camp with the University of London OTC. (RNP) LEFT: Professor Amoroso, known to all and sundry as 'Amo'. RIGHT: Professor John George Wright, who taught at the College from 1928 until 1941, when he became professor of veterinary surgery at the Liverpool school.

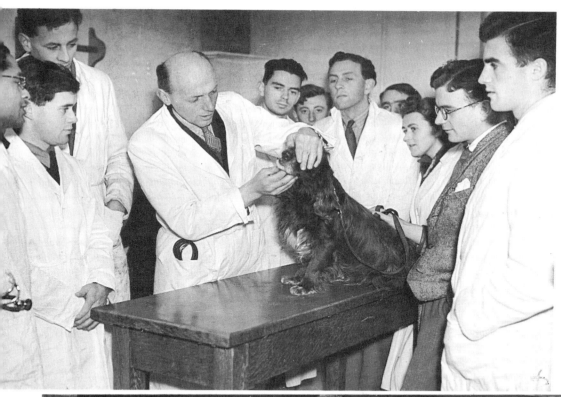

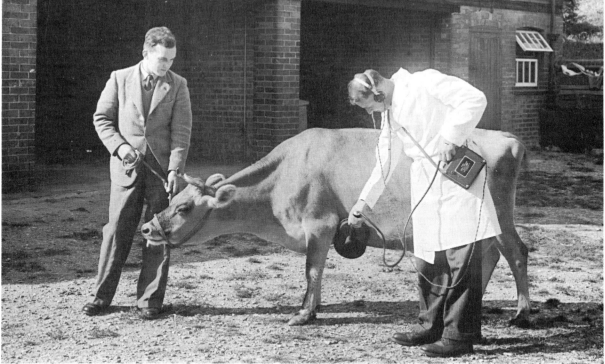

ABOVE: Albert Messervy examines a patient in the small animal clinic at Streatley. He later became professor of veterinary surgery at the Bristol school. BELOW: Professor Clifford Formston using the Cintel metal detector on a cow with traumatic reticulitis, assisted by Peter Bennet, at the Coombe, 1941.

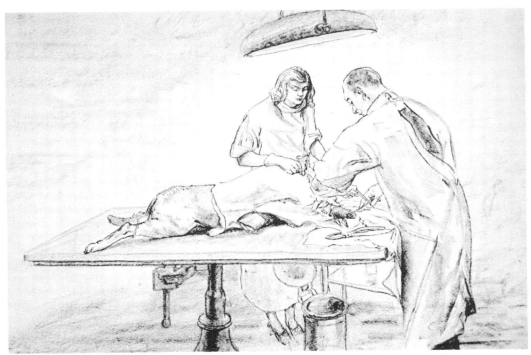

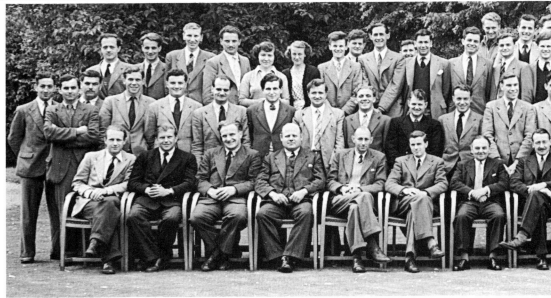

ABOVE: Illustrations drawn by William P. Moss, who qualified from the College in 1923, to illustrate his articles on The Modern Veterinary Surgeon in *Sport & Country*, 1946, showing an operation at the Beaumont and 'the path lab'.

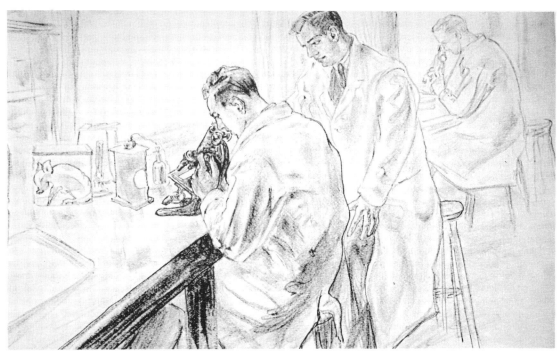

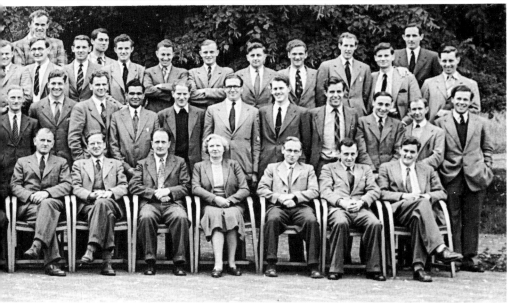

BELOW: Final year students 1952-53; left to right, from the back: Jordan, Godfrey, Menard, Russell, Neal, Whitaker, Martin, Walter, Fell, Berry; Eden, Douch, Keywood, Basinger, Miss Tucker, Miss Hooker, Evans, Dickens, Samuel, Box, Smith (G.R.), Biggs, French, Rabbich, Hawkins, Rodgers, Stockwell, Shaw, Williams, Townsend, Stear, Reid, Richards, Berwyn-Jones, Hayes; Pepper, Cochran Dyet, Larkin, Jones, Hunter, Kirby, Hall, Tuckey, Morris, Malone, Carter (J.B.), Lane, Morgan, Thomas, Barley, Gillett, Smith (P.L.F.), Asghar, Anderson, Carter (H.E.), Manton, Clay, Hullis, Michael, Mackay; Froyd, Tew, Haxby, E.F. Lewis, J.C. Greatorex, P.W. Daykin, H.R. Allen, Prof H. Burrow, Prof J.B. Buxton, Prof C. Formston, G.H. Arthur, L.C. Vaughan, Miss Marshall, Mr P.L. Ingram, Mr J.J. Yeats, Bloomberg.

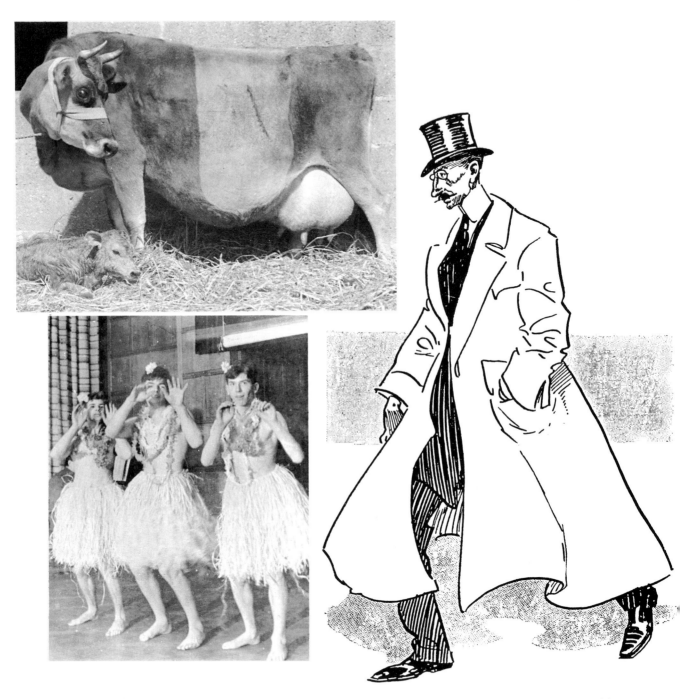

LEFT: 'Jenkyn Jane', the first cow in Britain to undergo a caesarian operation in the standing position, under paravertebral anaesthesia. Photographed immediately after the operation, performed by Clifford Formston, professor of surgery, in 1954. RIGHT: 'Uncle George' Wooldridge, complete with pince-nez and waxed moustache ends, as caricatured in *The Incisor*. BELOW: Students Martin, Jones and Wilson performing at a concert in Sonning, 1941. (LRT)

JAMES McCunn

Acting Principal 1954-1955

When Principal Buxton died, James McCunn, as the longest-serving professor of the College, became acting Principal on 10 June 1954. Qualifying from the College in 1918, he had been appointed professor of anatomy in 1926 and was popular both with the staff and the students.

A selection committee consisting of Lovatt-Evans, Burrell, McCunn, Bosworth, Cameron, Dalrymple-Champneys, Davies, Hamilton and W. R. Wooldridge was set up to look for a new Principal. A provisional list of those thought worthy of consideration included College academic staff, F. Blakemore (of Bristol veterinary school), R. E. Glover, L. P. Pugh, W. R. Wooldridge and J. G. Wright. On 1 December 1954 R. E. Glover was unanimously recommended as Principal, subject to a retiring age of 60, extendable to 65. McCunn was severely disappointed at being passed over, but he declared he would give the new Principal every loyalty, as indeed he strove to do. At the council meeting at which the selection committee's decision was confirmed, two members abstained from voting, and a third (Burrow) handed a note (contents unrecorded) to the chairman.

The key development in the College during McCunn's acting principalship was the authorization of the purchase of Hawkshead and Boltons Park Estate on 27 October 1954; the completion date was 8 February 1955, the University Grants Committee grant of £100,000 being made on 5 January. On 19 January it was reported that the College had been granted a further period of five years' recognition as a school of the University of London.

H. E. Bywater, a lifelong colleague, recalled meeting Jimmy McCunn in 1914 before McCunn entered the College, when he was working with his elder brother Archibald, in the mainly equine practice originally owned by his father in West Ham, London. James McCunn was born on the Welbeck Estate of the Duke of Portland in 1895. After an outstanding academic career he qualified in 1918, joined the RAVC and served in Mesopotamia and Kurdistan. After demobilization, and while still contriving to work in his brother's practice, he studied for his MRCS/LRCP at the London Hospital Medical School. He subsequently worked in Professor Bulloch's laboratory at the school, and on foot-and-mouth disease at the Lister Institute. William Bulloch MD LlD FRS (1888-1941) was a great friend of McFadyean. He was bacteriologist at the London Hospital from 1897 to his retirement in 1934, and from 1919 was Goldsmith professor of bacteriology in the University of London. For many years a Royal College examiner in pathology, he had a high opinion of veterinary students, stating publicly that their knowledge and understanding of this important subject were superior to that shown by medical students.

After being appointed professor of anatomy in 1926, McCunn developed an extensive consultation practice in the College, and for a while was responsible for running his brother's practice after the latter's untimely death. He was veterinary surgeon at the West Ham greyhound stadium, and was particularly noted for his skill as an expert witness in courts of law. He edited new editions of Hobday's *Surgical Diseases of the Dog and Cat*, and (with C. W. Ottaway, once his junior colleague as lecturer in anatomy) Stubbs's *Anatomy of the Horse*. He was also a co-editor of the *British Veterinary Journal*.

McCunn served on the council of the NVMA for an exceptionally long period. He was a past president of the Central Veterinary Society, a recipient of its Victory Medal, and its honorary treasurer for over 30 years. He was elected an honorary fellow of the Hunterian Society in 1962 (hitherto only one other veterinarian, Sir Frederick Hobday, had received this honour). He also received the honorary diploma of fellowship of the Royal College of Surgeons.

McCunn had an extraordinary talent for making friends in every walk of life. He was one of the best-known veterinary surgeons of his day, and probably knew personally more members of the profession than any of his colleagues. He was a great helper of lame dogs over stiles: student and veterinarian alike turned to him in time of trouble, none was disappointed. He was a down-to-earth person — indeed, he loved to tease those of his colleagues whom he delighted to call 'academic' — yet his own reading in the professional literature was extensive, and he encouraged his departmental colleagues in their teaching and research work. The excellent anatomy museum at the College is witness to this. He radiated affection for his fellow creatures, human and animal. As a teacher of anatomy he was outstanding, and his blackboard drawings were, one felt, too good to be erased, demonstrating the value of the too-often disparaged 'blackboard and chalk' method of teaching. He entered to the full into student activities. He loved the old College, and his interest in its history was so great that it almost seemed that a contemporary of the great Principals of the Victorian era was still with us.

Some of his colleagues considered that McCunn would have made a first-class Principal. When he retired in 1961 at the age of 65, his anatomy chair remained vacant until the appointment of J. L. Hancock on 1 October 1967, the department coming under the care of the head of the department of physiology, E. C. Amoroso, in the interim. The students parodied McCunn's views on the student entry: 'These damn suburbanites coming to the College, the place is going to the dogs. Dammit, there isn't a self-respecting farm-hand in the place. Most students have their origin in their digs, from which they pass forwards, downwards and sideways towards the College body, where they cross the canteen and are supplied by the Tea, Coffee and Vitic Plexi. Their relations are the Wheatsheaf, College Arms and "Uncle's" (the local pawnbroker). Dammit, the students can't drive three or four horses, yet they seem able to drive the total of seven as manufactured by Austin's'.

When Glover assumed office, McCunn became Vice-Principal on 29 June 1955. He died at home at Larks Hall Farm, in Chingford, Essex on 2 April 1967, aged 72. His funeral was attended by a vast congregation, representing his innumerable friends and acquaintances. In place of flowers, his family had asked that donations be sent to the Victoria Veterinary Benevolent Fund, of which he had been honorary treasurer. His memory is perpetuated in the College by the McCunn memorial prize in anatomy.

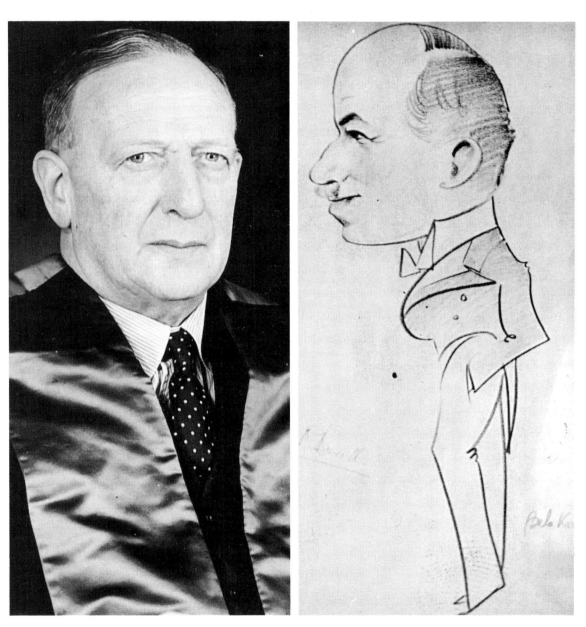

LEFT: Professor James McCunn. RIGHT: Cartoon of Sir Merrik
Burrell, chairman of the College governors from 1929-1946.

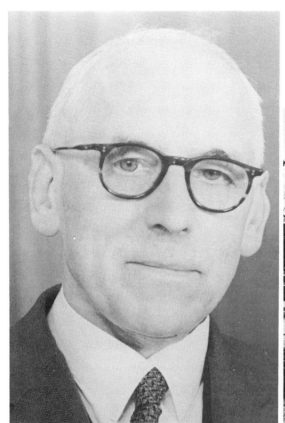

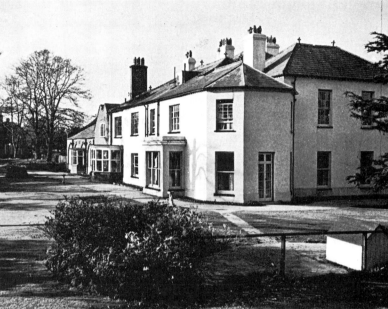

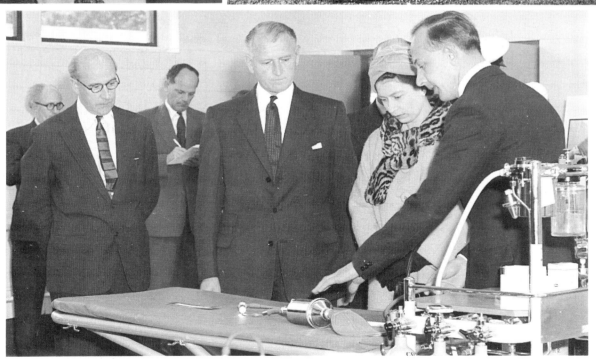

LEFT: R. E. Glover. RIGHT: Hawkshead House. BELOW: The Queen
in the small animal theatre at Hawkshead, 1959, with (from left) Gordon
Knight, Professor Formston and Derek Tavernor.

188

RONALD EVERETT GLOVER

Principal 1955-1965

The Hawkshead project became a triumphant reality during Glover's term as Principal. The 430 acre field station, comprising the Hawkshead House estate and Boltons Park Farm, was officially opened by the Queen in April 1959. Six years later, the students' hall of residence was opened by the Queen Mother, adding a new dimension to the life of the College. Sadly, Sir Merrik Burrell, who died in 1957, did not see the development of the field station for which he had striven so hard.

When the medicine and surgery departments moved to Hawkshead in 1958, Streatley House with about 13 acres of land was sold to Lt Col Richard Watt for £5,500. Childe Court, the Principal's residence, was also sold for £5,500.

Ronald Everett Glover was born on Christmas Day 1897 in London. He entered the College in 1915, but his studies were interrupted from 1916-1918 by war service in cavalry and infantry units, and he was for a time a prisoner-of-war in Germany. He qualified from the College in July 1920 and took his BSc in the University of London in December that year. After a period working under McFadyean in the research institute in animal pathology, and under Vallée at Alfort and in the Pasteur Institute, he was appointed in 1923 to the tuberculosis committee of the Medical Research Council, for work on the double intradermal tuberculin test. The following year he joined Buxton at the Institute of Animal Pathology at Cambridge, concentrating his work on tuberculosis. He was superintendent of the farm laboratories of the National Institute for Medical Research at Mill Hill from 1937 until 1947, when he became director of the newly-formed Laboratory Animals' Bureau of the Medical Research Council, which was housed in the College. In 1949 he was given the chair of veterinary pathology at Liverpool. He was appointed Principal and dean of the London College in December 1954, taking up his post in July 1955.

A few months after his appointment, on 23 February 1956, the College was granted its present charter, and the Duke of Gloucester, for many years president of the College, became patron.

When the Queen arrived to open the field station on 20 April 1959 she was met by the Lord Lieutenant of Hertfordshire, Hon David Bowes-Lyon, who presented Lovatt Evans, chairman of council, Principal Glover, and a group which included the vice-chairman of council, Sir Weldon Dalrymple-Champneys; the treasurer, Major Christopher York and Professor McCunn. The Queen unveiled the commemorative tablet, unlocked the door and declared the field station open. She toured the buildings under the guidance of Professors Formston and Burrow, saw students at work in the practical laboratory, asked numerous questions and heard about some of the work going on. The Queen also spent some time at the loose-boxes, meeting with obvious pleasure the equine inmates. On her return to the entrance hall others were presented, including Professors Amoroso, Laing and Lovell; H. W. J. Adams, secretary and bursar; I. E. Walker, president of the students' union society and Mrs P. Lorenzen, president of the women students' union society. Her Majesty then signed the visitors' book and received a bouquet from a first year woman student before leaving amid prolonged cheers.

The opening of the Northumberland Hall of Residence in 1965 is described in the students' magazine, *The Incisor*:

'It was perfect weather on the afternoon of Friday, 11th June when the Queen Mother came to open the new Hall of Residence at the Field Station, Potters Bar. The Principal, Governors, staff and students and the many guests poured into the Field Station and were shown to their various seats in the stand with its conspicuous blue and white awning. In front of the Hall the band of the Life Guards began its programme at 2.30 pm and played nobly through until 5.00 pm. To the right was the stretch of red carpeting (already bearing a number of dusty footmarks) from which the Hall was to be opened. Promptly at 3.00 pm the Queen Mother, Chancellor of the University of London, arrived. She received amongst others, the Principal of the University, Sir Douglas Logan, the Chairman of the College Council (Sir Weldon Dalrymple-Champneys, Bt) and Dr Glover, and was then conducted to the dais where other guests were presented. Sir Weldon introduced the Queen Mother and invited her to unveil the plaque commemorating the occasion and to declare the Northumberland Hall of Residence open. In reply the Queen Mother congratulated those responsible for the erection of "this fine building" and expressed her certainty that the students would find every incentive to work amid such surroundings. She then unveiled the plaque and declared the Hall officially open.

'A tour of the building followed during which the Queen Mother was accompanied by Mr Jackson (Warden) and was shown Dai Evan's room and Alison Leedale's room. It was hoped that she would not wonder why it was that the girls' and men's rooms were in such close proximity, for in actual fact Alison had 'borrowed' one of the men's rooms to save Her Majesty ascending another flight of stairs.

'After leaving the Hall the Queen Mother was driven round to the Medicine Block where she received Professor Bell who showed her round one of the laboratories in the teaching block where a number of students were engaged in practical work. She was then conducted by Professor Formston to the operating theatre where a dog was being anaesthetised prior to a routine operation. A demonstration of electroencephalography in the horse was seen in the Dutch barn, and finally Her Majesty looked round the horses in the loose boxes.

'Tea was laid on for the Queen Mother in the recreation room; before going in for tea she passed through the dining room where a number of students were assembled and stopped to talk to various groups as she walked through. The students having tea with Her Majesty were then presented and all sat down to the magnificent tea — the eight students a little nervously — each hoping that it would not be him or her who dropped a sandwich on the Queen Mother's lap. Fortunately all went well and the conversation flourished, the East Africa Expedition proved a great topic of conversation as was this year's coughing epidemic. When Derby Day was mentioned the Queen Mother stated emphatically that this should "certainly be a holiday for veterinary students". After twenty minutes or so of conversation, during which amazingly little was eaten, the Queen Mother was escorted to the entrance hall where she added her name to the Visitors' Book. As a parting gesture Kathy Steel presented her with a bouquet.'

The Queen Mother was told by Sir Weldon that the name 'Northumberland' had been chosen for the Hall because: 'This Hall . . . is the latest development of the Veterinary College founded in 1791 as the result of an enlightened campaign by a number of members of the nobility led by Hugh, second Duke of Northumberland, who was subsequently elected

President, a post which he held from 1791'. (This is a somewhat inaccurate account of the role of the Duke in the founding of the College.) Sir Weldon continued: 'It is his descendant, the present Duke, whose outstanding contributions to veterinary science as chairman of the Departmental Committee of Inquiry into Recruitment for the Veterinary Profession will be familiar to Your Majesty, who has honoured the College by permitting this new Hall of Residence to bear his name, and we are delighted to welcome him here today. The provision of this building, which will make such a difference to the life and teaching of our students, has been made possible by a grant from the University Grants Committee, covering the construction and equipment of the building. The Hall contains 63 study-bedrooms, dining facilities for staff and both resident and non-resident students, a recreation room, common-room, house surgeon's quarters, and changing rooms for athletics.'

The Northumberland report on recruitment to the veterinary profession, published in July 1964, described an inadequacy of staff and an insufficiency of buildings in the various British veterinary schools. The committee thought there should be no specialization at undergraduate level. A basic recommendation was that earmarked grants should be put at the disposal of the University Grants Committee so that the facilities for postgraduate training and research by teachers and research workers could be brought up to an acceptable level.

T. J. Bosworth (1893-1973) retired on 30 September 1960. Qualifying from the College in 1915, he returned in 1939 to succeed Minett as professor of pathology and director of the research institute. As a Royal College examiner, Bosworth had tried to raise the standard of pathology teaching throughout the country's veterinary schools. In a sense, he stood midway between the school of wide-ranging, almost polymath pathologists exemplified by McFadyean, whose disciple he was, and the present-day pathologist who, however able, is almost compelled willy-nilly to narrow his field of interest to make it manageable. Bosworth would take a shot at most problems of diagnosis, and it was a pleasure to watch him, eyebrows rising and scalp furrowing, as he searched his well stocked mind for the appropriate reference. He was succeeded as head of the department of pathology by Reginald Lovell (1897-1972). In his late 'teens Lovell had served in the First World War's closing stages and had taken part in the last cavalry advance under Allenby which wrested Palestine from Turkey. He qualified from the College in 1923, took the diploma in veterinary state medicine at Manchester University, and joined Topley and Wilson's bacteriology department, moving with them to the London School of Hygiene and Tropical Medicine. Lovell was involved in the early work on penicillin, and joined the College's department of pathology in 1933. Here he made his name, working with *Salmonella* and with *Corynebacteria*. He also studied *E. coli* infection in calves. He was a good lecturer, noted for his minuscule writing on the blackboard — students were advised to bring binoculars to lectures.

John Niven Oldham (1900-1968) qualified BSc (Forestry) in 1922, taking his PhD in 1926. He went to the Institute of Agricultural Parasitology to become senior assistant in 1935. In the same year he joined the College staff in the department of pathology, becoming university reader in parasitology in 1951, retiring in 1967. He will be remembered as a most lucid lecturer; generations of students recall his beautiful blackboard figures and gentle Scottish humour. He had an infallible memory for every student's name and face.

At the end of Glover's Principalship, a selection committee (Bell, Dalrymple-Champneys, Joseph Edwards, Gould, Hamilton, York and Lovell) recommended that Sir John Ritchie be appointed Principal and dean from 1 October 1965. Dr A. O. Betts, who was to succeed Sir John as Principal and dean in 1970, was appointed to the chair of veterinary microbiology and parasitology from 1 December 1965.

191

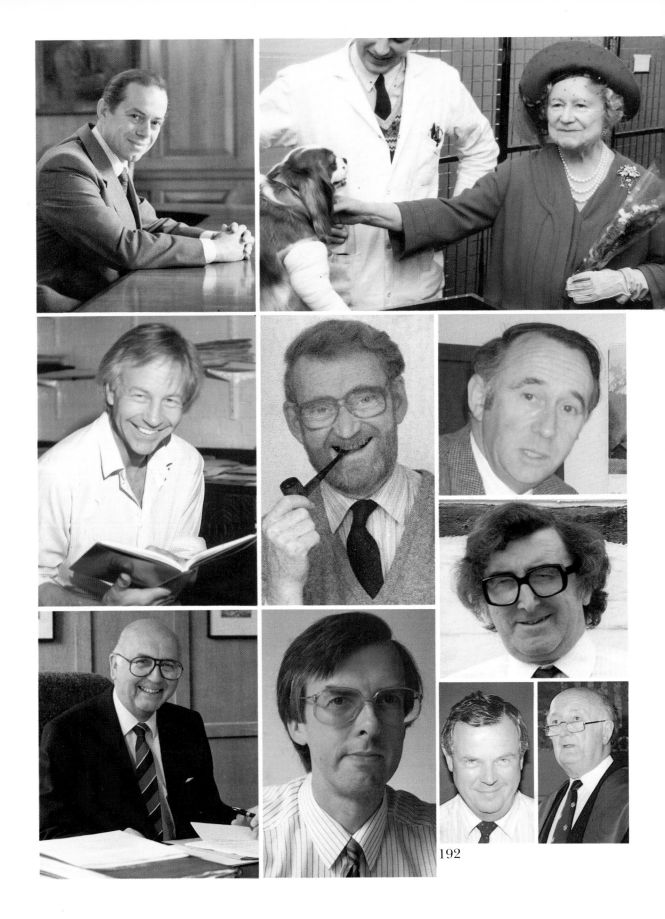

192

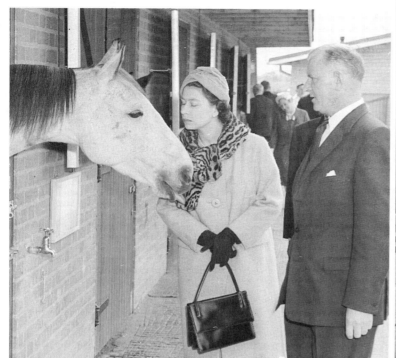

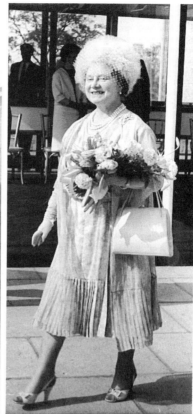

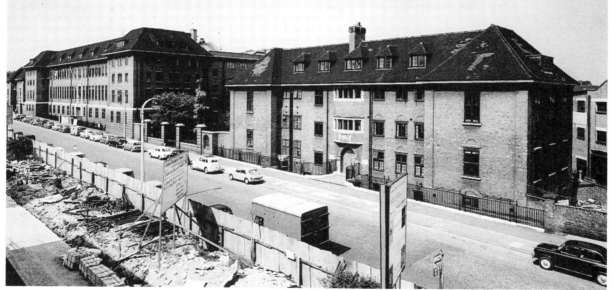

OPPOSITE ABOVE LEFT: Professor Lance Lanyon, Principal. (JF) RIGHT: The Queen Mother chats to a patient and members of staff, after opening the Queen Mother hospital in 1986. CENTRE LEFT TO RIGHT: Professor David Lodge; Professor Ian Smith; (JF) Professor David Noakes; BELOW LEFT TO RIGHT: Derek Gordon-Brown, College secretary; (JF) Professor Roger Batt; Professor 'JET' Jones; BELOW LEFT: Professor Lawrence Gerring. RIGHT: Professor Leslie Vaughan, Vice-Principal. LEFT: An enthusiastic welcome for the Queen, who obviously enjoyed touring the loose-boxes at Hawkshead. RIGHT: The Queen Mother at the official opening of the Northumberland hall of residence, 1965. BELOW: An impressive view of the Research Institute (right) and the main College building at Camden Town, taken in 1965 when the houses opposite had been demolished to make way for flats.

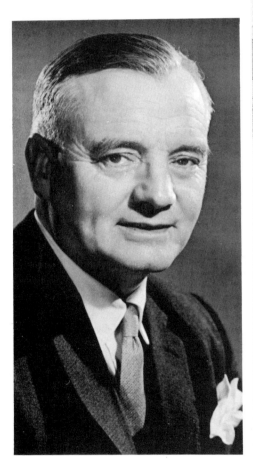

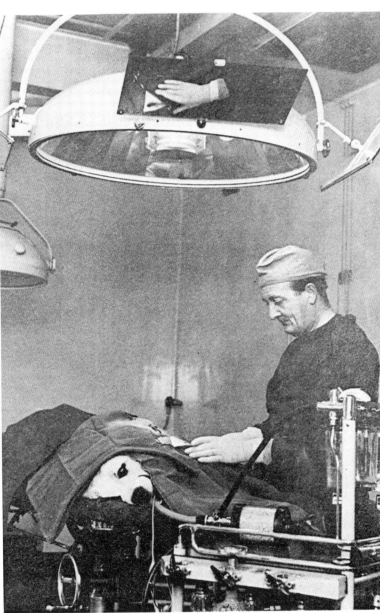

LEFT: Sir John Ritchie. RIGHT: Leslie Vaughan (then reader in veterinary surgery) operating in the Beaumont, 1970.

194

SIR JOHN RITCHIE

Principal and Dean 1965-1970

In 1960 the College was finally recognised as a school of London University, without time limit. The university abolished the BSc (VetSci) internal degree, and approved the award of a MVetMed degree. In 1966, the degree of DVetMed was approved, and the first course for the diploma in animal health (now the MSc in animal health) was initiated, followed in October 1969 by the MSc in veterinary pathology.

John Neish ('Joe') Ritchie (1904-1977) who became Principal of the College on 1 October 1965, was born at Turriff in Aberdeenshire. He was educated at Turriff secondary school and then at the 'Dick', qualifying MRCVS in 1925, DVSM in 1926, and BSc in 1927. He was clinical assistant at the Edinburgh school for six months, then became assistant veterinary officer in the veterinary service of the City of Edinburgh, and (in 1925) veterinary officer for Midlothian.

From 1935, when he was appointed senior veterinary officer in the department of agriculture, Scotland, John Ritchie became actively involved in the control and eradication of bovine tuberculosis. His achievements were recognised by the Bledisloe Veterinary Award of the Royal Agricultural Society of England in 1961. A succession of promotions within the state veterinary service culminated in his appointment as chief veterinary officer in 1952. From 1959-65 Ritchie was chairman of the European Commission for the control of foot-and-mouth disease, and there is no doubt that his efforts in this sphere contributed materially to the relative freedom from this disease which Britain has enjoyed over the years. He was created CB in 1955, FRSE in 1957 and was knighted in 1961.

Sir John was president of the Royal College for two consecutive years (1959-61) and from the time of his election to Royal College council in 1952 was actively concerned with all aspects of veterinary education. When he retired from the ministry in 1965 to become College Principal, he was chairman of the FAO/WHO expert panel on veterinary education. The recipient of honorary degrees from universities in Liverpool, Toronto and Edinburgh, he served on numerous national agricultural and scientific bodies.

Just before he retired, Sir John was instrumental in getting the College council to set up a committee to consider the future location of the College. He had presided over a period of further substantial building development at Hawkshead, including the transfer of the department of animal husbandry and veterinary hygiene to the Boltons Park site, and the construction of the medicine extension to the clinical block at Hawkshead. It was natural, therefore, that he saw the future of the College in terms of consolidation of all its activities in Hertfordshire. It was an expansionist period in universities generally, following the Robbins report of 1963 and new university campuses were springing up all over the country on green field sites. The urge for the College to follow suit, when funds for new building were to be had almost for the asking, must have been well nigh irresistible. There were many on the College council who held a similar view and so the scene was set for the conflict which was to trouble the College for the next 20 years, when those who believed in consolidation at Hawkshead were to be at loggerheads with those who had serious misgivings about the academic merits of such a move. In the paper which prompted the College council to establish its fact-finding committee in March 1970, Ritchie said:

'Having viewed the situation for a few years I incline to the belief that the best arrangement for the RVC, provided money and planning permission can be obtained, is that eventually the College should be on one site at Hawkshead, but that it must be recognised that efforts be made to —

  (i) allow staff to maintain contacts with colleagues and facilities in London
 (ii) allow students the same opportunities
(iii) provide multi-collegiate halls of residence in north London
 (iv) make contacts with nearby academic institutes
  (v) provide ample accommodation for postgraduate students in a variety of disciplines.'

Thus the period of Sir John Ritchie's principalship, though short, was, in a historical context, significant. He completed further steps of the development programme at Hawkshead planned by his predecessor, and his paper to the governing body of the College reveals him to be the architect of further substantial change. It fell to his successor, Alan Betts, to be the agent of this change.

Ritchie was noted for his unaffectedly dignified manner, his patent sincerity and his personal courtesy. He was flexible and imaginative in his approach to problems. He liked the students and they liked and respected him.

In 1968 Michael Jukes succeeded Amoroso as professor of physiology. Until the two preclinical departments were merged in 1987, he was head of the department of physiology, biochemistry and pharmacology. Appointed Vice-Principal (Camden) he had a genuine sympathy for generations of students. He died in office in January 1989.

Leslie Vaughan, who joined the surgery department as house surgeon when he qualified from the College in 1949, was appointed reader in veterinary surgery in 1968. His flair for orthopaedic surgery was obvious from the start and, while still at Streatley, he began carrying out disc fenestrations in dogs suffering from intervertebral disc protrusion, pioneering the technique in this country. He was awarded his FRCVS for this work, and went on to achieve another breakthrough by inserting hip prostheses in cats and dogs, initially using the same model as that employed in human surgery. Now an international authority on equine, bovine and canine orthopaedics, and a foundation diplomate in veterinary radiology, he has been professor of veterinary orthopaedics since 1972, and was appointed Vice-Principal of the College in 1982. Professor Vaughan was president of the Royal College in 1987-88. He has been awarded the RCVS Francis Hogg prize and the BSAVA Bourgelat and Simon awards.

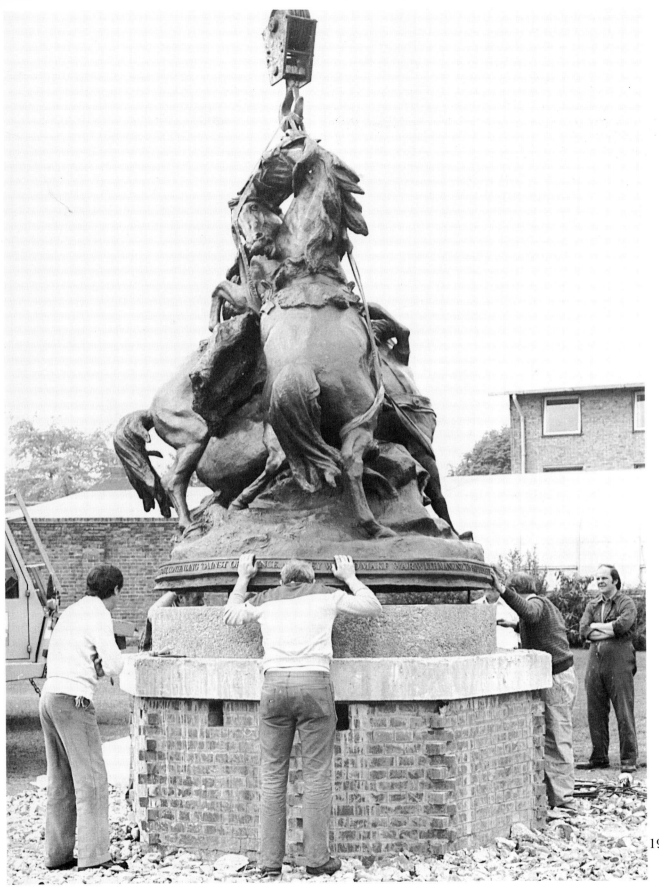

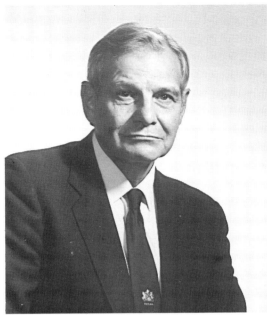

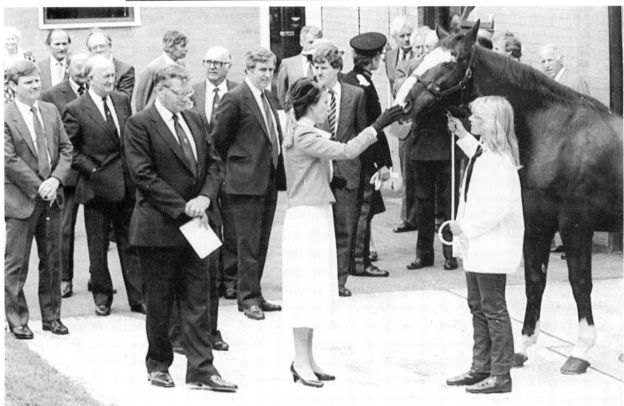

OVERLEAF: The massive bronze cast of Duncan's Horses is lowered into place at Hawkshead in 1985. ABOVE: Dr Alan Betts. BELOW: The Princess Royal (then Princess Anne) opened the Sefton wing of the equine hospital in 1986 and thoroughly inspected the patients. Also in the picture (on left) Professor Vaughan, Dr Alan Betts and Derek Gordon-Brown.

ALAN OSBORN BETTS —

Principal and Dean 1970-1988

When Alan Betts became Principal and dean in 1970, following the retirement of Sir John Ritchie, he suggested that his appointment should in the first instance be for five years only. The College council confirmed that they hoped he would serve until his retirement. However, when publication of the Riley committee's report became imminent, Betts announced that he intended to retire four years early to make way for a new Principal, who could have a reasonable expectation of serving long enough to guide the College through changing and perhaps difficult times.

Alan Betts was born on 11 March 1927 at Wroxham near Norwich. His father was a butcher and farmer. He was educated at Paston Grammar school, where Nelson was once a pupil. He became a student at the College in 1944, taking the BSc course in veterinary science to supplement the normal MRCVS course, so that in 1949 he graduated BSc in the University of London, and became a member of the Royal College. From 1949-1950 Betts was an assistnat in general practice. In 1950 he became a research student, with a scholarship of the Animal Health Trust, at Magdalene College, Cambridge. He graduated MA in 1952 and PhD in 1953. From 1952 to 1956 he was university demonstrator in bacteriology in the University of Cambridge School of Veterinary Medicine. He spent 1955-56 on sabbatical leave at Cornell University with a Commonwealth Fund Harkness Fellowship and, while in the USA, went on to enrol on an executive development programme at the Cornell Graduate School of Business and Administration.

From 1956-64 Betts was university lecturer in virology and in charge of the animal virus research laboratory in the Cambridge University school. In 1964, on the retirement of R. Lovell, professor of bacteriology, he became professor of microbiology and parasitology in the College. One of his major contributions as departmental head was the construction of a virus laboratory/gnotobiotic complex by conversion of the pathology museum, part of the former research institute in animal pathology, and the disused 'ride'.

Just before Betts became Principal, the College council set up a small committee 'to establish the facts and sound the opinion of the various interests of the College on the question of the removal of the whole College to Hawkshead and Boltons Park'. Urged on by a visit in 1971 by the veterinary sub-committee of the University Grants Committee, the council later that year voted in favour of consolidating the College at its field station site. It was noted that two important assumptions were the basis of the decision. Firstly, that it would not be possible to build a new Royal Veterinary College on a more suitable site in another university, and secondly, that the development of the Camden Town site for preclinical teaching in a single-faculty or multi-faculty school would not at that time be acceptable to London University or to the University Grants Committee.

After the College council's vote, the university, which may have been worried by the strength of conflicting opinions in the College, set up its own committee under the chairmanship of the dean of the London School of Hygiene and Tropical Medicine, Dr C. E. Gordon-Smith, 'to consider and report on the academic merit of consolidating the activities of The Royal Veterinary College at Potters Bar, or other possible arrangements, and on the academic priority to be accorded to the associated expenditure'.

Also in 1973, the Murray committee on the governance of the University of London suggested the integration of minor university schools. The College held talks with Westfield and Bedford Colleges, and staff from Queen Elizabeth College visited the field station on 26 March, but nothing concrete happened.

The Gordon-Smith report in 1973 was not particularly helpful, in that the College's recommendation of consolidation at Hawkshead was only supported by a minority of the committee; an alternative recommendation was that the possibility of moving the whole College to another university should be investigated. The majority advocated short-term improvements to the buildings at Camden Town, and the removal of parts of the department of pathology and the Beaumont animals' hospital, and indeed all clinical facilities to Hawkshead. The Camden Town site would be retained for preclinical studies.

Frustrated for years on the major issue of location, not least because of the lack of funds, Alan Betts continued to press the College forward with a number of other important initiatives. The establishment of the farm animal practice teaching unit, the continuing education unit, the laboratory animal science unit (with the first MSc course in this country in the subject), the clinical residency programme and the first chair of veterinary molecular and cellular biology were highly successful. It was an exciting era for the College, in spite of the general gloom in universities, and that excitement was stimulated largely by the restless energy of the Principal.

Betts saw the need for non-university funding to ensure survival and so established the RVC Animal Care Trust. He saw the importance of public relations and appointed the College's first public relations officer. He appreciated the need for specialisation, so that the College became the first UK school to have a substantial period for electives in the final year. He also enthusiastically supported the principle of clinical residencies so that on his retirement there were more residencies within the College than in the rest of the country's veterinary schools put together. Alan Betts also saw the importance of the European connection and seized the opportunity to attend meetings in Europe which it presented. In addition to participating in European committees he established the research and teaching connection between the College and the Munich veterinary school. His interest and vision encompassed more than the College itself and he played an important role in the university as deputy vice-chancellor, the first Principal of the College to hold such office.

However, it became increasingly clear that, if the College was to overcome financial problems arising from the obsolescence of many of its buildings and a shortage of funds from the university, it must do more to help itself. Much had been achieved by the successful pursuit of grants for research from trusts, commerce and industry, and by generous support for new buildings at Hawkshead, where the Home of Rest for Horses and the Horserace Betting Levy Board had been particularly generous. It now seemed worth exploring the possibility of tapping wider-based public resources. After a review of College priorities, a feasibility study reported in 1980 on the potential for a public appeal for funds to finance the building and endowment of a new small animal hospital. The College then proceeded to establish a registered charity, the Royal Veterinary College Animal Care Trust. Its aims are to provide facilities for the relief of pain and suffering in animals, and to establish teaching posts in the general field of animal care and welfare; to educate animal owners in matters of animal health, care and welfare, and to provide continuing education for veterinary graduates; to reduce the number of animals used in experiments through improved training of those responsible for laboratory animals, and the development of alternative methods of experimentation.

The Queen Mother agreed to become patron of the Trust, which was launched in March 1982. Its first function was to establish a pet animals referral hospital on the Hawkshead campus, and the initial phase of the hospital, which cost £1.25 million, was declared open and named after herself by the Queen Mother in November 1986. Next, the equine and surgical facilities at Hawkshead were modernised and expanded in a new equine hospital. The Princess Royal (then Princess Anne) opened the Sefton surgical wing of the equine hospital in June 1986. The cost was £500,000 of which £300,000 was generously provided by the Home of Rest for Horses to mark their centenary and as a tribute to one of their inmates — Sefton, a retired army horse who was badly injured by terrorist action, but restored to health by veterinary skill.

Betts also had the satisfaction of presiding at a ceremony on 26 June 1985 when the Duke of Edinburgh, patron of the College, unveiled the bronze cast of Duncan's Horses in front of Hawkshead House. Adrian Jones, the veterinary surgeon turned sculptor produced this masterpiece in 1892, inspired by Shakespeare's description in Macbeth. The plaster cast of the statue went on show at the Crystal Palace where it was damaged — fortunately not seriously — in the disastrous fire which destroyed in 1936. The following year, Adrian Jones offered the group to the College, and an appeal initiated by Major G. W. Dunkin raised enough money for the plaster cast to be repaired. There was talk of an appeal to cover the cost (at that time estimated at £900) of a bronze cast, but the war intervened. Duncan's Horses languished in Maples depository in Camden Town until 1967, when the group was transported to Hawkshead, coated with polyester resin and placed on a plinth on the lawn.

Unfortunately the cast did not stand up to damage by wind and rain, and by 1983 the College was faced with a major problem of rescue and restoration. A second appeal was launched, with the Duke of Edinburgh as patron. Adrian Jones's great-nephew, James Cunningham (who qualified from the College in 1953), organised the first-ever exhibition of the sculptor's works at the Sladmore Gallery in London — whose director Edward Horswell generously donated all profits to the appeal fund. The animal sculptor Geoffrey Tiney carried out the restoration, and the life-size bronze casting, which weighs about three tons, was made by Burleighfield Arts Foundry. The major contribution to the appeal fund by an American benefactor, Paul Mellon (former president of the National Gallery of Art, Washington) is commemorated on the plaque at the base of the statuary group. Mr Mellon was present at the unveiling, and was presented with a scroll by Prince Philip to mark his election as a fellow of the College.

During Alan Betts's period as Principal, the loyalty of former students to the College was demonstrated by the growing strength of the Royal Veterinary College Alumnus Association. Founded in the mid-1950s as the RVC Association, the organisation was reconstituted in 1978, with Betts's vigorous support, as the RVC Alumnus Association under the leadership of Michael Young. Since then, with a succession of presidents and council members, the association's activities, membership and influence have all grown. The objectives have been widened to promote contact between past graduates, present staff and students and to foster a variety of activities for the general benefit of the College.

Members of RVCAA council have become members of College council, the association nominates some members of the curriculum committee, it has been active in promoting the London-Munich exchange symposia and it provided vital support for the Animal Care Trust and the Unit for Veterinary Continuing Education in their formative stages. On the ceremonial side, the association provided the College mace and gowns for the Students' Union president and vice-president. Support for student activities has included financial help for a number of ventures, notably a casebook medal, research team expeditions, individual overseas projects, and a new racing eight. Not least, the association has been active in helping to organise the celebration of the College's bicentenary.

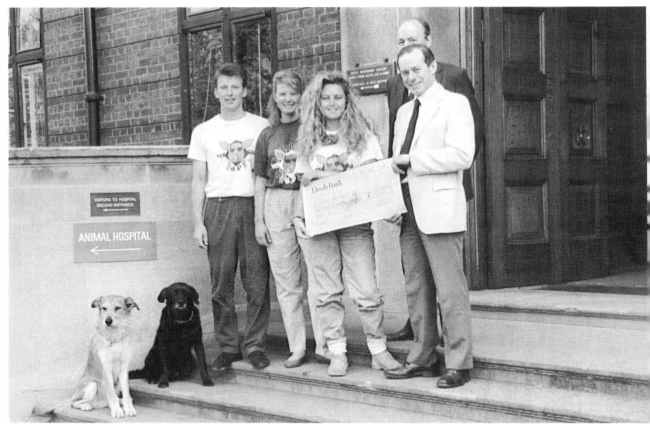

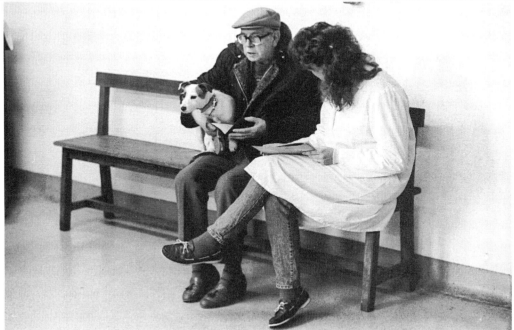

ABOVE: Professor Lance Lanyon receives a cheque for £2,200 raised for the RVC Animal Care Trust in student Rag Week, from Michael Griffith, Julie Johnson and Liz Forbes, January 1989. (JF) BELOW: A student in a clinical undergraduate duty group takes a case history at the Beaumont hospital. (JF)

PART V

Facing the Future

LANCE EDWARD LANYON

Principal and Dean 1989-

When Alan Betts retired, he was succeeded in January 1989 by Professor Lance Lanyon, the head of the department of veterinary basic sciences. His tenure as Principal has, as yet, been short but filled with activity. A major review of the curriculum has been undertaken, the long vacant chair in veterinary medicine has been filled, and the clinical departments restructured from the old divisions of medicine, surgery and animal husbandry, into small animal studies, large animal studies, and animal health. The building programme has increased in pace, over £2 million being spent in 1990 to upgrade research laboratories at both Camden Town and Hawkshead, to start the second phase of the Queen Mother hospital, and to build a new 30-bed student hall of residence. This will be named Odiham Hall in recognition of the College's origins. His activity has not been confined to the College, since he has also been appointed to the Court of the University of London. His representations to the university may have had some effect because, for the first time in many years, the annual Court grant has allowed a year in which the College has not had to make financial cuts.

Lance Lanyon represents the generation of veterinarians who grew up after the war and graduated from one of the six veterinary schools recommended by the Loveday Report. Lanyon was born in south London in 1944. His father, a cable engineer, had been a manager of various cable stations in the Pacific for Cable and Wireless, and when he died in 1948 the family was poor. At the age of 10 Lanyon went as a boarder to the City of London Bluecoat school, Christs Hospital, at Horsham. His holidays were spent mostly with family friends in Wiltshire. It was there, working on a dairy farm and attending John Parsons's practice in Trowbridge, that he decided to become a veterinarian, entering the Bristol school in 1961.

He qualified in 1966, and in 1972 married a fellow Bristol graduate, Mary Kear. After qualifying he returned to the anatomy department to do a PhD supervised by R. N. (Dick) Smith. He became an assistant lecturer in 1967 and progressed through the academic ranks to reader in 1978. However, in 1977 he had taken a sabbatical year to work at the Museum of Comparative Zoology at Harvard. He found both Boston and America irresistible and, when Tufts University founded their veterinary school, he left Bristol to join it. While there he was promoted to full professor, but nevertheless left in 1984 to join the RVC as head of the department of anatomy, later becoming head of the combined basic sciences department.

Lanyon's research interests have always centred around the mechanisms by which the structure of the skeleton is maintained appropriate for its functional loadbearing. Soon after gaining his own PhD he began maintaining a research team, and continues to do so despite his duties as Principal.

In the rest of this chapter Professor Lanyon gives an account of the College's recent history.

The 1960s were a time of unparalleled opportunity. Money for education was freely available and the establishment of a substantial national role for the Royal Veterinary College should have been attainable. Alas, periods of plenty rarely encourage the same enterprise and fertility of thought as when resources are hard to find. It is easy for those trying to lead the College in the institutional austerity of the late 1980s and early '90s to be critically envious of those who led it in the lotus years of the 1960s. However, the RVC entered the 1980s without a uniformly strong internal research base and without any associated supporting institutions such as the veterinary investigation centres at Cambridge and Bristol, the centre for tropical diseases at Edinburgh, and the tsetse fly research institute and food research institute at Bristol.

Alan Betts's principalship saw the development of the 'field station' into the 'Hawkshead campus'. The clinical facilities were vastly improved including, by the time he left, the Sefton equine hospital and phase 1 of the Queen Mother hospital for small animals. These developments were established using funds from a variety of sources including the university, the College's own resources, and money raised by the Animal Care Trust. The upgrading of Hawkshead was a substantial achievement but was only part of Betts's overall plan. His overriding objective was to complete the plans put forward by John Ritchie in 1970 and abandon the College's premises at Camden Town, consolidating everything on one site at Hawkshead. The consolidation policy never received the wholehearted approval of the academic staff, although Academic Board did approve the move 'preferably in association with a multifaculty institution'. As so often happens with such provisos this one became diluted and then buried. By backing the scheme for consolidation the College council set the scene for the difficult situation where council and Principal were seeking a radical solution which many in the academic community thought undesirable. Those most strongly of this latter view were not unnaturally the preclinicians who occupied the campus at Camden Town.

The strongest preclinical department was that which between 1946 and 1968 had been led by Professor Amoroso. It was a strength his successor was unable to sustain. The anatomy department, which never had a strong research base, also lost influence as the personalities with which it was populated, retired or left. This decline in preclinical influence in the 1970s and early '80s was accompanied by deterioration of the buildings at Camden Town. The increasing cost of the maintenance backlog, the perceived inconvenience and the general undesirability of the Camden Town location tended to reinforce attempts to get the College moved to Hawkshead. In 1987 Richard Barlow, Ernest Cotchin's recently appointed successor as professor of pathology, agreed that the pathology department's future was at Hawkshead. This move was immediately put into effect and the pathologists quit the building which McFadyean had established some 60 years before, leaving it sparsely populated by microbiologists.

What proved to be the final throw in the campaign to move from Camden Town was to put the premises on the market. This was done in 1987. The last nurses were removed from the Beaumont hospital to the Queen Mother hospital at Hawkshead, and bids were awaited.

At the same time as these developments were occurring within the College, the government was vigorously pursuing its policies of cost-effectiveness in higher education. It had been decided by the University Grants Committee (at that time the organ through which the government funded the universities) that each of the UK veterinary schools was too small to be cost-effective, and that they should be rationalised into larger single or co-operative units. Two schools were not to be allowed to continue in Scotland. In England, the geographical pairs of Bristol and Liverpool, and London and Cambridge were to come to an arrangement which preferably (from the UGC point of view) would involve the voluntary liquidation of one in each pair. The RCVS would act as midwife to these unlikely events.

The one certain result of this sabre-rattling from the UGC was that the profits of British Telecom soared, as old friends and enemies discussed improbable alliances and schemes by which as much as possible could appear to happen with minimal actual change to the *status quo*. The first meeting between senior academics of the London and Cambridge schools occurred at Hawkshead. Fired by the urgency and seriousness of the situation it was agreed by the senior staff of both schools to proceed on the basis of a single school for the south-east. The head of the Cambridge school, Professor Lawson Soulsby, demurred and the scope of the negotiations declined from that moment.

For the preclinicians of the London school, the choice was not straightforward. Although all favoured retention of both preclinical and clinical departments at the RVC, a number now considered that a single school in the south-east, in which the preclinical departments would be at Cambridge and the clinical departments at Hawkshead, was more viable than the situation in which preclinical departments were isolated by being moved to the College's clinical campus. In other words, for a preclinician, Cambridge was a better academic option than Hawkshead.

This message was scarcely popular within the College but was nevertheless relayed quietly to Cambridge, where it received support at least from the middle ranks of the academic staff and those intimately connected with veterinary teaching. It was however, not accepted by the heads of the Cambridge preclinical departments, who did not want the disruption to the medical tripos that more veterinary students might entail. As soon as this veto became apparent the chances of any meaningful collaboration between the two schools ceased, because the solution which would have played to the strengths of both schools, namely a preclinical course at Cambridge and a clinical course at London, was no longer available.

The level of agreement at the end of this RCVS-sponsored attempt at rationalisation stretched only to some joint teaching and swapping of expertise on matters in which few at that time were interested, such as poultry and food hygiene. The Bristol and Liverpool schools could only agree that they had nothing meaningful to say to one another. However, Edinburgh and Glasgow, faced with the written statement from the UGC that there should be no more than one school in Scotland, produced a scheme whereby a single cohort of students would spend two years in Edinburgh and two years in Glasgow, with one year between the two. It was political expediency written large and commonsense written small. Nevertheless, it was a definite agreement between two of the six schools. If Cambridge had seized their opportunity to make an offer that London could not have refused, four schools out of six would have reached a voluntary agreement, the subsequent phases of the process might never have happened, and the largest single change in the Royal Veterinary College's history might now be under way. As it was, faced with the reluctance of all the English schools to negotiate any significant diminution of their sovereignty, the UGC appointed a working party under the previous secretary of the Agricultural and Food Research Council, Sir Ralph Riley, to resolve the situation. Despite the agreement reached in Scotland, this working party was to visit all the UK schools, take evidence from them, and make its report.

After the appointment of the Riley working party it was obvious that the members within each school would have to present a united front, since the name of the game was no longer co-operation but individual survival. It was also obvious that, if the College's preclinical departments were in any case set to leave Camden Town for Hawkshead, Riley might well recommend they keep going northward to Cambridge, regardless of the reservations of their prospective hosts. Since the sale bids for the Camden Town premises were inadequate to fund the removal of the whole College to Hawkshead, the scene was set for a revision of the consolidation policy.

Some months before this, the University of London had asked Sir James Lighthill, provost of University College, to set up a working party to produce the liaison with Cambridge. When this phase was superseded by the establishment of the Riley committee, the Lighthill working party stayed in being. They deliberated long enough for Sir James and his committee to recommend that the academically sensible solution for the RVC was to remain on two sites. He gained his committee's acceptance for this proposal by suggesting that relevant elements of University College could share the Camden Town premises and occupy the space which had been vacated by the pathologists a few months earlier. At a stroke, Lighthill had contributed to solving his own problem of accommodation at UCL, thrown a cloak of respectable association over the Camden Town campus which had always been criticised for isolation, and placed the University of London firmly on the side of continued two-site operation.

In January 1988, only weeks before the submission to the Riley committee had to be made, the College's academic board met to debate a motion proposed by Professor Smith (head of the department of pathology) and Professor Jones (head of the department of medicine and animal husbandry). This motion stated that 'the College's policy, which will be put to the Riley Committee, shall consist of development both at Camden Town and Hawkshead campuses, the Camden campus to be occupied in part by components of the RVC and other relevant biomedical units from the University, principally University College'.

It was the best attended academic board meeting for years. The motion was supported by a paper from Lance Lanyon, the professor and head of the department of anatomy. Following this paper, member after member spoke in favour of two-site operation. The final vote was 27 in favour, none against. The only abstention was from Professor Leslie Vaughan, the Vice Principal of the College and himself a member of the Riley committee. This vote, which Council had to endorse, was an absolute rejection of the existing consolidation policy at a time when equivocation would have been dangerous. The policy placed before the Riley committee was for two site operation. Alan Betts announced his resignation in the summer of 1988. In the autumn of 1988, with no whisper of how the Riley deliberations were going, the College faced the task of recruiting a new Principal with the fate of the College still in doubt. It was not surprising in these circumstances that it was an internal candidate, Lance Lanyon, who became the College's 15th Principal on 1 January 1989. Twenty days later the Riley report was published.

The basis of the report was how to maintain standards in schools with too few students to command the necessary resources. The recommended solution was a reduction in the number of schools, to be achieved by the formation of a single Scottish veterinary school on the Edinburgh site, and closure of the clinical part of the Cambridge school. The uproar, particularly in Scotland, was predictable. No other school could have mounted a campaign like that put on by Glasgow, although the Cambridge school was scarcely less energetic. The RCVS, which only months before would have been relieved to have attained Riley's recommendations from the schools voluntarily, now trumpeted its disapproval. 'Support Glasgow Veterinary School' stickers appeared on thousands of cars, and within months 700,000 people had signed a petition to save Glasgow and 400,000 a similar one to save Cambridge.

The government's response was as predictable as that of the profession's, namely to establish another working party. This group, under the chairmanship of Dr Ewan Page (vice-chancellor of Reading University) was directed to examine one of the prime constraints accepted by Riley, that of the total number of veterinary students needed in the university system. Unfortunately, included within its terms of reference were the implications for the public purse of the high cost of veterinary education.

The three-man Page committee contained no veterinary educationalists, took no written education evidence and visited no veterinary schools. Just before Christmas 1989 the report was submitted to the Secretaries of State for Agriculture and Education, who had commissioned it. It was published on 31 January 1990, one year and eleven days after the Riley report.

The Page report was seen as unsatisfactory in many respects to the veterinary profession. It pronounced that the nation required a core of 400 students annually (a five-school solution by Riley standards) and yet it recommended the continuance of six schools. This recommendation was seized upon and accepted without delay by the Universities Funding Committee, which had replaced the UGC. How then to support six schools with the student capacity for only five? Page's answer was simple. Pay less for each student and, if the schools had to take more students (to cover their shortfall in income), then let them charge all the students an appropriate amount. This was a departure from the existing arrangements in many ways. It removed veterinary education from manpower planning constraints and gave influence over the numbers entering the profession to the schools, rather than the government. However, this could only be achieved by departure from one of the fixed points in higher education policy, which was that tuition fees should be paid from the public purse, through the block grant to the universities from the UFC, and from student fees from the local education authorities.

In its initial response to the Page report, the Royal Veterinary College rejected the proposal to charge students for tuition, as did the University of London and all the other veterinary schools except Bristol. At the time of the report's publication, the government was under heavy fire for introducing a bill to change the basis of students' maintenance funding from grants to loans. Consequently, there was hesitation all round in grasping the particular nettle of simultaneously introducing a means for charging students for tuition. This suggestion by Page may remain just a proposal, but it remains embedded in the paperwork of higher education bureaucracy, ready to be activated when the time is ripe.

The local problem of veterinary education, while achieving a public prominence disproportionate to its size or importance, is only a component of the national shake-up in higher education as a whole in 1990. The Royal Veterinary College is not, and will not be immune from these national pressures.

As a small specialist school within the federal University of London, the College leads a precarious if exciting existence, understaffed academically in the face of increasing professional demands, understaffed administratively to deal with both the 'opportunities' of freedom and the constraints of accountability. Its place never seems quite secure in the university federation, because there are always those who assume that small schools cannot cope, and would be cheaper if they were part of larger units. Efforts to achieve this 'rationalisation' have up to now been frustrated because the College is inconvenient enough in its requirements of using large, live animals, dissecting rooms, hospitals, farms etc. to make amalgamation with another college within London impracticable.

Assuming that this state of affairs continues, and that the College maintains its independent existence, the preferred policy is that which provides the optimum conditions for both its clinical and preclinical components; namely continued two-site operation. In this the College is only following the same path as all the other UK veterinary schools except Glasgow. However, for the College to capitalise fully on its opportunities there must be a greatly enhanced concentration on the basic sciences at one end in order to fill the Camden Town buildings with home-generated activity, and increased research activity at the clinical end, which at present relies more heavily on its clinical service role than on research. Unfortunately, although the research activity must increase, this cannot be at the expense of clinical work, since this must also increase in order to pay for the numbers of staff and quality of facilities which the public purse refuses to finance. How to achieve this expansion and at the same time enhance quality in all these areas, with only a limited number of students inadequately funded by the public purse, is the challenge for the 1990s.

Again and again in the College's history, despite severe economic pressure, it has managed not only to survive but to advance. Such is the present situation. In 1986 a chair in molecular biology was established at the College, followed in 1990 by a chair in laboratory animal science and welfare. Both of these were firsts for any UK veterinary school. Also during that period, three titles of professor, those of veterinary surgical science, veterinary pharmacology and veterinary parasitology were conferred on members of the College staff. This level of achievement is not characteristic of an institution in decline; quite the reverse. One reason why such advances can be made despite economic difficulty is that a small, single-subject school can concentrate all its efforts on a relatively narrow front, and can then make significant progress in that direction.

In 1990 the College is in a period of rapid internal change. The clinical departments are being reconstructed to focus attention in the main functional areas of veterinary concern — animal health, small animal studies and farm animal studies. Whether these divisions will prove to be more enduring or relevant to modern times than the original divisions of medicine, surgery, and animal husbandry remains to be seen, but over the period 1989-1992 the total leadership of the College will alter. New leaders need to initiate change in order to unfreeze the institutional *status quo* which often prevents them making improvements. The College is in that stage of creative upheaval at the moment. It is an upheaval which is not confined to the academic side of the house.

For much of the College's history, the council or board of governors was a glittering array of the aristocracy, chosen presumably to guarantee influence in high places. There is little tangible evidence that during this century much real benefit resulted. In the post-war period, the character of the council changed from the glittering to the worthy. Until the early 1980s the College's financial position was secure and completely dependent upon central government funds. Meeting some three or four times a year, the council's role in such times was little more than to ensure that the Principal and his colleagues did not plunge the College into debt. As times grew harder in the late 1980s, it became increasingly important for the College to have influential friends willing to further its interests wherever they could.

In December 1989 the term of appointment on council of John Moss, the current chairman, was due to expire, and it was decided to approach Lord Prior to succeed him. Jim Prior had a long record as a cabinet minister before he finally quit national politics to become chairman of GEC. A farmer and a former Secretary of State for Agriculture, with a sharp business sense, and all the connections resulting from his many years in high office, he seems an ideal choice to lead the College. We hope his appointment marks the beginning of a new active phase for the council, in which its members will increasingly act as effective agents, friends, and advocates for the College in the political, financial and business arenas of the country.

The celebrations surrounding the bicentenary, for which this book is being written, will undoubtedly enhance the College's reputation and emphasise its position in the veterinary world. As 1990 draws to a close, these events are still in the future. However, if the plans are fulfilled there will be three days of active celebrations, followed like a comet by a summer of events no less important, but with a lower profile.

The most symbolic event of the bicentenary celebrations will be an honorary degree ceremony at Camden Town. This is the first time that any such event within a constituent college has been celebrated in this way by the University of London. Since the Princess Royal is both a Fellow of the College, and the Chancellor of the University, it was a delight that she agreed to confer the degree of Doctor of Veterinary Medicine on four graduands.

Two graduands were chosen from the profession, Henry Carter and Professor Bill Jarratt. Both men are eminent in their own right but also represent respectively the practising and scientific components of the veterinary profession.

Henry Carter qualified from the College in 1953 when entry into the profession was still gained by taking the examinations of the Royal College of Veterinary Surgeons, and not by a university degree. He worked in practice in North London but was always active in professional politics and interested in new professional opportunities, in particular those related to public health and Europe. At the time of the degree ceremony he will be senior vice-president of the RCVS, having been president the previous year.

Bill Jarrett's work on retroviruses in cats leapt into prominence with the advent of human AIDs. The research team he built in the Glasgow veterinary school, where he is professor of pathology, is probably the largest research unit in any veterinary school in the country. Although he has received honorary degrees from many other universities, the College hopes that to receive one on this particular occasion will be a tribute of singular significance for him.

The choice of Paul Mellon KBE is also a particularly happy one. A philanthropist, racehorse owner and art connoisseur, he has already provided the College with the funds to cast in bronze the Adrian Jones statue of Duncan's Horses which now stands at Hawkshead. A fellow of the College he represents the important sporting, cultural and artistic place held by animals within society. In an imaginative gesture to mark the bicentenary he has offered the College, as a gift, not only his painting of Eclipse by George Stubbs, but also a two-thirds size statue in bronze of this uniquely successful horse. The dimensions for the statue were derived from those in Vial de St Bel's book, written after he conducted the post-mortem and detailed dissections in 1789. It has been suggested that the attention St Bel received as a result of his association with Eclipse contributed to his being offered the appointment as first Professor of the College. If so, it is truly appropriate that the statue and the only Stubbs painting of Eclipse reputed to be made from life should find their way to the College two centuries later.

The fourth honorary graduand, Her Majesty Queen Elizabeth the Queen Mother, accompanied her husband, King George VI, to open the current Camden Town buildings on the last day of Hobday's principalship in 1937. Formerly Chancellor of the University of London, she also opened Northumberland Hall in 1965, and as patron of the College's Animal Care Trust Appeal she opened phase 1 of the Queen Mother hospital in 1986. In honouring her, the university is recognising the royal links of the Royal Veterinary College, as well as taking a unique opportunity to formally express its affection and gratitude to this gracious lady, who was born when the College was only nine years past its first centenary.

Addressing the opening session of the College on 1 October 1891, some two weeks before the official centenary celebrations the Principal, Professor Brown, said 'I am extremely happy to meet you at the conclusion of the 100th year of our existence as a profession, and I venture to express a hope — it may be a futile hope, but it is at any rate a pleasant one — that we may start a second century with the determination to do the best we can for the profession, so that those who celebrate the second centenary in the history of the College will be able then to say in reference to the progress of the veterinary profession, that it far outshone in brilliancy the advance of the first century'.

The loud cheers which, according to *The Veterinarian*, greeted his remarks should be echoed by all those who celebrate the bicentenary of the College in 1991. The progress achieved by the veterinary profession has been remarkable. The academic standard of the student intake is the highest in the university system, the profession's influence and responsibilities are increasing year by year, and its contribution to science reaches the same peaks as those in medicine. It is undoubtedly one of the most highly regarded of all professions in the United Kingdom. All those associated with the Royal Veterinary College can take pride in the knowledge that their College has played a unique part in achieving this status, by providing the greatest single contribution to veterinary science and practice during the life of the profession in this country.

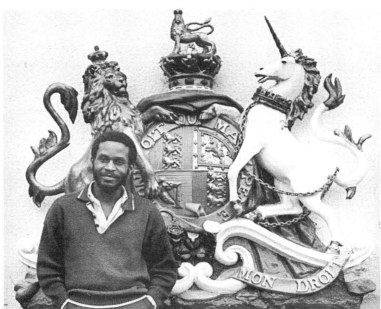

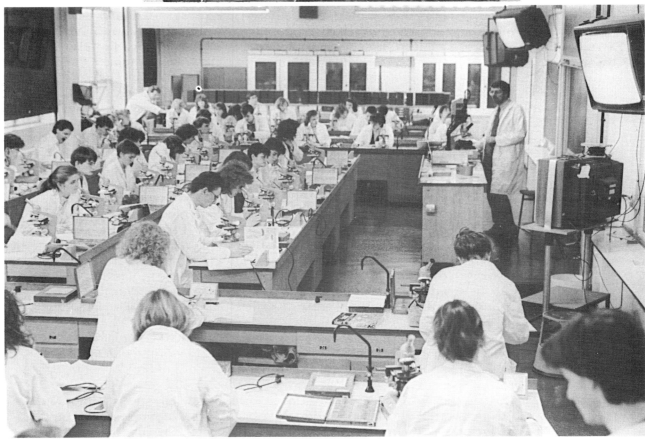

ABOVE: Cedric Lazarus (Jamaica), an MSc postgraduate student in animal health at Boltons Park, with the Coat of Arms rescued from the old Camden Town building. (JF) BELOW: Practical class in the histology teaching laboratory. (JF)

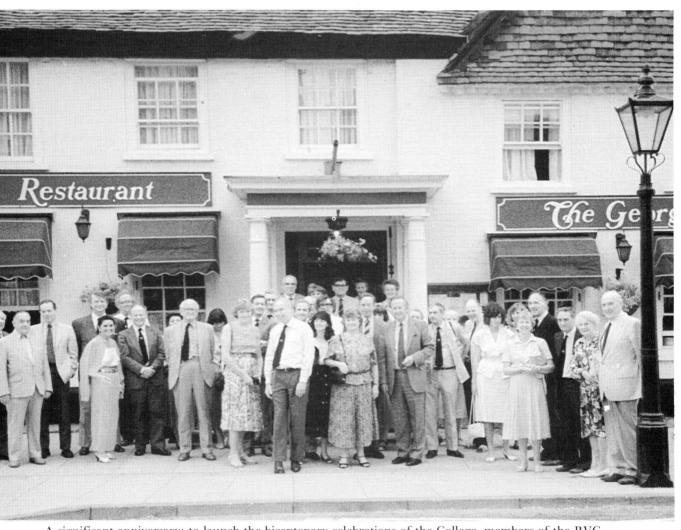

A significant anniversary: to launch the bicentenary celebrations of the College, members of the RVC Alumnus Association met at the George Hotel, Odiham, on 5 August 1990. It was on 5 August 1790 that the Odiham Agricultural Society, meeting in the same building — then the George Inn — reported the receipt from Vial of 10 copies of his plan for establishing in London 'an institution to teach veterinary medicine'. Following this meeting, events gathered momentum, culminating in the founding of the College the following year. Members of the Alumnus Association pictured above include Dame Olga Uvarov, Sir Gordon Shattock, Professor Clifford Formston, Professor Lance Lanyon, Professor J. E. T. Jones, Dr A. R. Michell, Miss Mary Brancker, Miss Connie Ford, Dr D. R. Lane, Dr H. Read, Dr D. D. Tyler, Miss S. Guthrie and Messrs A. Edney, H. E. Carter, M. Samuel, T. Turner, J. Heath, J. Brazier, O. Swarbrick, J. Cleverly, F. Trawford, K. Aspinall, J. Oliver and J. Broberg.

211

Academic staff

August 1990

DEPARTMENT OF VETERINARY BASIC SCIENCES
Head of Department — Professor D. Lodge

ANATOMY

Professor of Veterinary Anatomy	vacancy
Visiting Professor of Veterinary Anatomy	K.M. Dyce DVM&S BSc MRCVS
Senior Lecturer	N.C. Stickland BSc PhD
Lecturer	J.A. Bee BSc MSc PhD
Lecturer	Gurtej K. Dhoot BSc PhD
Lecturer	P.T. Loughna BSc PhD
Lecturer	P.J. O'Shaughnessy BSc PhD

BIOCHEMISTRY

Reader in Biochemistry	P.A. Mayes PhD DSc MIBiol CChem FRSC
Lecturer	Kathleen M. Botham BSc PhD
Lecturer	D.D. Tyler MA PhD

MOLECULAR AND CELLULAR BIOLOGY

Professor of Veterinary Molecular and Cellular Biology	G.E. Goldspink BSc PhD ScD CChem FRSC

PHARMACOLOGY

Professor of Veterinary Pharmacology	P. Lees BPharm PhD HonAssocRCVS
Lecturer	Fiona M. Cunningham BSc PhD
Lecturer	J. Elliott MA VetMB MRCVS

PHYSIOLOGY

Professor of Veterinary Physiology	D. Lodge BVSc DVA PhD MRCVS
Senior Lecturer	Jenifer M. Plummer JP BSc PhD
Senior Lecturer	P.F. Watson BVetMed BSc PhD MRCVS
Lecturer	S.D. Carrington BVM&S PhD CertOphthal MRCVS

DEPARTMENT OF VETERINARY PATHOLOGY
Head of Department — Professor I.M. Smith

MICROBIOLOGY AND PARASITOLOGY

Professor of Veterinary Microbiology and Parasitology	I.M. Smith MSc PhD MRCVS
Visiting Professor of Veterinary Microbiology	P.M. Biggs CBE DSc FRCVS FRCPath FIBiol FRS
Reader in Veterinary Virology	N. Edington BVSc PhD MRCVS
Senior Lecturer	P.H. Russell BVSc MSc PhD MRCVS
Lecturer	Mary E. Holt BSc BVetMed PhD MRCVS
Lecturer	J. Lida BVM&S PhD MRCVS

LABORATORY ANIMAL SCIENCE

Director	J. Bleby TD JP DVetMed DLAS FIBiol MRCVS
Lecturer	Nora Rozengurt MV MSc MRCVS
Lecturer	H.T. Donnelly BSc PhD

PARASITOLOGY

Professor of Veterinary Parasitology	D.E. Jacobs BVMS PhD MRCVS
Lecturer	M.T. Fox BVetMed PhD MRCVS

PATHOLOGY

Professor of Veterinary Pathology	R.M. Barlow BSc DVM&S DSc MRCVS
Reader in Veterinary Pathology	E.C. Appleby BSc PhD MRCVS
Lecturer	D.J. Humphreys BSc PhD CChem FRSC
Lecturer	Deborah J. Middleton BVSc MVSc PhD DipVetClinStud MRCVS
Lecturer	J.B.A. Smyth MVB MSc PhD MRCVS

Clinical Departments

Vice-Principal — Professor L. C. Vaughan DSc FRCVS DVR, Professor of Veterinary Surgery

DEPARTMENT OF ANIMAL HEALTH
Head of Department — Professor J.E.T. Jones

Courtauld Professor of Animal Health and Production	J.E.T. Jones PhD FRCPath MRCVS
Reader in Animal Husbandry	H.Ll. Williams BSc(Agric) MSc PhD FRAgS NDDH MIBiol
Senior Lecturer	A.J. Madel BA VetMB DipAH DipTCDHE MRCVS
Senior Lecturer	A.J. Wilsmore BVSc PhD MRCVS DipAH
Lecturer	J. Carr BVSc MRCVS CertPM
Lecturer	Mary Lanyon BVSc PhD MRCVS
Lecturer	Heather G. Pidduck BSc PhD
Lecturer	J.A. Stedman BSc PhD DipNutr

DEPARTMENT OF FARM ANIMAL AND EQUINE STUDIES
Head of Department — Professor E. E. L. Gerring

Professor of Veterinary Surgical Science	E.E.L. Gerring BVetMed PhD MRCVS
Professor of Veterinary Obstetrics and Diseases of Reproduction	D.E. Noakes BVetMed PhD FRCVS DVReprod
Reader in Veterinary Medicine	A.R. Michell BVetMed BSc PhD MRCVS
Senior Lecturer	W.E. Allen MVB PhD MRCVS
Senior Lecturer	A.H. Andrews BVetMed PhD MRCVS
Senior Lecturer	Kathleen W. Clarke MA VetMB DVetMed MRCVS DVA

Senior Lecturer	A.M. Johnston BVMS MRCVS
Senior Lecturer	P.M. Webbon BVetMed PhD MRCVS DVR
Lecturer	J.J. Covarr BSc BVSc MRCVS
Lecturer	R. Kyle MA BVSc MRCVS
Lecturer	D.G. White MA VetMB PhD MRCVS

DEPARTMENT OF SMALL ANIMAL STUDIES
Head of Department — Professor R. M. Batt

Professor of Clinical Veterinary Medicine	R.M. Batt BVSc PhD MSc MRCVS
Reader in Veterinary Ophthalmology	P.G.C. Bedford BVetMed PhD FRCVS DVOphthal
Senior Lecturer	B.M. Bush BVSc PhD FRCVS
Senior Lecturer [Director of Queen Mother Hospital]	D.G. Clayton Jones BVetMed MRCVS DVR
Senior Lecturer	D.H. Lloyd BVetMed PhD MRCVS
Lecturer	Serena E. Brownlie BVM&S PhD MRCVS
Lecturer	D.H. Scarff BVetMed MRCVS CertSAD
Lecturer	F.J. McEvoy MVB MRCVS DVR

UNIT OF VETERINARY CONTINUING EDUCATION

Director	Jennifer Poland OBE BVSc PhD MRCVS

COLLEGE SECRETARY	D.W. Gordon-Brown BA DMS
LIBRARIAN	Linda D. Warden BA ALA

BIBLIOGRAPHY

As far as we have been able to ascertain, the main sources used by Professor Cotchin were:

Archives, minute books and other documents owned by the Royal Veterinary College.

The Veterinarian published monthly 1928-1902.

The Veterinary Record, founded 1888 and still published weekly.

The Journal of Comparative Pathology & Therapeutics, published quarterly, 1888-1948, now in publication as *The Journal of Comparative Pathology.*

Minutes (in manuscript) of the Odiham Agricultural Society.

The Farrier & Naturalist 1828-29, vols 1 and 2.

Alder, Garry *Beyond Bokhara:* The life of William Moorcroft, Asian explorer, Century Publishing 1985.

Blaine, Delabere *The Outlines of the Veterinay Art* vol 1 Printed by A. Straham for T.N. Longman, London 1802.

Clark,, James *Treatise on the prevention of diseases incidental to horses,* James Clark, Edinburgh 1788.

Clark, James *First lines of veterinary physiology and pathology,* Vol 1, London 1806.

Clark. Bracy *A short history of the celebrated racehorse Eclipse* 1835.

Gray, Ernest *The Trumpet of Glory,* Robert Hale 1985.

Higgs, Edward *A Treatise on the best management of draught horses in the metropolis,* Highley & Son, London 1815.

McFadyean, J. *Recollected in Tranquility,* Pall Mall Press 1964.

Pattison, Iain *The British Veterinary Profession 1791-1948,* J.A. Allen 1984.

Pattison Iain *John McFadyean: A Great British Veterinarian,* J.A. Allen 1981.

Pugh, Leslie *From Farriery to Veterinary Medicine 1785-1795,* Heffer 1962.

Simonds, James Beart *The Foundation of the Royal Veterinary College 1790-1 with biographical sketches of St Bel, Edward Coleman, William Sewell and Charles Spooner,* Adlard & Son 1897.

Smith, Sir Frederick *The Early History of Veterinary Literature and its British Development,* (4 vols) Balliere, Tindall & Cox 1919 (reprinted 1976).

Taplin, William *The Gentleman's Stable Directory or Modern System of Farriery,* Robinson, London 1803.

An Account of the Veterinary College since its Institution in 1791, James Phillips, London 1793.

The Royal Veterinary College and Hospital commemorative brochure, The Royal Veterinary College, London 1937.

Veterinary History summer 1984 new series vol 3 no 3 (Sherwin A. Hall: The skeleton of Eclipse).

KEY TO CAPTION CREDITS

RCVS	Royal College of Veterinary Surgeons
JF	John Fisher
CL	Country Life Library
JC	John Clewlow
RNP	R.N. Phillips
UL	University of London Library
LBC	London Borough of Camden Local Studies Library
GLRO	Greater London Record Office (maps and prints)

ENDPAPERS — FRONT: Part of John Cary's map of London, c1790, before the College was built just north of Fig Lane; BACK: Laurie and Whittle's New Map of London, 1809, with the Veterinary College clearly shown. (UL)

Appendix 1

BIOGRAPHIES

Benoit Charles Marie Vial (1750-1793)
Much of the history of the College's first Principal remains uncertain. His own rather short firsthand account of his life appears in the *Preliminary Discourse* to his lectures, while the *Memoirs* of his life were prepared after his death, partly it seems from manuscripts in the hands of his widow, partly from the observations of the editor of the memoirs, and partly from information from Vial's admirers. The name of the editor of the memoirs is not directly stated, but Granville Penn, so active in the foundation of the College, is one strong possibility, as is another foundation governor, John Gretton MP. Some parts of Vial's own account of his life are open to serious doubt. He was approaching 40 when he came to England, and his widow, the Englishwoman he married in 1788, had no direct knowledge of his previous life in France.

Perhaps the most certain fact about our first Professor is that his family name was Vial. His name in full, as it appears in his widow's application for letters of administration (he died intestate), was Benoit Charles Marie Vial. His place of birth was almost certainly the village of Sain-Bel, some 12 miles north-west of Lyons, although the memoirs state that he was born in Lyons itself. Nothing seems to be known of his parents.

The statement in the memoirs that the Vial family had long had an estate called Sainbel and had, according to the custom in France before the 1789 Revolution, added this cognomen to that of Vial, is open to doubt. It is incompatible with information provided by Bracy Clark, who knew Vial well in England. He stated that Vial told him he had adopted the cognomen Sainbel himself. Whatever the truth of the matter, Vial, either by descent or by self-appointment, had acquired a cognomen, presumably based on the name of his birthplace — a village which for at least a century has been known as Sain-Bel, and which appears as such in the *Times World Atlas*, and was perhaps known as Sain-Bel in the late 18th century although in a published letter written in 1818 by Vial's niece Jeanne-Marie, she (or the printers) used the form Saint-Bel. It is curious that, while there are a large number of variations of the cognomen, only two writers appear to have used what would seem to be the then correct form of 'de Sain-Bel' — the anonymous author of an article entitled *Introspect and Retrospect* in the College students' union society magazine in 1932, and Dr Ernest Gray (who however, chose to use the form Sainbel).

The following list of variants of Vial's cognomen is largely based on a detailed letter from J. Barber-Lomax to the College, which had sought advice from him on the correct form to use when it was decided in 1963, at the prompting of Professor F. R. Bell, to commemorate Vial by a clinical prize. Apart from the 1932 magazine, the nearest approach to Sain-Bel is seen in the 1793 *Account of the Veterinary College*, where he is called Mr Sain Bel; the same spelling is found in a letter to Pitt from John Gretton MP, dated 25 July 1796, enquiring whether the copy of the memoirs sent to Downing Street had been read by Pitt — it had. The memoirs were published on behalf of Vial's widow, Mrs Sain Bel. In the *Sporting Magazine* of 1794 and 1795, the variants Sain Bel and Sainbel were used. The next closest variant is de Sainbel, which appears in Vial's *Lectures on the Veterinary Art*, in the memorial edition of his works, on the engraving from the original painting in the possession of Mrs Sainbel, in Bracy Clark's short history of the racehorse Eclipse, in Joseph Gamgee's *History of Horse-shoeing* (1864) and in Equus's letter on Eclipse. This form, Sainbel, is preferred by Smith, and (with some reservations) by Barber-Lomax himself. (The form Saenbel, in the index to Pugh's book, must be a printing error.)

As was pointed out at the end of the last century by Cornevin, the prefix 'Sain' in the cognomen had inexplicably acquired in Vial's lifetime an unwarranted final 't', as perhaps had the name of his native village. While 'Bel' figures in Assyro-Babylonian mythology as 'Lord of the World', it has not been possible to trace any saint called 'Bel'. This mutation has given rise to what may be called Saint Bel or St Bel variations: Vial-de-Saint Bel; Vial de Saint Bel; Mr Saint-Bel; Mr Saint Bell; Saintbel; Vial de St Bel; Viall de St Bel; M St Bel; St Bel; Charles Vial de St Bell; Viel de St Bel. In a letter to Huntingford, dated 12 January 1791, the signature appears as Vial De Saint Bel. On the other hand, Blaine is said to have had a letter signed simply St Bel, and this is now perhaps the most widely used form of Vial's name: indeed, the College decided to call the award the St Bel Prize. The name certainly has an undoubted (if spurious) romantic air. However it is spelt, the common pronunciation, putting stress on the second part of the name, is apparently incorrect (Cornevin) for the name of the village should in fact carry the stress on the first syllable, thus rhyming with 'handbell'. (It is of passing interest to note the death of Lionel St Bel Golledge, veterinary surgeon, in 1962.)

Anyone writing about Vial has thought it necessary to adopt one or other of the forms listed above. Throughout this work I have called the man 'Vial' *tout court*, as this was undoubtedly his surname.

Uncertainty continues when we come to the date of Vial's birth. The register of the veterinary school in Lyons, which he entered in August 1769, shows him as born in 1750, while the memoirs give his birthday as 28 January 1753. When Vial was three years old, both his parents and his grandfather died, and he came under the care of the guardian appointed by his father, a M de Flesseille, whom he looked upon both as patron and friend, and with whom he stayed until he was 16. Being interested in comparative anatomy, Vial went one day to the Lyons veterinary school (which had opened on 1 January 1762) to see the museum. He was led to ask the professor, M. Pean, to be allowed to attend lectures as a non-resident pupil. This was against school regulations, so he became a student, either at his own expense or at that of the town, on 6 August 1769. Professor Sewell said later that he was only an 'amateur student' — that is, not a full-time student. His studies introduced him to the outward conformation of the horse, a subject which largely occupied his interest, and to the skin diseases of the horse's legs. Vial soon won a prize for an essay on grease in horses. The prize was attributed by Vial to the (French) Royal Society of Medicine, but it may merely have ranked as one of a series of occasional class prizes. This essay earned the following severe comment from Delabere Blaine: 'The prize dissertation on grease, which we are informed gained the medal at Lyons, would induce me to regard the institution it was granted by, with some degree of contempt'.

At about this time, M de Flesseille settled on Vial an annuity of 500 livres. At the end of two years, Vial became lecturer and demonstrator to a class of 16 students (which sounds a grander appointment than it possibly was). A year later, he was appointed upper student, assistant surgeon and a public demonstrator, which gave him experience in practical veterinary matters and (a foretaste of his days in England) the opportunity of obtaining patrons, which would be most essential in an age in which rich patrons carried out functions analogous to those of grant-giving bodies today. About a year later, an epidemic disease broke out among horses in many French provinces. With five students of his choice, Vial set out on provincial visits to assist in combatting the disease.

216

He concentrated on human ophthalmology, graduating FRCS in 1870. He became a noted ophthalmic surgeon, operating successfully on Gladstone for cataract. In 1912 he was elected FRS.

In the veterinary field, he made some observations on albinism in dogs, and studied blindness in cattle due to optic neuritis. From the case reports by Nettleship and Hudson, and in the light of investigations into the causes of blindness in cattle (particularly the Channel Island breeds) at Streatley and subsequently at Hawkshead by Formston and Ingram, there can be little doubt that Nettleship was confronted with a Vitamin A deficiency. (It is a pleasure to record that this history was typed by Anna John, her father's great-uncle being Edward Nettleship.)

Appendix 2

SENIOR STAFF AT THE COLLEGE

PRINCIPALS: 1791 Vial de Saint Bel, 1793 Edward Coleman, 1839 William Sewell, 1953 Charles Spooner, 1872 James Beart Simonds, 1881 William Robertson, 1888 Sir George T. Brown, 1894 Sir John McFadyean, 1927 Sir Frederick T.G. Hobday, 1937 James B. Buxton, 1954 James McCunn [Acting], 1955 Reginald E. Glover, 1965 Sir John N. Ritchie, 1970 Alan O. Betts, 1988 Lance E. Lanyon.

VICE PRINCIPALS: 1937 George H. Wooldridge, 1955 James McCunn, 1963 Clifford Formston, 1974 Ernest Cotchin, 1982 Leslie C. Vaughan, 1987 Michael G.M. Jukes.

PROFESSORS: 1839 William Sewell, 1839 W.J.T. Morton, 1839 Charles Spooner, 1853 James Beart Simonds, 1860 R.V. Tuson, 1862 G.W. Varnell, 1872 William Pritchard,

1872 T.S. Cobbold, 1875 J.W. Axe, 1880 William Robertson, 1881 John Penberthy, 1881 Sir George Brown, 1886 E.W. Shave, 1888 J. Baynes, 1890 George Murray, 1892 Sir John McFadyean, 1893 F.T.G. Hobday, 1895 W.B. Bottomly, 1895 J. Macqueen, 1900 H.A. Woodruff, 1903 G.D. Lander, 1903 T.G. Brodie, 1906 H.W. Marrett-Tims, 1908 G.A. Buckmaster, 1908 G.H. Wooldridge, 1916 T.J. Evans, 1916 E.B. Reynolds, 1920 B. Gorton, 1920 J.T. Edwards, 1920 W. Legge Symes, 1920 G.W. Clough, 1922 A.B. Mattinson, 1923 E.G. Langford, 1926 James McCunn, 1926 A.R. Smythe, 1927 T.G. Hobday, 1927 Tom Hare, 1929 J.G. Wright, 1930 S.E. Wilson, 1933 F.C. Minett, 1934 W.C. Miller, 1938 Yule Bogue, 1939 T.J. Bosworth, 1943 C. Formston, 1944 H. Burrow,

1944 O.G. Edholm, 1946 N.J. Scorgie, 1947 E.C. Amoroso, 1953 R. Lovell, 1958 J.A. Laing, 1963 E. Cotchin, 1963 F.R. Bell 1964 A.O. Betts, 1965 G.H. Arthur, 1967 J.L. Hancock, 1968 E.C.G. Clarke, 1971 W. Plowright, 1972 R.H.C. Penny, 1972 L.C. Vaughan, 1977 D.E. Noakes, 1978 D.G. Harvey, 1981 I.K.M. Smith, 1984 L.E. Lanyon, 1984 J.E.T. Jones, 1984 D. Lodge, 1985 R.M. Barlow, 1986 E.E.L. Gerring, 1986 G.E. Goldspink, 1988 P. Lees, 1990 D.E. Jacobs.

READERS: 1937 H.R. Allen, 1938 H.F. Rosenberg, 1938 J.N. Oldham, 1938 J.H. Jackson, 1960 F.A. Holton, 1962 J.C. Greatorex, 1962 R. Hill, 1967 P.C. Trexler, 1967 R.H. Nisbit 1975 R.R. Ashdown, 1975 P.A. Mayes, 1976 C.A. Finn, 1978 H.Ll. Williams, 1980 E.C. Appleby, 1984 A.R. Michell,

1986 N. Edington, 1987 P.G.C. Bedford.

SENIOR LECTURERS: 1953 E.F. Lewis, 1954 J.T. Abrams, 1955 J.D. Biggers, 1956 A.E. Harrop, 1963 K.M. Dyce, 1964 P.L. Ingram, 1964 A.L.C. Thorne, 1964 R.F.S. Creed, 1968 O.G. Jones, 1969 G.B. Edwards, 1972 R.C. Frost, 1975 W.P. Beresford Jones, 1975 L.R. Thomsett, 1978 R.H. Marchant, 1978 I.K.M. Smith, 1978 P.A. Mullen, 1979 A.H. Andrews, 1979 M.G.A.D. Scott, 1980 D. Lodge, 1980 B.M. Bush, 1983 A.H.S. Hayward, 1983 D.G. Clayton Jones, 1983 P.M. Webbon, 1984 N.C. Stickland, 1984 A.J. Wilsmore, 1985 A.M. Johnston, 1986 P.F. Watson, 1987 W.E. Allen, 1987 J.V. Davies, 1987 D.H. Lloyd, 1987 P.H. Russell, 1988 Kathleen Clarke, 1988 A.J. Madel.

Appendix 3

THE COLLEGE COAT OF ARMS

Heraldic description of the official coat of arms of the College which came into use with the Charter of 1875:

Arms:— On a fesse, Gules, an Imperial crown between two anchors, Or. In chief, Or and Argent, on a band, Azure, an arrow entwined by a serpent, Or, between a poppy-head, proper, in dexter, and a ram's head erased, Sable, holding a trefoil in the mouth, erect, in sinister. In base Or and Argent; on a Pale, Azure, a hand holding a broken dart, Argent, between a greyhound's head, erased, Sable, collared, Or, in dexter, and an aloe, Proper, in sinister.

Crest:— A demi-horse, Argent.

Supporters:— Dexter, a horse Argent, and sinister a bull Proper.

Motto:— *Venienti occurrite morbo*.

An interpretation of terms used in the heraldry of the College may be helpful: Fesse — a band across the shield, filling a third part of it. In chief — upper part of shield. In dexter — right. Erased — torn away with a ragged edge, pleasantly conventionalised. Or — yellow (gold). Argent — white (silver). Proper — in its own natural colours. Pale — a broad stripe running the length of the shield. Trefoil — always has stalk left hanging.

The College motto, *Venienti occurrite morbo*, is from Persius, Satires, iii, line 64, AD 58. Aulus Persius Flaccus (34-62) was a Roman satirical poet. The motto, with its original context, has been translated as follows: 'It is too late to ask for hellebore [black hellebore was given in dropsies] as you see men doing, when the skin is just getting morbid and bloated. Meet the disease at its first stage, and what occasion is there to promise Cratorius [the name of a doctor, taken from Horace, Satires, 11, iii, 161] gold-mines for a cure?.' The motto has also been translated as 'Meet malady on its way', 'Meet the disease on its way', 'Meet the malady on its way, and then what need to promise big mountainous fees to Cratorius?'. According to Smith, the motto was used by James White, who graduated at the College in 1797, and was attached to the Royal Dragoons in April that year. After seven years' service, he left in June 1804 to go into practice (Exeter, Bath, Wells). 'The prevention of disease was ever uppermost in his mind; there is hardly a chapter of his works where the subject escapes notice; the title page of the later editions bears the motto.'

The motto, in an age of classical education, had the status of an adage. It was used, for example, by Henry Fielding in *The History of Tom Jones* (published in 1740) '. . . for surely the gentlemen of the Aesculapian art are in the right in advising, that the moment the disease is entered at one door, the physician should be introduced at the other; what else is meant by that old adage: venienti occurrite morbo? "Opposite a distemper at its first approach". Thus the doctor and the disease meet in fair and equal conflict; whereas, by giving time to the latter, we often suffer him to fortify and entrench himself, like a French army; so that the learned gentleman finds it very difficult, and sometimes impossible, to come at the enemy'.

The phrase is also appropriately echoed in the motto of the No 6 Maintenance Unit of the Royal Air Force — *Venienti occurrere casu*: To meet the occasion when it arises.

Appendix 4

THE REGULATIONS ORDERED TO BE PUBLISHED

Veterinary College, London, Established April 8, 1791, for the Reformation and Improvement of Farriery, and the Treatment of Cattle in General. London: Printed by James Phillips, George Yard, Lombard Street. MDCCXCI

Veterinary College. Regulations for the Interior Discipline of the Resident Pupils.
  Concerning the hours of rising, retiring to bed, and meals.
   I. The Pupils are to rise at six in the morning, from Lady-day to Michaelmas: and at seven from Michaelmas till Lady-day.
   II. The hour of breakfast is eight, of dinner two, and of supper in the summer nine, and winter eight o'clock.
   III. Immediately after supper, the Pupils are to retire to the common sitting-room till ten o'clock, at which hour each is to retire to his bedchamber.
   IV. No Pupil will be permitted to burn candle in the night under pretence of study; the lights are to be extinguished before the pupils go to bed, and none are to remain up after eleven o'clock.
   V. The Pupils are to take their places at table according to the order of precedence in their several classes.
   VI. No commons are to be carried into any private room but in case of sickness, and with leave of the Professor.
   VII. No provision but the commons, are to be dressed in the kitchen for any of the Pupils, nor to be introduced into their apartments from any other quarter. Wine and spirits are absolutely prohibited.
  Concerning the Studies
   I. Every Pupil is required to attend his studies and the Lectures regularly, according to the appointment of the Professor.
   II. The studies of the morning are to commence at nine o'clock and conclude at one o'clock; and in the afternoon are to commence at four o'clock, and conclude at seven o'clock; the afternoons of Thursday and Saturday excepted.
   III. The Professor is to keep a book, in which he is to record the attendance or non-attendance of the Pupils in their respective classes, which book is to be produced to the Committee at their meetings.
   IV. There will be a vacation, commencing the fifteenth of August, and ending the thirtieth of September, except with those Pupils who are in the third year of their studies.
  Concerning the Library
   I. Every Pupil who takes a Book out of the Library for his private use, is to make an entry of it in the Library Book, and is to be accountable for it.
   II. Every Pupil is to return the Books to their proper places in the Library by four o'clock on Saturday afternoon.
   III. No Book belonging to the Library is to be left in any public room, or passage; but must be carefully kept in the possession of the Pupil who takes it from the Library.

IV. No Pupil shall take Pens, Ink or Paper, the Library Book, or the Catalogue of Books, out of the Library; nor write in any Book belonging to the Library, except the entry of the Books he takes from hence.

Concerning absence from the College, and Return, and the time of shutting the gates.

I. Nothing but illness will be admitted as an excuse for any of the Pupils absenting themselves from some place of public worship.

II. No Pupil will be permitted to go to London, except by the desire of a Parent, Guardian, or persons properly authorised by them, expressed by a letter to the Professor, unless on some particular emergency, of which the Professor shall judge and report to the Committee at their next meeting.

III. No Pupil is to go beyond the boundaries of the College after the gates are locked in the evening, without permission from the Professor; and every Pupil who has leave of absence for the day, is to return to the College before the gates are locked.

IV. The gates are to be locked from Lady-day till Michaelmas at eight o'clock and from Michaelmas till Lady-day at seven o'clock.

V. Every Pupil who enters or leaves the College premises, by any other way than the gates, is guilty of a misdemeanour; and if this offence be committed after the gates are locked, it will be considered as a high aggravation.

VI. No Pupil shall interrupt the studies of the other Pupils, by quarrelling or playing; nor will any improper language or conversation be tolerated on any account, either in the hours of study, or at any other time; and the only distinctions in the College will arise from regular behaviour and diligent application.

VII. Every Pupil shall punctually attend to the fore-going Regulations, and also to the directions of the Professor. Every act of disobedience will incur, on the first offence, the reprimand of the Professor; on the second offence, the Professor is required to make a report to the Committee, who may either impose fine, or, if they think proper, report the matter to the Council at their first meeting, with whom remains the power of expulsion.

Payment of fines is not considered as in any degree an adequate compensation for an habitual breach of any of the laws; and as the Professor is expected to make a regular report to the Committee, with regard to the observance or violation of them: they will be strictly supported, as well for the reputation and improvement of the Pupils, as for the general credit and benefit of the Institution. The money arising from fines to be appropriated to the purchase of books for the Library.

VIII. Every Pupil who passes the night out of the College, without leave from the Committee (except as requested in No. II) will be expelled, or suffer such other punishment as the circumstances may require.

Miscellaneous

I. There shall be no intercourse between Pupils and the domestic servants; nor shall they go into the kitchen, or those parts of the houses where the servants are occupied in their necessary employments.

II. Whoever breaks, or in any respect injures, the utensils or furniture belonging to the College, shall pay for or replace the articles.

III. No visitors shall be admitted but in the intervals of study, and the Pupils shall not be allowed to entertain them, or each other, with any thing but tea or coffee.

IV. No Pupil shall on any pretence whatever take from the College, or lend to any person, any copy of the Professor's manuscripts; or any notes or memorandums of his Lectures.

Subscribers

Presentation Copies

I HRH the Prince Philip, the Duke of Edinburgh
Patron of the College
II HM Queen Elizabeth, the Queen Mother
Patron of the Royal Veterinary College Animal Care Trust
and Fellow of the College
III HRH the Princess Royal
Chancellor of the University of London and Fellow of the College
IV Paul Mellon KBE
Fellow of the College
V Mr Henry Carter
VI Professor William Jarrett

1 The Royal Veterinary College London
2 Professor Lance Lanyon
3 Derek Gordon-Brown
4 Valerie Carter
5 Mrs Hilda Cotchin
6 Clive & Carolyn Birch
7 Prof D.G. Whittingham
8 S.C. Reeve
9 E.C. Straiton
10 Professor J.O.L. King
11 M.J. Henigan MRCVS
12 Paul B. Rossiter
13 Dr Peter Roeder
14 John Gallagher
15 Abigail Drake
16
17 Bishopsgate Institute
18 Fred Gulson
19 Dr W.A.G. Charleston
20 Mrs Sheila K. Nichols
21 Miss Kay Oliver
22 Mrs C.A. Lawson
23 Mrs C. Deasy
24 Belinda A. Woodhouse
25 Carol Standy
26 Joy M. Hall
27 H. Travers
28 Audrey C. Hassan
29 D.M. Taylor
30 Derek W. Gordon-Brown
31 Mrs Marjorie Scott
32 Polly Curds BSc
33 David P. Clarke
34 Capt R.N. Phillips
35 Janet L. Pickstock
36 Rachel Burrow
37 Professor L.E. Lanyon

38 Stewart M. Womar BVet Med MRCVS
39 Miss Julia Fry
40 E.E. Herrod-Taylor
41 B.R. Herrod-Taylor
42 Louise E. Alcock
43 Edward Charles Best
44 Nancie May (née Spencer)
45 Mr & Mrs G.T. Birks
46 Louis L. Goodwin CEng MIMechE
47 Corporation of London
48 R.J. Bradley
49 R. Williams MRCVS
50 Mrs J. Greenwood
51 J.D. Nightingirl
52 Mrs Maureen Burrell
53 Jonathan Borchard
54 Miss S. Guthrie
55 Jean Pound
56 Thomas Henry Hewins
57 Miss Lesley Burgess
58 Elizabeth Allen
59 Andrew Scott
60 C.E. Kelly
61 Mrs M. Spriggs
62 J.W. Barber-Lomax
63 John Clewlow
64 Roger Ewbank
65 Institute of Agricultural History, University of Reading
66 Joseph A. Allen
67 R.D. Locke
68 Kenneth W. Aspinall
69 Mr & Mrs Peter Nelkin
70 Lt Col P.C. Koder RAVC
71 R.J.M. Franklin
72 Professor T.K. Ewer

73 Miss Sharon Webley
74 D.R. Lane
75 E. Norman Sinclair
76 C.J. Hillidge
77 Graham George Hudd
78 V. Grenfell
79 Dr J.C. Greatorex PhD FRCS FRSH
80 Andrew J. Fleetwood
81 Mrs A.J. Teasdale
82 E. Barbour-Hill
83 Clifford Formston
84 W.J.C. Donnelly
85 Jean Sainsbury Charitable Trust
86 H.W. & A.L. Allsop
87 Mass N'Jie
88 Barry Johnson
89 John McCaig
90 Library of the Faculty of Veterinary Medicine, State University, Utrecht
91 Mr & Mrs B.M. Evans
92 Norwegian College of Veterinary Medicine
93 D.C. North
94 Mrs Ann Hillier
95 E.B. Wain
96 Dr J.R. Fisher
97 Dr Robert I. Taylor
98 A.D. Stephens
99 Dr P.J. Lane
100 Kay White
101 Mountain Animal Sanctuary
102 Robert Gascoyne Mares
103 University of Guelph
104 Minerva
105 In Memory of Mr R.M. James, presented to the K.C. by Leicestershire Gundog Society

106 Lana & Hedy Watts
107 Stanley Stuart Kay
108 C.J. House & J.D. Jackson
109 University of Illinois Library
110 Leila Kooros
111 Mrs Jan Rowe
112 Librairie Marqueste
113 Prof Dr Wolfgang Jochle
114 Connie M. Ford
115 John T. Gunner
116 Dr P.S. Jackson
117 P.M. Biggs
118 Miss V.D. Marchant
119 Myra L. Clarke FRCVS
120 Dr P.G.C. Bedford
121 Jane Linsey Terry
122 Jean Humphrey
123 Mrs Tania Davies
124 Mrs Wendy Stacey
125 The Odiham Society
126 Margaret Sanderson
127 Dr Susanna Williamson
128 Miss Denise Copeland
129 Roy Hunter
130 Miss Jane Lyons MRCVS
131 Sheila Wall
132 The Croft Family
133 C.L. Burnett
134 Mrs Jenny Parrish
135 Mr & Mrs P.D. Tedder
136 Colin & Linda Silverton
137 Mrs S. Jenkins PhD
138 Mrs J.D. Hawtin
139 Mrs I.S. Bradbury
140 Miss M.B. Booth
141 Mrs D. Elizabeth M. Weston LDS
142 L.C. Vaughan

143 Miss M. duMont
144 G.R. Hewett
145 Mrs Esther M.H. Denham MRCVS
146 John Adamson
147 Sir Barry Cross
148 David T. Coffey BVetMed MRCVS
149 A.D.R. Hilbery
150 Anthony Cole Loftus
151 J.B. Tuckey
152 Brian Beardsall
153 G.S. Allen
154 Peter Fry
155 William Shipley
156 M.G. Davies
157 S.J.A. Woodger
158 Walter Dodd
159 M.J. Hoad
160 Roger Wickenden
161 N.F. Tebbutt
162 P.V. Allen
163 John B. Sutton
164 D.F. Shrimpton
165 Robin T. Pepper
166 Dr W.E. Allen
167 Howard A. Tribe
168 Mrs A.S. Davies
169 Robert W. Westhead
170 Joan A. Joshua
171 Mrs L.J. King
172 Thomas W. Dukes
173 J.F.A. Carver
174 K.G.D. Evans
175 Roger Freeman
176 Dr T.D. Grimes
177 J.E. Beach
178 John D. Millett
179 N.G. Buck
180 P.J.L. Hermette MRCVS
181 R.G. Gough
182 Kevin J. Whiting BVetMed MRCVS
183 John R. Hudson
184 W.E.R. Cook
185 Dr H.L.L. Williams
186 Professor E.I. Williams
187 D.H. Roberts
188 R.D. Hollands
189 Catherine O'Callaghan
190 M.A. Wright MRCVS
191 The Danish Veterinary & Agricultural Library
192 W.J. Gooden MBE FRSH
193 Dr R.M. Griffin
194 J.B. Tutt
195 D.J. Belford
196 Dr Stuart G. Lake
197 David Williams
198 T.D. White
199 N. Snodgrass

200 Colin R. Sitford
201 Roger Wickenden
202 T. Van Laun
203 Paul John Eager
204 J.J. Oliver
205 Peter Rixson
206 Michael St G.N. Drewitt
207 Louisiana State University
208 A.L.C. Thorne
209 Dexter Smith
210 Ecole Nationale Veterinaire
211 R.D. Lewis
212 Robert Durham Strang
213 Dr A.G. Warren
214 Michael Allen Gordon
215 W. Mary Brancker
216 L.R. Thomsett DVD FRCVS
217 Allan P. Berry
218 M.L. Hawken
219 W.P. Beresford-Jones PhD MA MRCVS
220 P.J. Underwood
221 Dr Jeremy V. Davies
222 R.C. Davidson
223 J.B. Derbyshire
224 Ms G.M. Ford
225 Mrs Hilda Cotchin
226 Dr P.J. Lane
227 (Mrs) Betty S. Sugden
228 E.J.A. Garner
229 Trevor Turner
230 Stuart Mackay Holland
231 C.A.G. Felgate MRCVS
232 Virginia Polytechnic Institute
233 H. Reynolds
234 David Sutton
235 Sir Gordon Shattock MRCVS
236 Dr John R. Pascoe
237 Purdue University
238 Raymond Lewis Williams
239 Philip James Throssel
240 John O. Broberg
241 Maurice V. Polley
242 Mrs M.J. Case
243–Royal College of Veterinary
244 Surgeons
245 Dr Colin R. Wilks
246 Nigel R. Taylor
247 John S. Heath
248 John Stratton
249 B.T. Lawrence
250 C. Charlesworth
251 A.B. Orr

252 Veterinary Medical Library, University of Missouri
253 Dr Andrew Higgins
254–Messrs Taylor &
255 Leas
256 Andrew James Madel
257 A. Boothroyd
258 Kenneth Chadwick Sykes
259 Clive Woodham
260 L.H. Rutherford
261 Andrew T.B. Edney
262 P.M. Attenburrow
263 David Mason
264 C.J. Dearlove
265 J.A. Vanderplank
266 Dr T. Morris
267 Miss K.F. Morris
268 R.B. Griffin
269 G.P. Wilding
270 K.S. Malone
271 Robert Henry Irwin
272 David Sainsbury
273 Barry Johnson
274 Alan John Bartram BVetMed MRCVS
275 I.S. & K.E. Mason
276 F.G.A. Thompson
277 D.H. Lloyd
278 Ernest A. Gill MRCVS
279 Dr J.H. Marston
280 Peter John Bircher
281 Robert McNeill
282 John W. Anderson
283 Dennis L. Smith
284 Mrs Penelope Robinson
285 Dr Ian F. Keymer
286 Miss A.J.M. Robson
287 Dr John N. Howse
288 Colin R. Sitford
289 Keith R. Reed
290 H.H. Skinner
291 R.A. Doncaster
292 A.C. Palmer
293 A.P. Woodford
294 T.F. Tunney
295 A.J. Manfield
296 John A. Moffitt
297 Felicity Williams
298 F.C. Ball
299 W. Ashwynne Jones
300 John R. Drew
301 Paul & Tina Davey
302 J.R. Robson
303 J.A. Dyson
304 B.M. Stocks MRCVS
305 J.E. Herrod-Taylor
306 Dr Paul A. Mullen
307 John Douch
308 Clive Jordan
309 Norman Comben
310 Patrick de Ville
311 Miss Lynn Crimlisk
312 John Carr

313 A.P. Trivan
314 Bernard J. Walsh
315 Professor E. Gerring
316 Michael J. Durrant
317 Michael Davies
318 Ernst Mehnert
319 R.H. Balkwill MRCVS
320 Lt Col J.A. Tanner MBE MRCVS
321 Walter Plowright
322 Mrs P. Chambers
323 A.E.G. Markham
324 John David Walker
325 D.G.H. Jones
326 George Dickinson
327 H.N. Green
328 Hilda & Graham Jackson
329 W.E.F. Hockenhull
330 Nelson Lester Rufus Bowden
331 J.G. Lane
332 Jalal-ud-Din Shuja OBE MRCVS
333 Andrew Clarke
334 Michael G. Jones
335 Anne Blackburn
336 Catherine Sharpe
337 S.W.R. Mitchell
338 Professor W.I.M. McIntyre FRCVS
339 Iowa State University
340 Unlisted
341 J.B. Kerry
342 Miss S.A. Ambler
343 Collin W. Willson
344 D.G. Clayton Jones
345 Peter S. Clark
346 Mrs Vanessa M. Dixon
347 Kevin R. Kerr MRCVS
346 C.J.G. Shawcross
349 Kim June Allcock
350 M.V. Dale
351 Brian R. Ray
352 Dr Simon Wheeler
353 Martin Routledge BVetMed MRCVS
354 D.S. Babington
355 Peter G. Wilkins
356 J.N. Wright
357 Geoffrey Thorpe
358 Donald A. Rutty
359 M.R.W. Lewis MRCVS
360 Lt Col I.G.C. Cochrane-Dyet
361 David Fields
362 A.C. Matthews
363 Jane Elizabeth Godbeer
364 Sarah Haynes
365 Sylvia C. Jones
366 Ronald Cotchin

367 R.W.M. Gover
368 Jeremy P.C. Giles MRCVS
369 D.J. Collyns
370 Derek Morath
371 M.P. Bennett
372 J.C. Buxton
373 Peter John Harley
374 F.J.O. Anthony
375 Richard Griffiths
376 Bruce V. Jones
377 Dr F.G. Startup
378 Derek Stoakes
379 B.H. Mackay
380 Dr J. Ishmael
381 J.B. Sargeant
382 E.C. Straiton
383 Bryan Montague
384 Michael Minns
385 Robert D. Thurlow
386 R.J.L. Williamson
387 R.G. Roberts
388 Mrs K.A. Colman
389 John G.G. Saxton
390 Ian E.T. Sladden
391 Edward Button
392 David B. Morton
393 P.R. Jenkerson
394 C.W. Watkins
395 John Cowie Whitney
396 B.R. Howard
397 Professor T.K. Ewer
398 G.A. Embleton
399 H.L.L. & L.P. Salmon
400 W.A. Scott
401 Roger C. Fox
402 David Charles Davies
403 Barry Birchall
404 Roger Birchall
405 David H. Soldan
406 L.W. Hall
407 F.C. Hammond
408 Mrs Gillian S. Knowland
409 Clifford George
410 Gurth C.M. Scriven
411 David Owen Hobbs
412 R.S. Pinniger
413 Dr P.G.C. Bedford FRCVS
414 S.H. White
415 Martin Leith
416 J.E.T. Jones
417 M.J. Nagele
413 David Hendry Shearer
419 M.W. Baker
420 W.H.G. Rees
421 Frederick P. Pingram
422 Dr G.H. & Mrs M. Singleton
423 W.J. Starr
424 Raymond E. Burnside
425 David Brian Townley
426 Charles Frank Coleman

427 Jane E. Alexander
428 Dr B.A. Sommerville
429 J.G. Hollands
430 M.H.A. Townley
431 A.C. Talbot
432 L.N. Payne
433 Robin Collins
434 G.R.F. Crouch BVetMed MRCVS
435 Godfrey Torr
436 Kevin Patrick March
437 S.M. Russell
438 Neil Rudram BVetMed MRCVS
439 J.N. Prescott
440 Robert I.M. Elliott MRCVS
441 Patricia Sutton
442 Brian Mason
443 Keith H.B. Wood
444 Dr E.B. Davies
445 Peter J. Clark
446 R.S. Broadbent
447 M.A. Wright MRCVS
448 N.G. Kingston
449 James H. Seed
450 Ian Palmer
451 Michael St George Napier Drewitt
452 Diana Mewha-Williams
453 David Sillars
454 John Christopher Parlane Granger
455 John Trevor Blackburn
456 Colin Ellis
457 John W. Penfold
458 Denis Blaxland
459 Peter H. Lonnon
460 W.E.S. Evans
461 R.S. Murdoch
462 H.A. Crawshaw
463 David Ian Grant
464 Andrew Edgson
465 Stephen A. Lister MRCVS
466 J.B. Sutton
467 Dr Alastair Michell
468 Mr & Mrs L.J.C. Pilling M's RCVS
469 E.F. Hilder
470 Philip S. Parker
471 Dr Gavin Anthony Cullen FRCVS
472 J.L. Crooks MRCVS
473 T.B. Smithson
474 Dr R.R. Ashdown
475 L.C. Geeson
476 D.J. Simmonds MRCVS
477 J.L. Stuart
478 Peter A. Cockett
479 Paul Farrington
480 Clive S. Reid
481 Michael L. Howe
482 S.C. Reeve

483 A.L.M. Shepherd
484 P.W. Hunt
485 E.P. Mount
486 Clifford L. Wright
487 Dr P.M. Headley
488 G.T. Bowler
489 H.W. Symonds
490 David W. Barfoot
491 E.A. Chandler
492 Prof Eric I. Williams
493 Michigan State University Libraries
494 Frederick Cotchin
495 Mrs Alison Hall
496 Anna Nolan
497 Betty Murray
498 Peter C. Koder MSc
499 Jonathan P.P. Harwood
500 M.R. Minns
501 Tony Flint
502 Clare Hogston
503 C.J. Gregson
504 Mrs E. Thomas
505 John D. Mackinnon
506 Guy G. Freeland
507 John Edward Cox
508 David R. Ellis
509 Dr P.J. Goddard
510 W. Eaton-Evans
511 F. Lloyd Griffiths
512 Andrea Shaw McMillan
513 W.G.A. Penhale
514 F. Smith
515 Alan P. Carter
516 Neil T. Hubbard
517 John L. Fagan
518 Edward John Davidge
519 Graham Davies
520 M.S. Wilson
521 Col J. Hickman MA FRCVS
522 Walter John Downes
523 Stewart D. Sutherland
524 Peter Smitherman
525 Dr Richard A.S. White
526 Richard M. Newey
527 Anthony Basher
528 Dr M'Hamed Sedrati
529 William R. Potter
530 Brian John Cox
531 Leonard Gaunt
532 J.A.G. Jack
533 Charles Ryan Hartley
534 H.E. Carter
535 J.B. Walsby
536 Professor Geoffrey H. Arthur
537 David Pope
538 Michael Samuel MRCVS
539 Aubrey I. Thomas

540 B.P. Viner BVetMed MRCVS
541 Dr Michael J. Dunkley
542 Mrs M.G. Hignett
543 Donald J. Skinner
544 Margaret & Robin Perkins
545 Mary Dyer
546 Dr D.H.L. Rollinson
547 Paul R. Greenough
548 Paul Malin
549 Dr Roger C.K. Stevens
550 Judy Habbitts
551 Dr G.R. Thomson
552 David Sandwith
553 Cynthia M. Trim
554 Dr W. John Herbert
555 A. David Weaver
556 D.J. Tansley Thomas MRCVS
557 Librairie Marqueste
558 Annabel Irwin
559 John C.S. Head
560 Peter Saville
561 Michael J.H. Rogers MRCVS
562 W.M. Wadman Taylor
563 John E. Lancaster
564 Dr B.A. Baldwin
565 Ronald Greenwood
566 Kenneth David Parkinson
567 John Henry Lewington
568 Robert Anthony Bradley
569 Professor F.W.G. Hill
570 Dr Francis Testoni
571 J.D. Hawkins
572 John A. Mason MRCVS
573 Charlotte Briscall
574 Randal McDonnell
575 Ellis Cledwyn Griffiths
576 Dr John Alexander Quinane
577 Marco Mezzabotta 1969
578 Mrs B.J. Dudley
579 Mike Jessop MRCVS
580 Dr Terence J. Drake
581 Mr & Mrs Jon Cotchin
582 Michael Kingdon
583 D.I.B. Hoare
584 George Edward Bradley
585 Dr L.W. Greenham
586 D.H. Scarf
587 Christopher M. Wilkins BVSc MRCVS
588 C.D. Mackenzie
589 C.M.J. Field

231

590 T.G.G. Herbert
591 A.R. Woodward
592 Robert Joseph McEnery
593 S.H. Langford
594 Allatorvostudomanyi Egyetem
595 W.B. Swift
596 Geoffrey Raymond Oliver
597 Josephine Palmer
598 Douglas Bruce
599 Dr Alan K. Bater
600 S.J. Livesley
601 J.B. Tutt FRCVS
602 Alan E. Pierce
603 J.B.A. Smyth
604 D. Catherine McCarthy
605 Stuart Marston
606 Geoff Robins
607 Linda Warden
608 Cheryl A. Blaze
609 Ho Mah Soon BVetMed MRCVS
610 Brendan W. Furlong MRCVS
611 Wayne Lester Berry
612 H.C.A. Duffin
613
614 Jane Maxwell King Heron
615 John Herring
616 Martin R. Gough
617 B.W. Eagles
618 Robert Pashen
619 Brian Sorrell DVM
620 David Killoch Blackmore
621 Dr B.A. Summers
622 David Burrows
623 Merensky Library, University of Pretoria
624 Robert Edward Cottam
625 Michael Pay
626 Prof K.P. Baker
627 Vanessa Miller
628 Douglas F. Gray
629 University Library, Bristol
630 John Tasker
631 R.W. Betty
632 H.P. Dawkins
633 Julia Tetley
634 Mrs M.J. Case
635 Nichola Saunders
636 Dr Samuel Jakovljevic
637 Mrs Brenda Collins
638 Dr Alan G. Warren
639 J.T.R. Evans BSc MRCVS
640 F.M. Ellerd-Styles

641 Bryan Sayle
642 Dr Glen Clarke
643 Roger A. Drew
644 Mrs Janet M. Owen
645 John M. Lifton MRCVS MACVSc
646 Dr C. Perumal Pillai FRCVS
647 E.L. Caspari
648 John Rhodes
649 Dr R.A.S. White
650 Mrs Julia E. Marr
651 Neville Gibson Japp
652 Phillip Watson
653 Mrs Rosemary Ann McGrigor
654 Paul Kane
655 Ivan Katic
656 Claire S.L. Shorthose
657 L.B. McNaught
658 M.C. Schramme
659 D.L. Smith MRCVS
660 M.H. Woodford
661 David J.C. Cuffe MVB MRCVS
662 John Brown
663 Roger S. Windsor
664 J.P. Sheridan
665 T.R. Ayliffe
666 Mrs C.E. Cawte
667 Stephen P. Dean BVetMed MRCVS DVR
668 E.C. Hulse BSc MRCVS
669 Prof D.E. Jacobs
670 J.R. Bainbridge BVSc MRCVS
671 Clive S. Reid
672 David Grant
673 Richard Newey
674 Mrs B.A. McIrvine
675 Dr Rufus Creed
676 Clifford Formston
677 Malcolm Holliday
678 R.J.A. Packer BVet Med MRCVS
679 B.R. Philps
680 William T.
681 Nutter
682 John Verstegen
683 Norman Comben
684 R.S. Murdoch
685 David C. Lawler
686 Gillian S. Knowland
687 Brian R. Ray
688 Dr Jenny Remfry
689 Roman Smelhaus
690 Graham Davies BSc BVet Med MRCVS
691 John R. Drew
692 G.S. Peyton
693 L.A. Harries
694 Ian Sanderson Kynoch

695 Norman Comben
696 Keith L. Thoday
697 Jack Heptinstall
698 MRCVS
699 Michael D. Kock
700 Gerald N. Woode
701 London Borough of Camden, Local
703 Studies Library
704 Mary Katharine Southwell
705 K.B.A. Hurst
706 Anthony Mackrill
707 Josephine Palmer
708 The Higher Institute of Zootechnics & Veterinary Medicine
709 Colin R. Tedman
710 Rosemary & Allen Scott
711 Heather Hawkins
712 Doreen Wootton
713 G.E. Underwood
714 Clifford Crush
715 Mr & Mrs J.M. Crane
716 Derek & Eileen Adams
717 Jose Dawson
718 Mrs Diana Parkin
719 J.R. Bartholomew
720 Katherine Woolman
721 John R. Moss CB
722 Eric A. Holt
723 Dr Paul F. Watson
724 Prof Peter Lees
725 Dame Olga Uvarov
726 Dr Peter A. Mayes
727 Miss Valerie A. Downes
728 D.E. Noakes
729 Jenifer Plummer
730 J.E.T. Jones
731 David Tyler
732 Neil Stickland
733 Mrs Coral Weaver
734 Mrs P. Yealland
735 Miss Phillipa Shepherd
736 Catherine L. Buckett
737 Mrs Hilary Drew
738 Keith S. Malone
739 R. Edgar
740 Miss L. Adams
741 Mrs Nora Rozengurt
742 Dr Harry Donnelly
743 Miss E.J. Pegg
744 The Department of Veterinary Pathology, The Royal Veterinary College, London
745 Dr J. Bleby
746 The Veterinary Library, Bangkok

747 Pam Evely
748 John Chitty
749
750 Mrs J.I. Bailey
751 J. Pengelly & M.O.A. Pengelly M'sRCVS
752 Miss Sarah Louise Dawkins
753 Antonio Jose Almeida Ferreira
754 Paul Walden
755 Marion Joan Anstee Wooldridge
756 Dennis Hayes
757 Jill Butterworth
758 Richard C. Broad
759 David Leslie Brown
760 Peter Faulkner
761 R.J.C. Beeton
762 T.H. Jones
763 Royal (Dick) School of Veterinary Studies
764 Dr M. Tirgari
765 Roger C. Fox
766 D.A.K. Thornton
767 Medical Sciences Library, Tamu
768 Gail K. Robertson
769 Mrs Jane Frances White
770 Ms Durdica Stubican
771 D.G. Hogger
772 Roger G. Eddy
773 Oliver Angus Garden
774 David Long
775 Michael M. Toes
776 Mrs Beverley Piejus
777 Christopher P. Mann
778 The Revd Jeremy Caddick
779 Andrew Hayes
780 Mrs Diana Parkin
781 Unlisted
782 Henry A. Robertson
783 James Swanson
784 Franz J. Peritz
785 David John Evans
786 Peter J. Irwin
787 King Edward VI School, Southampton
788 Mrs J.M. Owen BVetMed MRCVS
789 Sidney Harry Adams
790 P.L. Chitty
791 Marian Hawkes
792 George F. Bunting
793 R. Churchill Frost
794 A.R. Tribble
795 Lorraine Waters
796 Mrs J. James

Remaining names unlisted

232

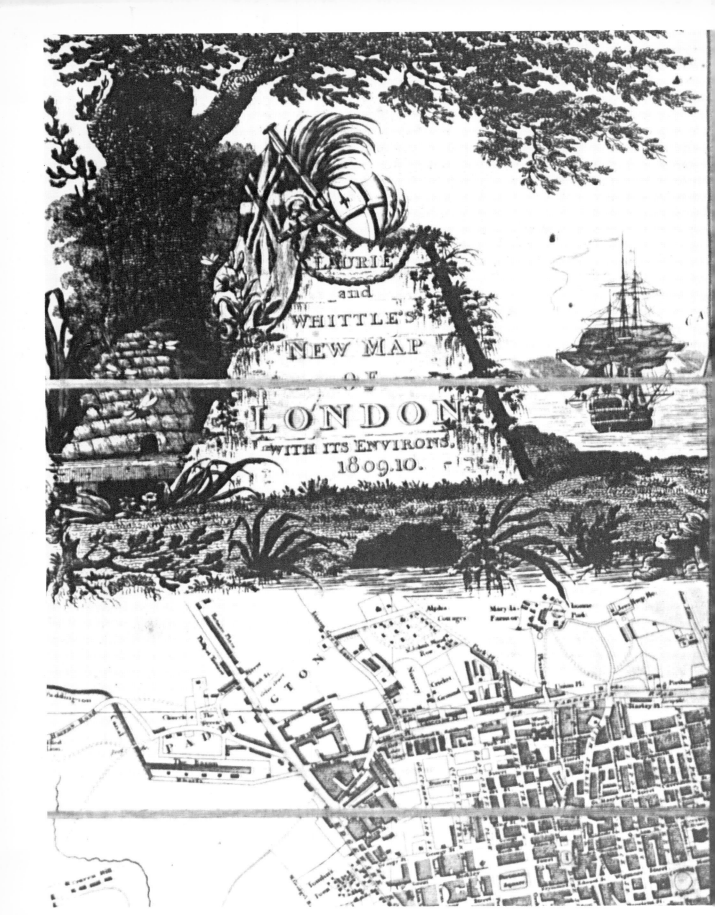